Nephrology

CLINICAL CASES UNCOVERED

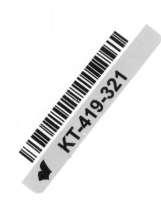

Nephrology
CLINICAL CASES UNCOVERED

Menna Clatworthy

BSc, MBBCh, PhD, MRCP

University Lecturer in Renal Medicine and
Honorary Consultant Nephrologist
University of Cambridge
Addenbrooke's Hospital
Cambridge, UK

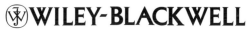

WILEY-BLACKWELL

A John Wiley & Sons, Ltd., Publication

Library of Congress Cataloging-in-Publication Data

Clatworthy, Menna.
  Nephrology / Menna Clatworthy.
  p. ; cm. – (Clinical cases uncovered)
  Includes indexes.
  ISBN 978-1-4051-8990-3
  1. Kidneys–Diseases–Case studies.   2. Kidneys–Diseases–Examinations, questions,
etc.   I. Title.   II. Series: Clinical cases uncovered.
  [DNLM: 1. Kidney Diseases–Case Reports.   2. Kidney Diseases–Problems and Exercises.
WJ 18.2 C614n 2010]
  RC903.C5525 2010
  616.6'10076–dc22
  2009018584

ISBN: 9781405189903

A catalogue record for this book is available from the British Library

Set in 9 on 12 pt Minion by Toppan Best-set Premedia Limited
Printed and bound in Malaysia by Vivar Printing Sdn Bhd

2   2010

Contents

Preface

Renal medicine is often viewed as a complex, 'hard-core' medical specialty, mastered by a small minority of intellectual physicians. The lasting impression of many medical students (and indeed non-renal specialists) is of a list of glomerulonephritides (GNs), which have random and difficult names and blur into one incomprehensible mass. In reality, nephrology is actually relatively simple and logical.

In the first section of the book, I have provided a broad introduction to nephrology. Where possible, I have tied together a clinical presentation with underlying pathology and immunology, using diagrams to distil the important points. I have also provided an 'ABC of GN', which offers a simple framework in which to place the GNs so that they can be understood.

The main part of this book consists of 31 cases, which have been chosen because they reflect the bread and butter of day-to-day life as a nephrologist. Nephrology is a fantastic specialty which allows the physician to deal with a wide variety of clinical problems, ranging from the critically unwell patient with acute renal failure to those with multisystem immune-mediated disease or tubular dysfunction, and those with chronic disease who we sometimes look after for decades on dialysis or following transplantation. For the junior doctor on a 4-month renal attachment (or even the junior renal trainee), the cases I have presented will be surprisingly similar to those which you see (and the questions that follow will reflect those which your consultant will ask). For the purposes of clarity, the cases are divided into seven sections according to clinical presentation: those presenting with acute renal failure, nephrotic syndrome, hypertension, urine dipstick abnormalities, acid–base disturbances, chronic kidney disease/dialysis-associated problems and renal transplant-related problems.

The kidneys are often involved in diseases which are primarily the remit of other specialties, for example, infectious diseases, oncology or haematology. Thus, the renal physician needs to maintain a breadth of medical knowledge, and is perhaps one of the few remaining generalists. This is deliberately reflected in some of the cases, whose presentation begins with a symptom or sign which appears unrelated to the kidneys. As a result, this book will also help you polish up on some basic general medical facts.

Another concept which I have tried to convey in this text is that the kidneys are 'sensitive' organs, and can frequently become acutely dysfunctional in the context of a variety of pathologies. Thus, all doctors, regardless of their specialty or career choice, will encounter patients with acute renal failure (acute kidney injury). On the average 'medical take' or surgical/orthopaedic ward, there will always be a handful of patients with acute renal failure. These patients can be very unwell but if managed promptly and appropriately, may regain their renal function. These are typified by the 10 cases of acute renal failure, starting with common causes and moving to rarer, to illustrate the principles of investigation, management and diagnosis of this important problem.

Chronic kidney disease (CKD) is now widely diagnosed, due to the increased availability of measurements of renal function, in particular eGFR. General practitioners need to be aware of the complications associated with CKD and the appropriate time for referral to nephrology services. I have therefore presented a number of cases of patients with CKD, which touch upon the practicalities of managing associated complications and of providing renal replacement therapy for the increasing number of patients diagnosed with CKD. For those with CKD reaching end-stage renal failure, dialysis and renal transplantation are no longer limited to the lucky, 'fit' few but are available to all. Very few textbooks provide practical advice on the management of these patients and I hope that students (and junior doctors) asked to deal with these chronic nephrology patients will find the cases in this book of genuine practical use. On a more pragmatic note, patients with CKD are often well with stable clinical signs and are therefore frequent attendees at student clinical examinations (with an arteriovenous fistula, palpable kidneys or a transplanted kidney). This text should allow you to really fly through those stations of the exam. The MCQs, EMQs and SAQs also provide practical help to test your nephrology knowledge prior to examinations.

In summary, nephrology need not be feared and can be understood. Over the last 10 or so years, I have taught many students clinical medicine at the bedside. There is no substitute for this but in this text, I have tried to recreate some of these cases in an attempt to convey some of the important concepts and, I hope, to make renal medicine accessible to all.

Menna Clatworthy
Cambridge

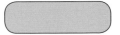 # Acknowledgements

There are a number of people to whom I owe a great deal of thanks. First and foremost to the many patients and students who have been involved in my teaching sessions over the last decade, who have provided a stimulus to clarify some of the more tricky aspects of renal medicine for the purposes of teaching. In terms of direct assistance with this book, my sincere thanks go, in particular, to Dr Meryl Griffiths (histopathologist, Addenbrooke's Hospital, Cambridge) for the many renal biopsy pictures featured in this book. To the patients who consented to photographs, especially those in the transplant clinic and dialysis unit at Addenbrooke's Hospital, Cambridge. To Dr Liz Wallin, for tirelessly tracking down and retrieving a number of radiology images, drug and fluid charts for illustrations, as well as proof reading Part 1. To Dr Lisa Willcocks (for assistance with renal biopsy pictures), to Sister Angela Green (for help in gathering PD-related pictures), to Mr Chris Watson (for formatting assistance and general wisdom) and to Sarah Harford (for cheerfulness, encouragement, tea and scanning skills). To many of the renal SpRs at Addenbrooke's for proof reading and providing comments on the cases contained within this book, including Dr Lisa Willcocks, Dr Eoin McKinney, Dr Andy Fry, Dr Thomas Heimstra, Dr Elaine Jolly and Dr Sharon Mulroy. Finally, to my family back in South Wales, who tolerated a whole Christmas holiday of writing with patience and provided a constant source of support and encouragement.

How to use this book

Clinical Cases Uncovered (CCU) books are carefully designed to help supplement your clinical experience and assist with refreshing your memory when revising. Each book is divided into three sections: Part 1, Basics; Part 2, Cases; and Part 3, Self-assessment.

Part 1 gives you a quick reminder of the basic science, history and examination, and key diagnoses in the area. Part 3 contains many of the clinical presentations you would expect to see on the wards or cropping up in exams, with questions and answers leading you through each case. New information, such as test results, is revealed as events unfold and each case concludes with a handy case summary explaining the key points. Part 3 allows you to test your learning with several question styles (MCQs, EMQs and SAQs), each with a strong clinical focus.

Whether reading individually or working as part of a group, we hope you will enjoy using your CCU book. If you have any recommendations on how we could improve the series, please do let us know by contacting us at: medstudentuk@oxon.blackwellpublishing.com.

Disclaimer

CCU patients are designed to reflect real life, with their own reports of symptoms and concerns. Please note that all names used are entirely fictitious and any similarity to patients, alive or dead, is coincidental.

List of abbreviations

AAA	abdominal aortic aneurysm		CAD	coronary artery disease
AAV	ANCA-associated vasculitis		CAH	chronic active autoimmune hepatitis
ABG	arterial blood gas		CAPD	continuous ambulatory peritoneal dialysis
ABPI	Ankle Brachial Pressure Index			
ACE	angiotensin-converting enzyme		cCa	corrected calcium
ACEI	angiotensin-converting enzyme inhibitor		CCF	congestive cardiac failure
			CCPD	continuous cyclic PD
ACR	albumin/creatinine ratio		CI	confidence interval
ADH	anti-diuretic hormone		CIN	contrast-induced nephropathy
ADPKD	autosomal dominant polycystic kidney disease		CIT	cold ischaemic time
			CK	creatine kinase
AF	atrial fibrillation		CKD	chronic kidney disease
AGE	advanced glycosylation end products		CKD-BMD	chronic kidney disease-bone and mineral disorder
aHUS	atypical haemolytic uraemic syndrome			
AKI	acute kidney injury		CMV	cytomegalovirus
ALG	antilymphocyte globulin		CNI	calcineurin inhibitor
ALP	alkaline phosphatase		CO	cardiac output
ANA	anti-nuclear antibodies		COPD	chronic obstructive pulmonary disease
ANCA	anti-neutrophil cytoplasmic antibody		CPM	central pontine myelinolysis
ANP	atrial natriuretic peptide		CRP	C-reactive protein
APD	automated peritoneal dialysis		CSA	ciclosporin-A
APKD	adult polycystic kidney disease		CT	computed tomography
APTT	activated partial thromboplastin time		CVA	cerebrovascular accident
AR	atrial regurgitation		CVP	central venous pressure
ARB	angiotensin receptor blockers		CVS	cardiovascular system
ARF	acute renal failure		CXR	chest X-ray
ASO	anti-streptolysin-O		DGF	delayed graft function
ATG	anti-thymocyte globulin		DIC	disseminated intravascular coagulopathy
ATN	acute tubular necrosis		DKA	diabetic ketoacidosis
AVF	arteriovenous fistula		DM	diabetes mellitus
AVM	arteriovenous malformation		DVT	deep vein thrombosis
BCC	basal cell carcinoma		EBV	Epstein–Barr virus
BFT	bone function tests		ECG	electrocardiogram
BHS	British Hypertension Society		eGFR	estimated glomerular filtration rate
BM	basement membrane		EH	essential hypertension
BMI	Body Mass Index		EM	electron microscopy
BP	blood pressure		ENT	ear, nose and throat
BPH	benign prostatic hypertrophy		EPO	erythropoietin
bpm	beats per minute		EPS	encapsulating peritoneal sclerosis

ESR	erythrocyte sedimentation rate	MCGN	mesangiocapillary glomerulonephritis
ESRF	end-stage renal failure	MCP	membrane co-factor protein
FBC	full blood count	MCV	mean corpuscular volume
FFP	fresh frozen plasma	MDT	multidisciplinary team
FGF23	fibroblast growth factor 23	MEN	multiple endocrine neoplasia
FH	family history	MI	myocardial infarction
FMD	fibromuscular dysplasia	MM	multiple myeloma
FOB	faecal occult blood	MMF	mycophenolate mofetil
FSGS	focal segmental glomerular sclerosis	MPGN	membranoproliferative glomerulonephritis
GAG	glycosaminoglycans		
GCS	Glasgow Coma Score	MPO	myeloperoxidase
GBM	glomerular basement membrane	MR	mitral regurgitation
GFR	glomerular filtration rate	MRA	magnetic resonance angiography
GI	gastrointestinal	MRI	magnetic resonance imaging
GN	glomerulonephritis	MSU	midstream urine
HAART	highly active antiretroviral therapy	NAD	no abnormality detected
HD	haemodialysis	NBM	nil by mouth
HDU	high-dependency unit	NPBP	nephritis plasmin-binding protein
HELLP	haemolysis, elevated liver enzymes, low platelets	NIPD	nightly intermittent peritoneal dialysis
		NSAID	non-steroidal anti-inflammatory drugs
HHV	human herpes virus	NSAP	nephritis strain-associated protein
HIV	human immunodeficiency virus	NSF	nephrogenic systemic fibrosis
HIVAN	HIV-associated nephropathy	OCP	oral contraceptive pill
HLA	human leucocyte antigen	OPD	outpatients department
HPV	human papilloma virus	ORG	obesity-related glomerulopathy
HR	heart rate	PAAg	preabsorbing antigen
HS	heart sounds	PAMP	pathogen-associated molecular patterns
HSP	Henoch–Schönlein purpura	PAN	polyarteritis nodosa
HUS	haemolytic uraemic syndrome	PBC	primary biliary cirrhosis
IC	immune complex	PCA	patient-controlled analgesia
ICP	intracranial pressure	PCP	*Pneumocystis carinii* pneumonia
ICU	intensive care unit	PCR	polymerase chain reaction
IGT	impaired glucose tolerance	PCr	protein/creatinine ratio
INR	international normalised ratio	PD	peritoneal dialysis
IP	intraperitoneal	PE	pulmonary embolism
IPD	intermittent peritoneal dialysis	PEX	plasma exchange
ITP	immune thrombocytopaenic purpura	PKD	polycystic kidney disease
ITU	intensive treatment unit	PMH	past medical history
IVC	inferior vena cava	pmp	per million people
IVDU	intravenous drug use	PND	paroxysmal nocturnal dyspnoea
JVP	jugular venous pressure	POP	plaster of Paris
LAD	left axis deviation	PPI	proton pump inhibitor
LFT	liver function tests	PR	per rectum
LN	lymph node	PSA	prostate-specific antigen
LV	left ventricle/ventricular	PT	prothrombin time
LVH	left ventricular hypertrophy	PTH	parathyroid hormone
MAC	membrane attack complex	PTHrP	parathyroid hormone related-protein
MAHA	microangiopathic haemolytic anaemia	PTLD	post-transplant lymphoproliferative disorder
MAP	mean arterial pressure		

PVD	peripheral vascular disease	SOB	shortness of breath
RAA	renin-angiotensin-aldosterone	STEC	shigatoxin-producing *E. coli*
RAS	renal artery stenosis	SV	stroke volume
RBC	red blood cell	TCC	transitional cell carcinoma
RF	rheumatoid factor	TIA	transient ischaemic attack
RHF	right heart failure	TIN	tubulointerstitial nephritis
rpm	respirations per minute	TLR	Toll-like receptors
RR	respiratory rate, relative risk	TNF	tumour necrosis factor
RRT	renal replacement therapy	TPD	tidal peritoneal dialysis
RTA	renal tubular acidosis	TPR	total peripheral resistance
RVH	right ventricular hypertrophy	TTP	thrombotic thrombocytopaenic purpura
SAA	serum amyloid A	U&E	urea and electrolytes
SAH	subarachnoid haemorrhage	UF	ultrafiltration
SAP	serum amyloid P	URR	urea reduction ratio
SCC	squamous cell carcinoma	US	ultrasound
SIADH	syndrome of inappropriate antidiuretic hormone	UTI	urinary tract infection
		WBC	white blood cells
SLE	systemic lupus erythematosus	WG	Wegener's granulomatosis

Normal range for investigations

Haematology

Full blood count (FBC):

Haemoglobin (Hb) 11.5–16 g/dL (female), 13.5–18 g/dL (male)

White blood cells (WBC) $4–11 \times 10^9$/L

Platelets (plats) $150–400 \times 10^9$/L

Biochemistry

Sodium (Na) 135–145 mmol/L

Potassium (K) 3.5–5.3 mmol/L

Urea (U) 2.5–6.7 mmol/L

Creatinine (Creat) 50–120 μmol/L (varies according to muscle bulk and diet)

Corrected calcium (cCa) 2.18–2.6 mmol/L

Phosphate (PO_4) 0.8–1.45 mmol/L

Glucose (Glu) 3.5–5.5 mmol/L

Albumin (Alb) 35–50 g/L

Alkaline phosphatase (ALP) 30–300 iu/L

C-reactive protein (CRP) <6 mg/L

Creatine kinase (CK) 25–195 iu/L

Serum osmolality 278–305 mosmol/kg

pH 7.25–7.45

Bicarbonate (HCO_3) 24–28 mmol/L

Chloride (Cl) 95–105 mmol/L

Parathyroid hormone (PTH) <65 pg/mL

pO_2 10–13 kPa

pCO_2 4.9–6.1 kPa

Basic science

The structure of the kidney has evolved to effectively accomplish its main tasks, which include a number of functions that do not obviously relate to its main blood-cleaning role. They are:

• control of water balance
• control of electrolyte balance
• excretion of water-soluble waste
• control of acid–base balance
• control of blood pressure (through both control of water and electrolyte balance and production of renin)
• the production of active vitamin D (through the action of 1α-hydroxylase) and hence control of calcium-phosphate metabolism
• the production of erythropoietin, and hence control of haemoglobin level.

When the kidneys become diseased or dysfunctional, the symptoms with which a patient presents arise because of the failure to perform one or more of the above tasks. Before considering the clinical presentation of renal diseases, it is useful to put them in the context of basic renal anatomy, histology, physiology and biochemistry.

Anatomy

Most individuals have two kidneys, which lie in the retroperitoneum on either side of the midline (at vertebral level T12–L3). In adults, the kidneys measure around 10–12 cm in bipolar length and the upper poles are protected by the 11th and 12th ribs. The kidneys are pushed down into the abdomen during deep inspiration as the lungs expand and the diaphragm flattens. The adrenal glands rest on the upper poles of the kidneys and both organs are encased by two layers of fat (the peri- and pararenal fat) and a layer of fascia. The kidneys are surrounded by a tough capsule and are made up of an outer cortex and inner medulla. In older adults, cysts may form but these should number less than five per kidney.

Nephrology: Clinical Cases Uncovered. By M. Clatworthy.
Published 2010 by Blackwell Publishing.

Given that the kidneys play a major role in clearance of circulating waste products and drugs, it is unsurprising that they receive a large volume of blood (25% of cardiac output) via the renal arteries, branches of the abdominal aorta. Each renal artery divides into progressively smaller vessels (arcuate, interlobular, then afferent arterioles). Blood is drained via the renal veins into the inferior vena cava, and urine via the ureter, which winds through the retroperitoneum to the bladder. Here the urine is stored and finally expelled through the urethra, which is longer in the male, thus reducing the risk of bladder infections. In males the urethra is encircled by the prostate gland, which may become enlarged in later life, causing obstruction to the outflow of urine (Figure A).

The functioning unit of the kidney is the nephron (Figure B), of which there are about a million per kidney. The nephron is made up of a glomerulus, proximal tubule, loop of Henle, distal tubule and collecting duct. Each capillary loop within the glomerulus has a layer of fenestrated endothelium surrounded by the glomerular basement membrane, which is in turn enveloped by an epithelial cell, the podocyte (Figure C). Each capillary loop is supported by a mesangial cell with surrounding matrix. Inflammation of the glomeruli (glomerulonephritis (GN)) tends to cause proliferation of one or more of the component cells of the glomerular capillary loop; for example, in IgA nephropathy, there is proliferation of the mesangial cells, in cresecentic GN there is proliferation of the epithelial cells to form a cellular crescent. Basic descriptions of these histological changes are used to define the different types of GN (see later).

Physiology

An overview of tubular function is given in Figure D.

Glomerular function

Blood arrives at the glomerulus via the afferent arteriole and around 20% of the plasma (and none of the cellular components of blood) is filtered into Bowman's capsule

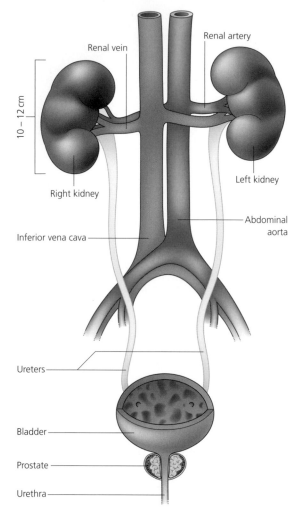

Renal vein

Renal artery

10 – 12 cm

Right kidney

Left kidney

Inferior vena cava

Abdominal aorta

Ureters

Bladder

Prostate

Urethra

Figure A Anatomy of the renal tract.

as it passes through the glomerular capillary loops. The filtered blood leaves the glomerulus via the efferent arteriole which subsequently divides to form the peritubular capillaries. Filtration is a passive process which is driven by the hydrostatic pressure acting across glomerular capillaries and is countered by the oncotic pressure exerted by circulating proteins such as albumin. It is also in part dependent on the permeability of the glomerulus (which can increase if the podocyte becomes diseased, leading to proteinuria, or decrease in many conditions, e.g. if there is thickening of the basement membrane). Glomerular filtration is a key requirement for the blood-cleaning and water-handling functions of the kidneys. Thus, the glomerular filtration rate (GFR) is the main measure of kidney function used by nephrologists. GFR varies but is

around $130\,\mathrm{mL/min/1.73\,m^2}$ in men and $120\,\mathrm{mL/min/}$ $1.73\,\mathrm{m^2}$ in women. GFR remains constant until around the age of 40 years, but thereafter gradually declines (by approximately $1\,\mathrm{mL/min/1.73\,m^2}$ per year) ($1.73\,\mathrm{m^2}$ is the average body surface area of an adult).

The simplest way of estimating GFR is to measure the serum creatinine. Creatinine is constantly being produced by muscle cells and is filtered by the kidney. If GFR declines, then serum creatinine will increase.

Tubular physiology (Figure D)

The normal GFR of $120\text{–}30\,\mathrm{mL/min/1.73\,m^2}$ requires the renal tubules to reabsorb vast quantities of water and electrolytes. For example, 180 litres of water are filtered at glomeruli per day. The total body (intracellular and extracellular) water volume is around 40 litres. If tubular reabsorption of water ceased, then the total plasma volume would be urinated in around 30 minutes.

Solutes such as Na^+, K^+, bicarbonate, and Cl^- and amino acids filtered at the glomerulus into Bowman's capsule need to be reabsorbed by tubular cells, or else they would all be lost in the urine (with severe consequences). Soluble waste products such as urea are also reabsorbed, but only partially, in contrast to the 'useful' solutes listed above, which are almost completely reabsorbed. In addition, tubular cells are involved in the secretion of waste products (such as creatinine, uric acid and H^+) into the urinary/tubular space. Thus, tubular cells express a number of surface pumps, allowing them to move molecules from the urinary space into the interstitium, and vice versa. These pumps require energy to function properly, so the metabolic needs of tubular cells are high and they are extremely susceptible to ischaemic injury, as seen in acute tubular necrosis (ATN).

The fine tuning of Na^+ and water balance is achieved in the distal tubule and collecting duct (via the influence of aldosterone and antidiuretic hormone (ADH)). Normal urine volume is around 1.5–2 litres/day.

Table A shows the average values of water and some electrolytes handled by the kidneys.

Proximal tubules

The main role of the proximal tubule is reabsorption of water and filtered electrolytes, glucose and amino acids, including:
- 60–80% of water
- 60–70% of filtered sodium (via the Na/K-ATPase)
- 90% of potassium
- 90% of bicarbonate

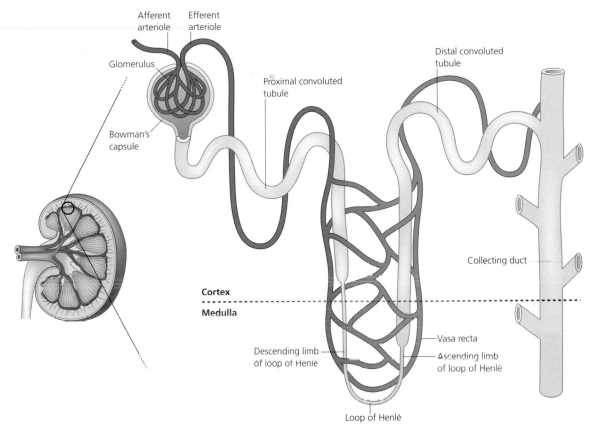

Figure B The nephron.

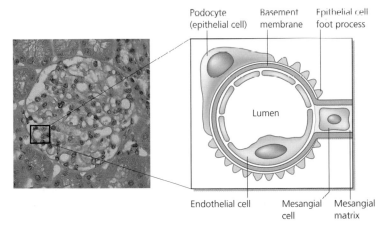

Figure C The glomerulus. Left panel shows typical histological appearance of the glomerulus. A single capillary loop is boxed and the structures within identified in the right-hand panel.

- 100% of glucose
- 100% of amino acids
- variable quantity of chloride, calcium and magnesium

- variable quantity of phosphate (dependent on parathyroid hormone (PTH) concentration).

Waste products secreted into the tubular space in the proximal tubule include creatinine and uric acid.

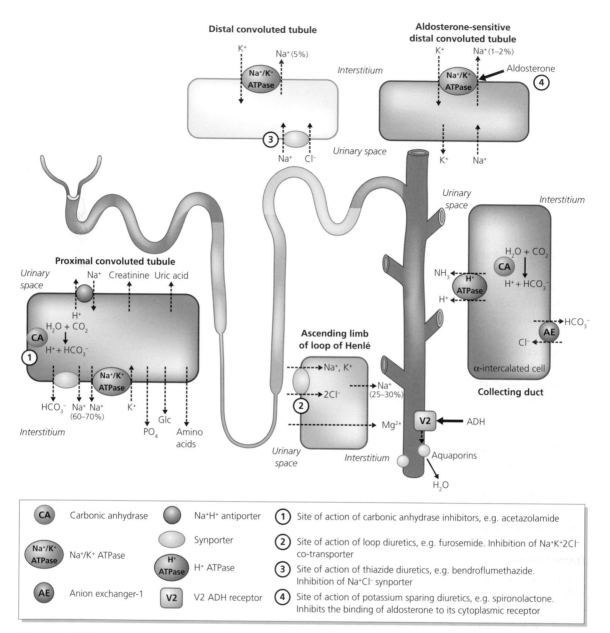

Figure D Tubular function (see text for detailed description).

Substance	Amount filtered/day	Amount excreted/day	% reabsorption
Water (litres)	180	1.8	99
Sodium (g)	630	3.2	99.5
Glucose (g)	180	0	100
Urea (g)	56	28	50

Table A Renal water and solute handling

If there is proximal tubule dysfunction (e.g. in type II (proximal) renal tubular acidosis) then there is glycosuria, aminoaciduria and acidosis (due to loss of bicarbonate).

Loop of Henle

The main role of the loop of Henle is to generate an interstitial sodium gradient between the cortex (low concentration Na^+) and inner regions of the medulla (high concentration Na^+). This concentration gradient is generated by virtue of the fact that the ascending limb of the loop of Henle is impermeable to water.

Twenty to 40% of sodium is reabsorbed from the tubular space into the interstitium in the loop of Henle by the NaK2Cl co-transporter and around 10% of filtered water. This generates a high concentration of Na^+ in the interstitium but water is unable to follow, due to the impermeable ascending limb. The high interstitial Na^+ concentration provides a gradient which allows urine to be concentrated as it flows through the collecting tubules (the permeability of which is controlled by ADH).

The NaK2Cl co-transporter is inhibited by loop diuretics, the effect of which is to reduce sodium reabsorption, and hence the concentration gradient generated, so that a more dilute urine is produced. In addition to sodium transport, the majority of magnesium is also absorbed in the ascending limb of the loop.

At the end of the loop of Henle, as it arrives back up in the cortex, lie the cells of the macula densa. These cells sense luminal sodium concentration and are involved in controlling the release of renin, and hence systemic blood pressure (see below).

Distal tubule

The distal tubule plays a role in fine tuning the final urine sodium concentration (and hence determines how dilute or concentrated it will be). Around 5% of sodium is reabsorbed here via the NaCl co-transporter, which is inhibited by thiazide diuretics.

Collecting duct

A further 2% of sodium is reabsorbed by the aldosterone-sensitive sodium channels found within the distal convoluted tubule and the collecting duct.

Acid secretion is performed by the α-intercalated cells of the collecting tubule and involves two pumps: $H^+ATPase$ and the basolateral $Cl^-:HCO_3^-$ anion exchanger 1 (AE-1) and an enzyme (carbonic anhydrase 2 (CA2); see Figure D for details.

Antidiuretic hormone (ADH) exerts its effects on this portion of the nephron, causing the insertion of aquaporins into the luminal membrane, thus facilitating the reabsorption of water, which travels from the tubular space into the interstitium as a result of the concentration gradient generated by the loop of Henle.

The physiology of blood pressure control

When considering the ways in which the kidneys are involved in blood pressure control, it is important to bear in mind the basic physiological principle that mean arterial pressure (MAP) is dependent on cardiac output (CO) and total peripheral resistance (TPR) (Box A). CO is affected by stroke volume and hence venous return. As tubular function declines in chronic kidney disease (CKD), the kidney retains fluid and the venous return increases, causing a rise in MAP. Thus CKD is often associated with hypertension.

Renin-angiotensin-aldosterone (RAA) pathway (Figure E)

Renin is released from the juxtoglomerular apparatus of the kidney in response to reduced renal perfusion or low sodium delivery to the distal part of the loop of Henle. Renin coverts angiotensinogen (made in liver) to angiotensin I. This is converted to angiotensin II by angiotensin-converting enzyme (ACE), found principally in the pulmonary vasculature. Angiotensin II is a potent vasoconstrictor and will thus increase TPR and MAP. It also causes the release of aldosterone from the adrenal cortex, which acts on the distal tubule to cause retention of sodium, and thus water, expanding volume and increasing venous return, CO and MAP.

In addition, angiotensin II leads to the release of ADH from the posterior pituitary. ADH increases permeability of the collecting duct by stimulating the insertion of water channels (aquaporins) into the apical (luminal) membrane of principal cells of the collecting duct. This is achieved through the action of ADH on V2 receptors, G protein-coupled receptors on the basolateral (intersti-

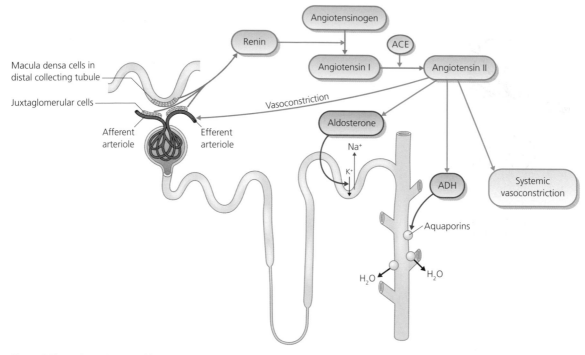

Figure E The renin-angiotensin-aldosterone system.

tial) membrane of principal cells. Following binding, activation of the cAMP cascade leads to the release of aquaporins from storage vesicles by exocytosis. The aquaporins are then inserted into the apical (luminal) membrane, allowing water to pass out of the distal convoluted tubules and the collecting tubules into the interstitium, and back into the blood. The net effect is to increase the concentration of urine and expand blood volume, causing a rise in MAP.

Biochemistry
Endocrine functions of the kidney
Vitamin D metabolism
Naturally occurring vitamin D requires hydroxylation, first in the liver to 25,OH-vitamin D and then in the kidney to $1,25(OH)_2$-vitamin D via the action of the enzyme 1α-hydroxylase. If the kidneys are diseased, there is a reduction in production of active vitamin D ($1,25(OH)_2$-vitamin D). This results in reduced absorption of calcium from the gut, impaired bone mineralisation and hypocalcaemia. The low levels of calcium and $1,25(OH)_2$-vitamin D (as well as high phosphate) are sensed by cells of the parathyroid gland, which increase

the production of PTH in an attempt to restore normocalcaemia, a state known as secondary hyperparathyroidism. If there is chronic kidney dysfunction and persistent hypocalcaemia, the parathyroid glands hypertrophy and begin to function autonomously, i.e. independently of blood calcium level, leading to hypercalcaemia (tertiary hyperparathyroidism) (Figure F).

Erythropoietin production
Endogenous erythropoietin (EPO) is produced by peritubular cells. It acts on erythroid precursors within the bone marrow, stimulating proliferation and maturation. Damage to the kidney leads to reduced EPO production and can be seen when GFR falls to <50 mL/min. Anaemia in CKD patients is exacerbated by impaired intestinal absorption of iron and reduced iron intake. Prior to the introduction of recombinant EPO, anaemia was a major cause of morbidity and mortality in patients with end-stage renal failure, and was associated with cardiovascular complications in particular. In some renal conditions, e.g. polycystic kidney disease or renal cell carcinoma, the production of EPO may increase, leading to polycythaemia.

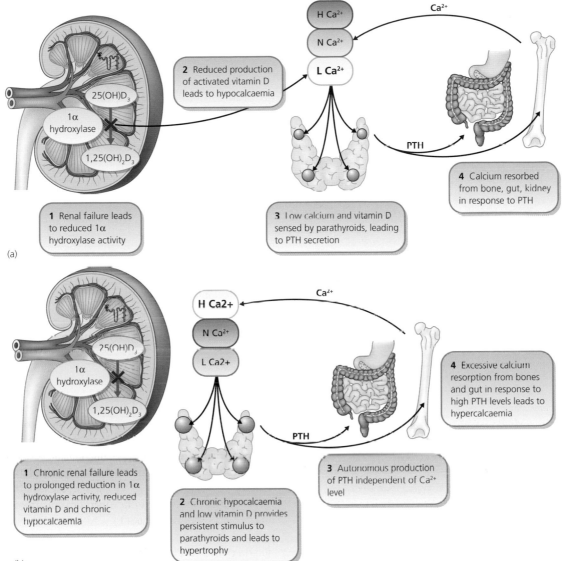

Figure F (a) Secondary hyperparathyroidism. (b) Tertiary hyperparathyroidism.

PART 1: BASICS

Approach to the patient

History
Specific features related to renal disease

1. Urine abnormalities
   - *Amount*
     - A reduced amount of urine (<300 mL/day) is termed oliguira.
     - An absence of urine production is termed anuria. Oliguria occurs in nephritic syndrome, acute renal failure (ARF) and chronic end-stage renal failure (ESRF). Absolute anuria suggests a complete obstruction to the outflow of urine (e.g. prostatic disease), a vascular catastrophe or acute cortical necrosis.
     - An increased production of urine is termed poly-uria (urine output >3 L/24 h). This may occur as a result of:
       - diuretic agents
       - reduced ADH secretion (cranial diabetes insipidus, alcohol)
       - insensitivity to ADH (nephrogenic diabetes insipidus)
       - psychogenic polydipsia
       - atrial natriuretic peptide (ANP) release (e.g. associated with cardiac arrhythmias, cardiac failure)
       - osmotic diuresis (hyperglycaemia, hypercalciuria)
       - chronic kidney disease (CKD) (inability of the diseased tubular cells to appropriately move Na and hence concentrate urine)
   - *Nocturia*: adults do not normally pass urine at night, although there is some variability. Nocturia occurs in CKD, in conditions where an osmotic agent is found in the urine (e.g. glucose in diabetes mellitus (DM), calcium in conditions associated with hypercalciuria) or in prostatic disease.

- *Urinary frequency* can occur in DM, hypercalciuria and urinary tract infections (UTI).
- *Poor urinary stream*: this is a symptom of prostatic disease or sphincter dysfunction.
- *Colour*: urine should be clear to light yellow in colour (depending on concentration). 'Coke-coloured' is seen in nephritic syndrome, where there is glomerular haematuria. 'Tea-coloured' urine is seen in myoglobinuria (usually secondary to rhabdomyolysis). Macroscopic haematuria (where urine is obviously blood-stained) may be due to bleeding in the upper (e.g. IgA nephropathy) or lower urinary tract (e.g. bladder cancer, renal calculi). Frothy urine is observed if there is heavy proteinuria. Other causes of discoloured urine include rifampicin or beetroot ingestion (pink-red) and cholestatic jaundice (bright/strongly coloured yellow). Discolouration of urine on standing may occur in alkaptonuria or porphyria.
- *Dysuria* (pain whilst passing urine): this classically occurs in UTI or in urethritis (e.g. in gonococcal infection).

2. Loin pain: this can occur due to renal calculi (stones), infection, IgA nephropathy, loin pain haematuria, and polycystic kidney disease. Renal colic (due to the passage of a renal calculus through the ureter) is usually agonisingly painful, and patients often require opiates to relieve the pain.
3. Oedema: occurs if there is volume overload (increased hydrostatic pressure) or in nephrotic syndrome where heavy proteinuria leads to reduced oncotic pressure.
4. Symptoms of hypertension, e.g. headache, blurred vision or fitting (if severe).
5. Symptoms of anaemia (secondary to erythropoietin (EPO) deficiency), e.g. tiredness, dyspnoea.
6. Symptoms of uraemia such as nausea/vomiting, chest pain associated with pericarditis or confusion due to uraemic encephalopathy.
7. Symptoms of hyperphosphataemia such as itchiness, lethargy.

Nephrology: Clinical Cases Uncovered. By M. Clatworthy.
Published 2010 by Blackwell Publishing.

Symptoms 4–7 occur if there is a decline in renal function such that the kidney cannot perform its basic tasks.

Past medical history (PMH)

Has the patient ever had any renal problems previously? Have they ever had their kidney function assessed? This is useful if trying to delineate between acute and chronic renal failure.

Is there a PMH of diseases which can cause chronic kidney disease?
- Diabetes mellitus (diabetic nephropathy)
- Hypertension (can be a cause of, or occur as a result of renal impairment)
- Vascular disease, including peripheral vascular disease, myocardial infarction, cerebrovascular disease. A past history of such diseases marks out the patient as an arteriopath who may also have renovascular disease
- Prostatic hypertrophy (obstructive uropathy)
- Recurrent UTI (chronic pyelonephritis)
- Recurrent renal calculi (nephrocalcinosis)

Is there a PMH of diseases which can cause acute renal failure?
- Systemic lupus erythematosus (SLE) (50–60% of patients with SLE have renal involvement)
- Vasculitis
- Infections (hepatitis B/C, HIV)
- Myeloma

Is there a PMH of diseases which can cause nephrosis (heavy proteinuria)?
- Diabetes mellitus
- SLE
- Amyloid
- Infections (hepatitis B/C, HIV)
- Myeloma

Systems review

It is important to ascertain whether the patient had any other illness prior to presentation, e.g. pharyngitis (which may be associated with IgA nephropathy or post-streptococcal glomerulonephritis (GN)), vomiting/diarrhoea/blood loss (all of which predispose to volume depletion and pre-renal failure), sepsis (risk factor for pre-renal failure/ATN) or back pain (which can be associated with myeloma).

Many autoimmune diseases are systemic and affect multiple organ systems. Thus, there may be non-specific symptoms such as fever, night sweats, lethargy and malaise. A failure to enquire about or recognise the importance of such relatively non-specific systemic symptoms can lead to a delay in diagnosis of some serious autoimmune diseases, particularly systemic vasculitis. In addition to systemic symptoms, there may also be evidence of inflammation in other systems such as joints (arthralgia), eyes (red eyes due to anterior uveitis, dry eyes due to keratoconjunctivitis sicca), gastrointestinal tract (mouth ulcers, abdominal pain), genitourinary ulcers, skin (photosensitivity rash, discoid lupus, purpuric rash of vasculitis) or symptoms typical of a systemic vasculitis (e.g. sinusitis, ear ache, hearing loss, shortness of breath, haemoptysis). The occurrence of pulmonary haemorrhage in association with acute renal failure secondary to a rapidly progressive glomerulonephritis is known as pulmonary-renal syndrome, and is important to recognise (the causes are described in detail in case 8).

Drug history

- Has the patient started on any new drugs? Such a history may suggest acute tubulointerstitial nephritis (TIN), particularly if associated with a rash. Some drugs are associated with the development of SLE (e.g. hydralazine).
- Is the patient taking any nephrotoxic medications? Angiotensin-converting enzyme inhibitors (ACEI), non-steroidal anti-inflammatory drugs (NSAID), ciclosporin-A (alter renal blood flow); gentamicin, lithium, amphotericin, cisplatin (directly toxic to tubules); NSAID, antibiotics, proton pump inhibitors (PPI) (associated with interstitial nephritis); gold, penicillamine (can cause proteinuria).
- Is the patient taking any drugs which are predominantly excreted by the kidneys, e.g. digoxin or allopurinol? In such cases, the dose of the drug should be reduced if there is a significant renal impairment. The *British National Formulary* (BNF) has a specific section indicating which drugs require a dosage adjustment in patients with renal impairment.

Social history

- Employment history: certain occupations are associated with an increased risk of developing diseases which can present with renal problems. For example, livestock and arable farming is associated with an increased risk of developing anti-neutrophil cytoplasmic antibody (ANCA)-associated vasculitis.

- Smoking history: smoking is a risk factor for renovascular disease and is associated with pulmonary haemorrhage in patients with Goodpasture's disease). In contrast, smoking is protective in pre-eclampsia.
- Intravenous drug use (IVDU) is a risk factor for hepatitis B/C/HIV, which are associated with a variety of GN.

Family history
Monogenic disorders which affect the kidneys
- The most common genetic disorder affecting the kidneys is adult (autosomal dominant) polycystic kidney disease (APKD). New mutations occur in only 5% of cases, although many patients will not be aware of a positive family history of disease. Closer questioning or discussion with older relatives may prompt recall of a family member who died of 'kidney trouble' or 'brain haemorrhage'. APKD is caused by mutations in one of two genes, PKD1 (chromosome 16p) and PKD2 (chromosome 4q), encoding polycystin 1 and polycystin 2 respectively. Mutations in PKD1 are more common than PKD2, accounting for 85% of cases of APKD.
- Alport's syndrome presents with a nephritic syndrome and is often associated wth sensorineural deafness. It occurs due to mutations in the genes encoding collagen chains (mainly type IV) and can be inherited in an autosomal recessive or X-linked fashion.
- Some forms of focal segmental glomerular sclerosis (FSGS) are also familial, occurring due to mutations in the genes encoding podocin or nephrin (components of the slit diaphragm of podocytes).

Polygenic disorders which affect the kidneys
Some disorders occur due to the presence of polymorphisms in more than one susceptibility gene. These polymorphisms are often found as relatively common variants in the general population, and it is the inheritance of a specific combination of a number of these susceptibility genes which predisposes to disease. Examples of such polygenic diseases include autoimmune conditions such as diabetes mellitus and SLE. Some genetic polymorphisms confer susceptibility to a number of different autoimmune diseases. Therefore a history of one autoimmune disease (e.g. rheumatoid arthritis) in a family member increases the likelihood of another family member developing a different autoimmune disease (e.g. type I diabetes mellitus).

Examination
General features
- Is the patient sick or stable? It is important to identify this early as some patients with acute renal failure

> **Box B The classic signs associated with inflammation**
>
> The first four were described by Celsus in around 30 BC. The fifth was added by Virchov in 1870.
> 1. Calor – Heat
> 2. Dolor – Pain
> 3. Rubor – Redness
> 4. Tumor – Swelling
> 5. Functio laesa – loss of /reduced function

may require high-dependency or intensive treatment unit (ITU) care.
- *Temperature*: a fever may indicate infection or systemic autoimmune disease.
- *Nails, hands, and feet*: examining for the presence of splinter haemorrhages, nailfold infarcts, necrotic areas (signs of vasculitis/endocarditis). Leuconychia (associated with hypoalbuminaemia which may be secondary to liver failure, nephrotic syndrome or chronic inflammatory disease). Small joints of the hands for signs of arthritis (heat, swelling, pain, erythema, the classic signs of inflammation; see Box B) which can occur in some systemic autoimmune diseases that affect the kidney, e.g. SLE, rheumatoid arthritis.
- *Skin rashes*: purpuric lesions (associated with vasculitis), photosensitivity rash (usually on sun-exposed areas such as dorsum of forearms, neck and face – seen in SLE), maculopapular erythematous rash (drug associated), petechial rash (associated with thrombocytopaenia, e.g. as seen in haemolytic uraemic syndrome).
- *Legs*: peripheral oedema (evidenced by swelling of the ankles/legs or by the presence of sacral oedema in bed-bound patients). Peripheral oedema may occur secondary to an increase in hydrostatic pressure (e.g. right heart failure or volume overload) or if there is a reduction in oncotic pressure (e.g. liver failure, nephrosis, malabsorption).
- *Eyes*: conjunctivitis and anterior uveitis both present with red eyes and can occur in autoimmune conditions which are also associated with renal involvement (e.g. rheumatoid arthritis can cause a keratoconjunctivitis and may be associated with amyloidosis). In addition, fundoscopy should be performed in order to assess whether there is retinopathy associated with hypertension or diabetes mellitus. The presence of diabetic retinopathy indicates significant microvascular disease, and such patients will usually also have diabetic nephropathy.

- *Mouth*: in a renal transplant patient, there may be gingival hypertrophy if the patient is on long-term ciclosporin. SLE and Behçet's disease are associated with mouth ulceration. Amyloidosis is associated with macroglossia.

Cardiovascular system

- Assess intravascular volume status, as volume depletion is a cause of ARF and fluid overload can occur as a consequence of oligoanuria. Volume status should be assessed by examining skin turgor, dryness of mucous membranes, jugular venous pressure (JVP) (elevated JVP suggests volume overload, low JVP suggests volume depletion) and blood pressure (BP) (if low or postural drop then it is likely that there is hypovolaemia). A high BP can cause CKD or may be associated with CKD of any cause.
- *Heart sounds*: murmurs may be audible in endocarditis (which can be associated with GN due to deposition of circulating immune complexes in the glomeruli). Mitral regurgitation or mitral valve prolapse is associated with APKD. An aseptic endocarditis can occur in SLE (Libmann Sachs endocarditis).
- Severe uraemia can lead to pericarditis and a pericardial rub (sounds like feet crunching in the snow).

Respiratory system

- Pleural effusion (ipsilateral reduced expansion, reduced breath sounds, stony dull percussion note) can occur in nephrotic syndrome and if there is fluid overload secondary to acute or chronic renal failure.

- Pulmonary oedema (increased respiratory rate, reduced oxygen saturations, bibasal crepitations) can occur if there is volume overload. Coarse inspiratory crepitations may also occur if there is pulmonary haemorrhage (seen in Goodpasture's disease and ANCA-associated vasculitis).
- Pulmonary fibrosis (reduced oxygen saturations, reduced expansion, fine end-inspiratory crepitations) can be associated with ANCA-associated vasculitis.

Abdominal system

- Hepatosplenomegaly may occur secondary to cirrhosis with portal hypertension secondary to hepatitis B/C (both associated with GN) or secondary to amyloidosis (can affect the kidney, causing nephrotic syndrome and renal impairment). Splenomegaly may be observed in SLE.
- *Palpable kidneys*: occurs in APKD or renal tumour, or occasionally in amyloidosis.
- Abdominal aortic aneurysm (associated with renovascular disease and retroperitoneal fibrosis).
- Renal bruits +/− femoral bruits: associated with renovascular disease.
- Renal transplant *in situ* (usually a palpable mass in the left or right iliac fossa, with overlying 'hockey-stick' scar) (Figure G). There may also be a scar visible from previous peritoneal dialysis catheter insertion.

Nervous system

- Uraemia can be associated with encephalopathy (i.e. impairment of conciousness +/− confusion).

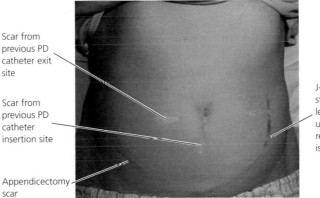

Scar from previous PD catheter exit site

Scar from previous PD catheter insertion site

Appendicectomy scar

J-shaped ('hockey stick') scar in the left iliac fossa, under which the renal transplant is palpable

Figure G Abdominal examination in a renal transplant patient. Other signs which should be specifically sought in a renal transplant patient include: blood glucose 'finger-prick' test marks (DM is one of the most common causes of ESRF); skin and gums for signs of long-term immunosuppression (e.g. gingival hypertrophy associated with ciclosporin); evidence of tunnelled line insertion in the neck/upper chest (used for temporary haemodialysis); evidence of arteriovenous fistula formation in the upper limbs; enlarged kidneys or liver (as seen in patients with APKD).

• Deafness (usually conductive) may occur in ANCA-associated vasculitis (particularly Wegener's granulomatosis). Sensorineural deafness is a feature of Alport's syndrome and some rare tubular diorders (where the same pumps are found in the ear as in tubular cells).

• Patients with long-standing diabetes with associated microvascular disease may have signs of neuropathy (peripheral or autonomic) as well as nephropathy.

• Vasculitides (particularly Churg-Strauss syndrome) are associated with peripheral neuropathy or mononeuritis multiplex.

• Some patients with SLE have neuropsychiatric features, including poor memory and depression.

• Systemic amyloidosis is associated with peripheral neuropathy (peripheral nerves may enlarge and become palpable) and/or autonomic neuropathy (evidenced by loss of heart rate variability and an increase in postural drop).

Clinical overview

Renal disease generally presents in three ways:
- hypertension
- urine dipstick abnormalities (proteinuria/haematuria)
- abnormal renal function tests/glomerular filtration rate (GFR).

These clinical features reflect a loss of the main roles of the kidney. Some patients present with only one of each of the features, but most will have a combination.

Clinical presentations
Hypertension
Asymptomatic hypertension
Hypertension may frequently be picked up at a routine work medical or in a 'well-person clinic' in individuals who are completely asymptomatic. Idiopathic/primary hypertension may cause chronic kidney disease (CKD) and is one of the most common causes of CKD in the UK, but hypertension may also occur secondary to CKD of any cause. Hypertension may also occur secondary to specific renal problems, e.g. renal artery stenosis.

Symptomatic hypertension
Hypertension may be associated with headache or blurred vision. Accelerated hypertension/malignant hypertension occurs when BP is acutely elevated, and is associated with papilloedema on fundal examination. Such patients may also begin to fit or be at risk of cerebral haemorrhage. Causes of accelerated hypertension include systemic sclerosis, haemolytic uraemic syndrome (HUS), and eclampsia.

Urine dipstick abnormalities
Proteinuria
The urine normally contains only small amounts of protein (<150 mg/24 h). This is because large molecular

Nephrology: Clinical Cases Uncovered. By M. Clatworthy. Published 2010 by Blackwell Publishing.

weight proteins (>40,000 Da) are not filtered at the glomerulus, provided there is an intact basement membrane/podocyte slit diaphragm. Smaller proteins, such as β2-microglobulin or light chains are freely filtered. Any filtered protein is normally catabolised in the proximal tubule. Any amino acids filtered are fully reabsorbed in the proximal tubule. Three causes of proteinuria are possible.

- *Glomerular proteinuria.* This occurs if there is failure of the glomerular filtration barrier, allowing inappropriate filtration of proteins. This may be due to damage to the basement membrane and/or podocyte or if there is a marked increase in glomerular capillary pressure (e.g. if there is excess angiotensin II).

- *Tubular proteinuria.* This occurs when there is a failure of tubular catabolism and may be due to tubular cell damage by toxins, e.g. aminoglycosides or heavy metals, or secondary to some congenital tubular disorders, e.g. Fanconi's syndrome.

- *Overflow proteinuria.* If there are inappropriately high levels of some proteins in the blood, then there will be some overflow filtration of these proteins. For example, high levels of light chain in multiple myeloma can lead to proteinuria, as can high levels of myoglobin (rhabdomyolysis) and haemoglobin (haemolysis).

If proteinuria becomes heavy enough, then the classic picture of nephrotic syndrome is observed (see later).

Haematuria
Normally there are only tiny amounts of red cells in the urine. Detection of blood in the urine, by dipstick or eye, occurs if there is a defect in the glomerular barrier allowing filtration of red cells (glomerular haematuria) or it may occur secondary to pathology in the lower urinary tract, e.g. urinary tract infection (UTI), bladder stone or malignancy (urological haematuria), all of which cause bleeding into the tubular/urinary space.

Microscopic haematuria

This is diagnosed by urine dipstick and the patient will not have observed any abnormality in the colour of their urine. There are a variety of causes of microscopic haematuria. If the patient is otherwise asymptomatic then IgA nephropathy or bladder tumours are common causes. All causes of macroscopic haematuria (see below) can also lead to dipstick abnormalities.

Macroscopic haematuria

Blood is visible in the urine. This may be bright red if it originates from the lower urinary tract (e.g. bladder carcinoma or renal calculi which may be associated with obstructive nephropathy) or may be 'coke coloured' if originating from the upper urinary tract/glomeruli (e.g. IgA nephropathy). In IgA nephropathy episodes of macroscopic haematuria often occur 3–4 days following the onset of pharyngitis. The causes of macroscopic haematuria are described in detail in case 6.

Abnormal GFR

Abnormalities of the filtering function of the kidneys lead to an accumulation of waste products which would normally be cleared by the kidneys, e.g. urea and creatinine. When physicians refer to a patient as having renal failure, this is usually based on the fact that they have an elevated serum creatinine value, and hence a suboptimal GFR. Renal failure, as evidenced by a decline in GFR, has tra-ditionally been classified in two ways, first according to its temporal progression, i.e. rapidly developing renal failure over a period of days or weeks is termed 'acute renal failure' (ARF) or 'acute kidney injury' whereas a decline in GFR occurring over months to years is termed 'chronic renal failure' or, more recently, 'chronic kidney disease' (CKD) (Figure Ha). The second way in which renal failure has been characterised is according to its cause. Thus the terms pre-renal, renal and postrenal failure have been coined, indicating the anatomical site at which the aetiological factor is acting (Figure Hb).

Acute renal failure (acute kidney injury)

Acute renal failure may be detected on routine blood tests in a patient who has non-specific symptoms such as malaise, lethargy or headache. Some present with oliguria and volume overload with shortness of breath due to pulmonary oedema. Other presentations depend on the cause. ARF implies by definition that the patient recently had normal renal function which has declined over a period of days to weeks. Hence, review of any previous renal function tests performed can be helpful in distinguishing between acute and chronic cases. As described above, causes of ARF can be divided into:

- *pre-renal causes*, e.g. hypotension of any cause, volume depletion, sepsis or renovascular disease
- *renal causes*, e.g. glomerular pathology, tubular pathology, interstitial pathology, vascular pathology

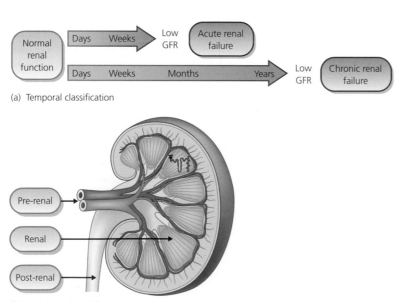

(a) Temporal classification

(b) Aetiological classification

Figure H Classification of renal failure.

Table B Classification of acute kidney injury

Stage	Serum creatinine criteria	Urine output criteria
1	Increase of >26.4 µmol/L (0.3 mg/dL) OR 150–200% of baseline (1.5–2-fold increase)	<0.5 mL/kg/h >6 h
2	Increase to >200–300% of baseline (2–3-fold increase)	<0.5 mL/kg/h >12 h
3	>354.4 µmol/L (4 mg/dL) with an acute rise of at least 44 µmol/L (0.5 mg/dL) OR >300% of baseline (3-fold increase)	<0.3 mL/kg/h for 24 h or anuria for 12 h

- *post-renal causes*, e.g. obstruction in the ureter (calculi), bladder (malignancy), urethra (prostatic hypertrophy or cancer).

The most common cause of ARF is pre-renal failure +/− progression to acute tubular necrosis (ATN) which accounts for between 50% and 80% of cases. Other causes include primary and secondary glomerulonephritis (GN) (5–10%), obstruction (5–15%), acute tubulointerstitial nephritis (<5%). This will be dealt with in more detail in the ARF cases in part 2.

More recently, ARF has been 're-badged' as acute kidney injury (AKI) in an attempt to provide more uniform standards for diagnosing and classifying AKI. The hope is that more accurate classification will improve management and outcomes for patients who develop an acute decline in their renal function. The classification system for AKI was devised by the first AKI Network Conference in 2005 and is summarised in Table B.

Chronic kidney disease

Chronic kidney disease/chronic renal failure can be completely asymptomatic until its very terminal stages. Eventually anaemia (tiredness/congestive cardiac failure (CCF)), uraemia (nausea, reduced appetite, confusion), phosphate build-up (itchiness), symptomatic hypertension (headache, blurred vision) may prompt the patient to seek medical attention where a routine blood test reveals high urea/creatinine, high phosphate and low haemoglobin, all in-keeping with CKD.

Causes include:
- diabetes mellitis with associated diabetic nephropathy
- hypertensive nephropathy
- obstructive uropathy (usually secondary to prostatic hypertrophy)
- chronic primary glomerulonephritis, e.g. IgA nephropathy or focal segmental glomerular sclerosis (FSGS)
- APKD
- chronic pyelonephritis
- renovascular disease.

Chronic kidney disease is now classified into different stages according to the patient's GFR and the presence of urine dipstick abnormalities. These have allowed the development of suggested management guidelines for patients with stable CKD, and facilitate the provision of consistent care in this patient group (Table C).

Combinations of the key presenting features

Many patients with renal disease do not present with isolated hypertension, urine dipstick abnormalities or abnormal GFR; rather, they have combinations of these features. Some typical presentations have been classified as syndromes, for example nephrotic and nephritic syndrome (Figure I).

Useful note: syndromes of any sort are usually defined by three or more typical clinical features rather than by the underlying causative pathology.

Nephrotic syndrome (Box C)

This is defined as a triad of proteinuria (>3.5 g/24 h), hypoalbuminaemia (due to renal protein loss) and oedema (due to low intravascular oncotic pressure associated with hypoalbuminaemia). Patients often lose other important proteins in the urine, for example, IgG (antibody) and proteins which control the clotting cascade. Hence patients with nephrotic syndrome are at increased risk of both infection (particularly spontaneous bacterial peritonitis) and thromboembolic disease. Patients will also have hypercholesterolaemia in addition to the above features. This is thought to be due to an increase in lipoprotein production by the liver in an attempt to maintain oncotic pressure. Renal function, as assessed by clearance of soluble waste products (i.e. urea and creatinine levels), is usually normal. Nephrotic range proteinuria is usually glomerular in origin.

Causes include:
- primary GN
  - minimal change GN
  - membranous GN (most common cause of nephrotic syndrome in adults)
  - FSGS
  - mesangiocapillary GN

Table C Classification of CKD

CKD stage	eGFR (mL/1.73 cm^2)	Other features	Suggested management
1	90+	Normal renal function but urine dipstick abnormalities or known structural abnormality of renal tract or diagnosis of genetic kidney disease	Observation, control of BP. Consider investigation for cause of urine dipstick abnormalities
2	60–89	Mildly reduced renal function plus urine/ structural abnormalities or diagnosis of genetic kidney disease	Observation, control of BP. Management of cardiovascular risk factors. Consider investigation for cause of renal impairment
3	30–59	Moderately reduced renal function	Observation, control of BP. Management of cardiovascular risk factors. Measure Ca^{2+}, PO$_4$, PTH, Hb and cholesterol. The patient may need treatment for anaemia or secondary/tertiary hyperparathyroidism
4	15–29	Severely reduced renal function	Regular observation, control of BP and CVS risk factors. Measure Ca^{2+}, PO$_4$, PTH, Hb and cholesterol. Management as for stage 3. Preparation for ESRF with an early decision on the preferred mode of RRT
5	<15	End-stage renal failure	Can be managed conservatively but RRT should be considered for most patients (i.e. provision of dialysis or transplantation)

BP, blood pressure; CVS, cardiovascular system; Hb, haemoglobin; PTH, parathyroid hormone; RRT, renal replacement therapy.

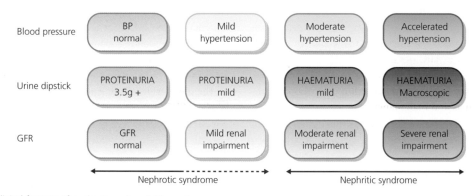

Figure I Clinical features of nephrotic and nephritic syndrome.

> **Box C Clinical features of nephrotic syndrome**
>
> - Proteinuria (>3.5 g/24 h)
> - Hypoalbuminaemia
> - Oedema
> - +/– Hypercholesterolaemia

- secondary GN
  - diabetic nephropathy
  - amyloidosis
  - systemic lupus erythematosus (SLE) (Class V, with a membranous pattern on biopsy)
  - hepatitis B/C (usually a membranous pattern, Hep C can cause a mesangiocapillary GN).

Box D Clinical features of nephritic syndrome

- Hypertension
- Haematuria (micro- or macroscopic)
- Acute renal failure
- +/− Oedema

Nephritic syndrome (Box D)

Defined as a triad of hypertension, haematuria (usually microscopic) and oliguria/acute renal failure. There may also be associated proteinuria and oedema.

Causes include:

- primary GN
  - IgA nephropathy
  - mesangiocapillary GN
- secondary GN
  - post-streptococcal GN
  - vasculitis
  - lupus nephritis
  - Goodpasture's disease
  - cryoglobulinaemia.

Special note: clinical presentation of glomerulonephritides

The glomerulonephritides are a source of much fear and confusion for medical students, and in fact many non-renal clinicians. An initial glance at the subject reveals a long list of oddly named GN but in fact they can be easily mastered if you bear in mind some basic facts, which I have labelled the ABC of GN.

- *Aetiology:* GN can be primary or occur secondary to four processes: infection, autoimmunity, dysgammaglobulinaemias and malignancy.
- *Biopsy findings:* glomerulonephritides are named according to the appearance of the renal biopsy (see discussion on renal biopsies and Figure Q). For example, in minimal change GN, there is no abnormality or change at the light microscope level; in membranous GN, there is thickening of the glomerular basement membrane; IgA nephropathy is characterised by the deposition of mesangial IgA, etc. Each of these biopsy-defined glomerulonephritides can be primary or secondary, as described above.
- *Clinical features:* some glomerulonephritides almost always present with nephrotic syndrome (for example, minimal change) and others with a more nephritic syndrome (for example, diffuse proliferative GN). IgA nephropathy has two major modes of presentation: some

patients are picked up on an employment screen or at well-person clinics when their urine is dipped or BP measured (I've termed this IgA nephropathy[1] in Figure Jb). The other main way in which these patients present is with episodic synpharyngitic macroscopic haematuria (I've termed this IgA nephropathy[2] in Figure Jb). The classic clinical features of the main glomerulonephritides are shown in Figure Ja–c.

Investigations

Blood tests which help you decide *if* the kidney is working properly

Serum creatinine is used as a surrogate marker of GFR and is therefore part of the work-up of any patient with suspected renal disease. There are a number of limitations to using creatinine to assess GFR: its production is dependent on muscle bulk, so if there is a decline in GFR and a simultaneous loss of muscle bulk, then there may be no change in serum creatinine. In addition, when there is relatively good renal function, a small rise in creatinine can indicate a large fall in GFR (see Figure K).

A more accurate way to estimate GFR is to measure creatinine clearance (Box E). This is done by collecting the urine for 24 hours and then measuring creatinine in both blood and urine. Creatinine clearance tends to overestimate GFR as creatinine is both filtered and secreted. Some drugs reduce tubular creatinine secretion (trimethoprim, spironolactone, amiloride) and will therefore lead to a fall in creatinine clearance and a rise in creatinine.

Glomerular filtration rate can be formally measured by assessing inulin clearance (a small molecule freely filtered at the glomerulus and not secreted) or chromium-labelled EDTA clearance. However, GFR is most commonly estimated rather than measured using formulas (Box F) which require input of the patient's creatinine, age, sex and weight, e.g. the Cockcroft–Gault formula (Box G) or the MDRD equation. Many labs will give an estimated GFR on the 'U+E' result form, as this has become important in classifying the different stages of CKD.

Urea is a waste product produced by the liver as the end product of protein catabolism. If renal excretion does not keep pace with liver production (e.g. if there is reduced GFR or abnormal tubular function), then urea levels will rise (although an elevation in urea can also be observed in some other conditions (Box H).

The kidney is important in managing the levels of electrolytes (Na^+, K^+, Mg^{2+}, Cl^- as described above).

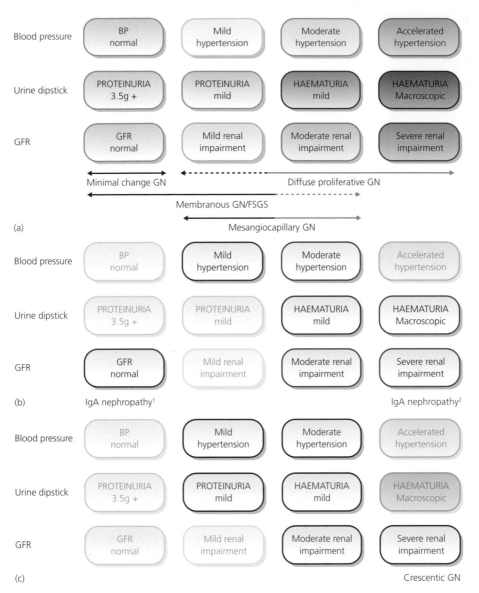

Figure J (a) Clinical features of different forms of GN. (b) Clinical features of different forms of IgA nephropathy. (c) Clinical features of crescentic GN.

In most hospitals, a basic 'U+E' test will give Na^+, K^+, urea and creatinine.
- Acid–base status (pH, H^+, bicarbonate, base excess)
- Calcium/phosphate/parathyroid hormone (PTH) elevated in CKD
- Haemaglobin: low if EPO deficiency

Blood tests which tell you *why* the kidney isn't working properly

These are mainly used if a 'renal cause' of renal failure is suspected.

Is there an autoimmune disease or primary GN?
Non-specific inflammatory markers

- C-reactive protein (CRP), an acute phase response protein made by the liver within hours of infection/inflammation.
- Erythrocyte sedimentation rate (ESR): assessed by allowing the patient's blood to stand in a tube and noting the rate at which red cells collect/sediment at the bottom of the tube, therefore described in mm/h. Red cells will sediment quicker if they are bigger/heavier. Thus, ESR is increased if there is increased fibrinogen or IgG in the

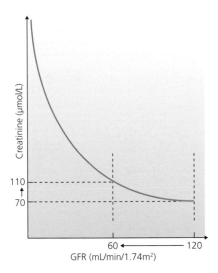

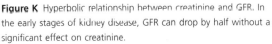

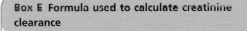

Figure K Hyperbolic relationship between creatinine and GFR. In the early stages of kidney disease, GFR can drop by half without a significant effect on creatinine.

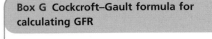

> **Box G Cockcroft–Gault formula for calculating GFR**
>
> $$GFR = \frac{(140 - \text{age in years}) \times \text{weight (kg)} \times 1.23\,(\text{men})\ \text{or}\ 1.04\,(\text{women})}{\text{Plasma creatinine (}\mu\text{mol/L)}}$$

> **Box H Causes of elevated urea**
>
> - Increased production:
>   - high-protein diet
>   - increased catabolism (infection, surgery, trauma)
>   - corticosteroids
>   - gastrointestinal bleeding
>   - tetracyclines
> - Reduced excretion
>   - reduced GFR (e.g. acute or chronic renal failure)
>   - tubulointerstitial nephritis

> **Box E Formula used to calculate creatinine clearance**
>
> $$\text{Creatinine clearance} = \frac{Ucr \times Uv \times 1000}{Pcr \times 24 \times 60}$$
>
> where U is urine, P is plasma, cr is creatinine concentration, and v is volume.

> **Box F Ways of estimating or measuring GFR**
>
> - Serum creatinine
> - Creatinine clearance (24-hour urine collection with blood sampling)
> - Calculated/estimated GFR (using Cockcroft–Gault or MDRD equation)
> - Measured GFR (inulin or EDTA clearance).

blood which causes red cells to clump together. Hence it is elevated in many inflammatory/autoimmune diseases (e.g. SLE) and in dysgammaglobulinaemias (e.g. multiple myeloma).

• Complement levels (C3 and C4): the complement system is composed of a number of proteins which are sequentially activated in a cascade which culminates in the formation of a membrane attack complex (MAC, Figure L). The MAC forms a pore in the membrane of the cell into which it is inserted (pathogen or host), disrupting the integrity of the membrane and causing cell lysis. The complement system can be activated in three ways; the classic pathway, the alternative pathway and the mannose-binding pathway. Diseases which are characterised by immune complex formation or deposition activate the classic pathway (e.g. SLE) and lead to a low C4 and C3. Diseases which activate the alternative pathway (e.g. mesangiocapillary GN type II, with C3 nephritic factor) lead to a low C3 level but preservation of C4. In some diseases, both pathways are activated, e.g. post-infectious GN.

Markers of specific autoimmune diseases (some are more specific than others)

• Anti-nuclear antibodies (ANA) and anti-double-stranded DNA antibodies (dsDNA), hypergammaglobulinaemia and hypocomplementaemia (low C3/C4) are associated with SLE.

• Anti-neutrophil cytoplasmic antibodies (ANCA) are associated with small vessel vasculitis (Wegener's granulomatosis, microscopic polyangiitis and Churg–Strauss syndrome).

• Elevated systemic IgA can occur in some patients with IgA nephropathy or Henoch–Schönlein purpura (HSP).

• Cryoglobulins or rheumatoid factor are associated with cryoglobulinaemia (which may occur in Hep C infections) and rheumatoid arthritis.

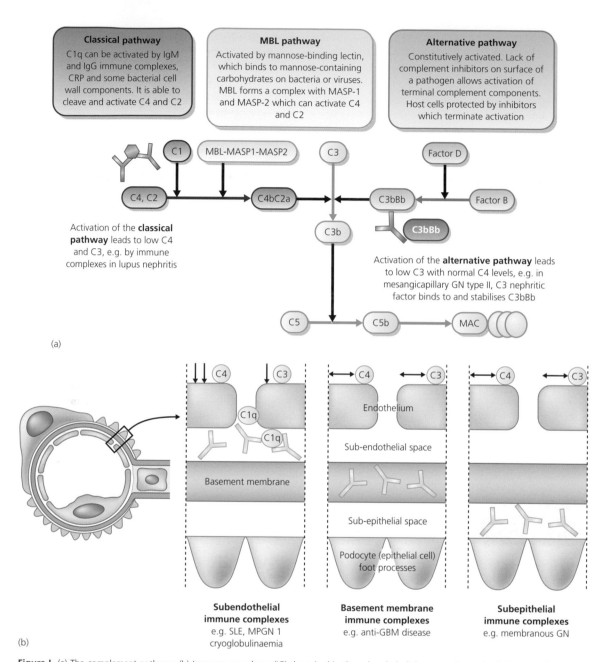

Figure L (a) The complement pathway. (b) Immune complexes (IC) deposited in the subendothelial space activate circulating complement via the classic pathway. IC deposited within the basement membrane or in the subepithelial space do not.

• C3 nephritic factor: an antibody which stabilises the C3 convertase C3bBb, causing persistent activation of the alternative pathway of complement with C3 consumption. This is associated with mesangiocapillary GN type II.

Does the patient have a dysgammaglobulinaemia?
• Serum immunoglobulins + paraprotein: the presence of elevated immunglobulins, with a specific monoclonal protein band on serum electrophoresis, suggests the presence of an abnormal plasma cell clone which is produc-

ing lots of a single type of protein. This may be an entire immunoglobulin molecule or part of it, such as the light chain. These proteins can become deposited in the kidney, causing light chain or cast nephropathy, or AL amyloid in other patients.

• Bence Jones proteins/urinary free light chains: as well as looking for the protein in serum, urinary light chains may also be detectable.

Does the patient have evidence of an infection or recent infection some of which can be associated with GN?

• ASO titres/anti-DNAse titres: the classic post-infectious GN is post-streptococcal GN. This typically occurs 2–3 weeks following a streptococcal pharyngitis and presents as a nephritic illness with haematuria, hypertension and renal impairment. Recent streptococcal infection can be confirmed by history and by measuring the titres of antibodies typically produced in response to streptococci, including anti-streptolysin O and anti-DNAse antibodies. A throat swab should also be performed in an attempt to isolate the organism.

• Some patients with IgA nephropathy experience flares of disease which appear to be precipitated by mucosal infections, typically occurring 2–3 days prior to presentation with macroscopic haematuria.

• Hepatitis B and C and HIV serology/polymerase chain reaction (PCR) should be performed, as these infections can be associated with a number of glomerulonephritides.

Urine tests which help you decide if the kidney is working properly
Urine dipstick and microscopy for protein, blood, leucocytes, nitrite, pH, specific gravity, casts, crystals (Figure M)

• The significance of the detection of blood and protein in urine is described under clinical presentation.

• The presence of white blood cells (WBC, leucocytes) in the urine (pyuria) may indicate infection or inflammation within the renal tract. Ten or more WBC per mm³ of unspun midstream urine on microscopy is considered abnormal and is commonly due to a UTI (in which case there are usually bacteria detectable in urine, either on microscopy or following culture). Sterile pyuria may occur in UTI if the patient has already received antibiotic therapy, or with tuberculosis, renal calculi, tubulointerstitial nephritis or chemical cystitis.

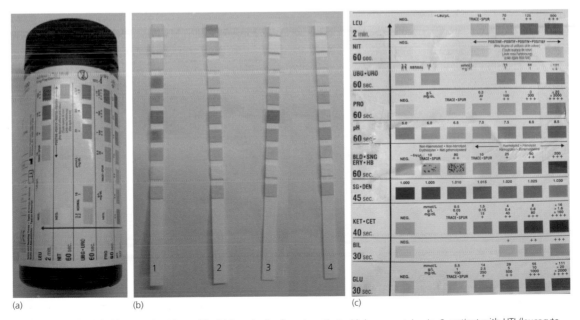

Figure M Urine dipstick. (a) Urine dipstick test kit. (b) Sample dips from 1. patient with heavy proteinuria, 2. patient with UTI (leucocyte and nitrite positive), 3. patient with microscopic haematuria, 4. normal individual. (c) Reference chart used for reading urine dipsticks (found on the side of the test kit pot).

Eosinophils may be identified in the urine using Hansel's stain and this classically occurs in acute tubulointerstitial nephritis.

• Nitrites are detectable in patients with UTI.
• pH abnormalities (typically alkaline urine which does not acidify) occur in renal tubular acidosis, where there is a failure to acidify urine in spite of an excess acid in blood.
• Urine specific gravity is a measure of the weight of dissolved particles in urine, which closely reflects urine osmolality (the number of particles in the urine). Its usefulness is limited but abnormalities can be suggestive of particular pathologies, e.g. specific gravity is low in patients with syndrome of inapproporiate ADH secretion.
• Casts are cylindrical bodies which are moulded or cast in the shape of the tubule in which they were formed (usually distal tubule). They may be hyaline, granular or cellular. Hyaline and fine granular casts represent precipitated protein and may be seen in normal urine (e.g. post exercise). More coarse granular casts occur with heavy proteinuria and in tubular disease. Red cell casts indicate renal inflammation. White cell casts may be seen in acute pyelonephritis.

Quantification of urine protein

Quantification of urinary protein is important and can be done in a number of ways. If the urine dipstick is positive for protein, then proteinuria should be quantified either by collecting the urine for 24 hours and assessing the total amount of protein excreted in the entire sample, or by measuring the protein/creatinine ratio in a one-off, preferably morning sample. The problem with 24-hour collection is a practical one, as it requires the patient to remember to collect every urine specimen. Even for catheterised in-patients, this can be a challenge.

The protein/creatinine ratio allows assessment of proteinuria on a single specimen and is therefore much easier to obtain. However, although it allows quantification of urine protein excretion over a shorter period of time, it may not be entirely representative of a 24-hour period. It is therefore advised that the protein/creatinine ratio is measured on at least two occasions, and ideally on the first morning void on both occasions. Proteinuria detectable on dipstick will usually give a minimum protein/creatinine ratio of 45 mg/mmol. A ratio of 50 mg/mmol is approximately equivalent to a 24-hour excretion of 0.5 g in 24 hours.

Microalbuminuria is defined as 30–300 mg/24 h and occurs in the early stages of renal disease. Patients with microalbuminuria will have a negative urine dipstick for protein using the regular dipstick kits. Microalbuminuria may be detected using a specialised (and more expensive) urine dipstick kit or can be quanitified by estimating the albumin/creatinine ratio (ACR) in a single urine sample. This has proved useful in monitoring patients with diabetes who are at risk of developing diabetic nephropathy. An ACR of >2.5 mg/mmol in males or >3.5 mg/mmol in females is indicative of microalbuminuria. An ACR of >30 mg/mmol indicates there is proteinuria which will be identifiable on regular dipstick. An ACR of 30 mg/mmol is approximately equivalent to a protein/creatinine ratio of 50 mg/mmol.

A number of factors can increase the protein detected in the urine in the absence of renal disease, including heavy exercise and acute febrile illnesses.

Special tests to look for abnormal electrolyte concentration in urine

Quantification of urinary electrolytes is not commonly performed in the day-to-day management of patients with renal disease, but there are some disorders in which it may be of use:
• distinguishing pre-renal failure from established ATN
• diagnosis of tubular dysfunction.

Tests of urine osmolality

This is used in the investigation of patients with hyponatraemia. A comparison of serum and urine osmolality allows the physician to determine whether or not the kidneys are appropriately concentrating urine. Urine osmolality is largely controlled by the effects of ADH on the collecting duct.

Imaging to investigate the cause of kidney dysfunction

• *Plain abdominal radiograph/kidney, ureter, bladder:* can be useful in identifying renal calculi given that around 90% of calculi contain calcium and are thus radio-opaque.
• *Intravenous urography:* less frequently used these days but can allow the identification of structural abnormalities of the urinary tract, for example, a bladder-filling defect indicative of a tumour.
• *Ultrasound:* this is probably the most common radiological renal investigation undertaken. It allows assessment of kidney size, presence of hydronephrosis, presence

of cysts, presence of tumours, the absence of a kidney or other developmental anomalies such as horseshoe kidney. In addition, the outer cortex and inner medulla can be differentiated. The cortex becomes thin in CKD. Loss of differentiation between the cortex and medulla can occur in many causes of ARF, including GN and tubulointerstitial nephritis (TIN). Ultrasound (US) also allows assessment of whether the kidney is being normally perfused, and the Doppler traces obtained from renal vessels can allow the diagnosis of renal vein thrombosis and renal artery stenosis. The main limitations are that it is only as good as the operator and the patient; in particular, it can be difficult to get adequate views in obese subjects. Some renal US images are shown in Figure N.

• *Computed tomography (CT) of the abdomen:* iodine-containing contrast agents can induce worsening renal function (contrast-induced nephropathy), therefore patients with CKD should only be given contrast if truly necessary and should be prehydrated (+/− given N-acetylcysteine or sodium bicarbonate prior to the procedure). CT scans can be helpful to define vessels, including renal artery stenoses, and to identify hydronephrosis in patients for whom US examination has been difficult. CT can also be used to more fully delineate renal masses identified on US examination, giving a better idea of whether they are benign or malignant. In addition, CT allows the visualisation of renal cysts, including those into which there has been recent haemorrhage. Some CT images are shown in Figure O.

• *Magnetic resonance imaging (MRI)/magnetic resonance angiography (MRA):* a non-invasive way of defining renal anatomy in more detail, particularly the vessels. However, the gadolinium-containing contrast agents used in MRA appear to be occasionally associated with the development of a systemic sclerosis-type illness in patients with impaired renal function (nephrogenic systemic fibrosis), so this investigation is now often avoided in patients with a GFR <60 mL/min.

• *Angiography:* this is the gold standard investigation for viewing the renal vessels and also allows intervention

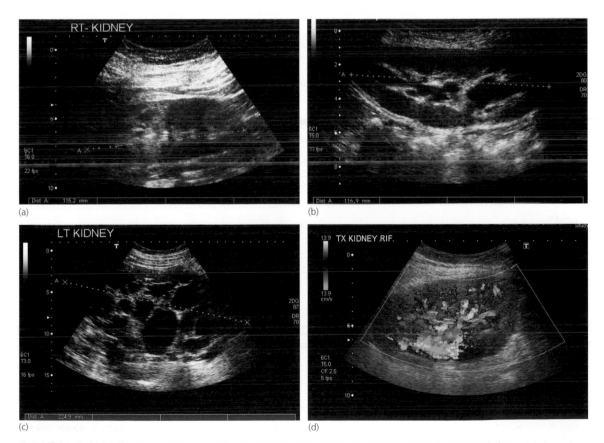

(a)

(b)

(c)

(d)

Figure N Ultrasound scans showing (a) normal native kidney, (b) hydronephrosis, (c) polycystic disease, (d) renal perfusion.

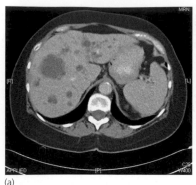
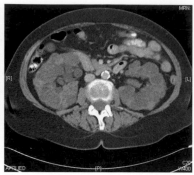

Figure O CT abdomen showing (a) cystic liver and (b) kidneys in a patient with polycystic kidney disease.

(a)   (b)

at the time of examination, including angioplasty and stenting. Angiography also involves the use of nephrotoxic contrast agents, so patients may require prehydration and N-acetylcysteine, as described for CT studies.

• *Nuclear medicine scans:* three radionuclides are used to investigate renal disease. They are injected intravenously and then their excretion through the kidneys is visualised.

　○ *DMSA* – these scans are useful to detect renal scarring in patients with chronic pyelonephritis.

　○ *DTPA and Mag-3* – these scans provide information on renal perfusion and also whether there is functional obstruction to urine outflow. The effect of the administration of an angiotensin-converting enzyme (ACE) inhibitor (captopril) on renal perfusion can also be assessed and can be useful in the diagnosis of renal artery stenosis. In practice, these days many patients will be referred directly for angiography if there is a high clinical suspicion of renal artery stenosis.

Renal biopsy

In order to confidently diagnose any GN, a biopsy is needed. It is a useful tool in any patient with ARF where the cause is unclear. All adult patients with nephrotic syndrome should also be biopsied to determine underlying cause and appropriate treatment.

A renal biopsy is performed under a local anaesthetic, using US to guide the biopsy needle to the correct position. This can be difficult if a patient is large. The patient is placed in a prone position and scanned to determine the depth of the kidneys from the skin. A mark is then placed with the patient in held inspiration. Ideally, the biopsy should be taken at the lower pole of the kidney. Local anaesthetic is placed in the skin and deeper tissues,

using a spinal needle until this rests on the renal capsule. This is usually obvious as there is a visible swing in the needle with deep inspiration and expiration. The biopsy is then taken by inserting the biopsy needle down the same tract as the spinal needle, and with the patient in held inspiration. Automated needles/guns are usually used and the operator will attempt to obtain a core of predominantly cortical tissue (Figure P).

The main risk following renal biopsy is bleeding. If an adequate kidney biopsy is taken, then some blood vessels will be sampled by definition. The deeper the sample is taken from the cortex and into the medulla, the greater the chance that a larger vessel will be damaged. Hence the physician performing the biopsy usually attempts to sample as far as the corticomedullary junction to minimise the risk of haemorrhage. Even with US guidance, almost all patients will experience some dipstick haematuria. Around one in 5–10 will develop macroscopic haematuria, which generally resolves spontaneously without treatment. In 1 in 200 patients, the bleeding is sufficiently serious to require a blood transfusion. In 1 in 1000 patients, some intervention is required to stop the bleeding; usually the interventional radiologist will place a coil or glue at the bleeding point. Very rarely, the bleeding is not amenable to radiological intervention and the patient may require surgical intervention, including a nephrectomy. Requirements to minimise biopsy risk are shown in Box I.

Once obtained, the core of tissue is placed in formaldehyde for mounting in paraffin, and in some units a core is also snap frozen to facilitate immunostaining. Renal biopsies are processed and examined in three ways.

• *Light microscopy:* biopsies can be rapidly processed and the initial H+E section can be viewed by light

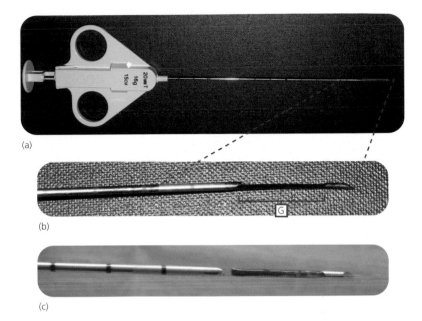

Figure P Renal needle biopsy. (a) An automated renal biopsy needle shown from above. A magnified, side profile of the needle tip is shown in (b); a core of tissue is collected in the groove (G) on firing the needle (c).

Box I Requirements for a safe renal biopsy

- BP <150/90 mmHg
- Platelets >100 × 10^9/L
- Normal clotting
- No low molecular weight heparin in past 24 hours

---

microscopy within 6–24 hours of collection. This allows the histopathologist to give a basic preliminary diagnosis by assessing the appearance of the glomeruli, tubules, interstitium and vessels in turn. This may allow the identification of abnormalities in the glomerulus; for example, thickening of the basement membrane, as seen in membranous GN, or segmental sclerosis, as seen in FSGS (Figure Qa). There may be casts visible within the tubules (as seen in multiple myeloma) or tubular atrophy and interstitial fibrosis (as seen in chronic TIN). The sections can be stained with different solutions, allowing visualisation of particular pathologies, e.g. a silver stain is good for identifying thickened basement membrane.

- *Immunostaining:* this is generally used to detect the presence of different components of the immune system within the kidney. It is performed using antibodies as a diagnostic tool. For example, an antibody which specifically recognises IgG via its variable region is incubated with the section. The specimen is then washed and any residual antibody bound indicates the presence of IgG within the section. This can be visualised either by using antibodies with fluorescent tags or with horseradish peroxidase tags (Figure Qb). This allows the detection of IgG, IgM, IgA, C1q, C3, C4, B cells, T cells, macrophages, etc. depending on which detection antibody is used. This additional information can help the histopathologist to confirm their initial light microscopic finding or may make them think of a different differential diagnosis. Immunostaining tends to take a few days to perform, so the result will come after the initial H+E.

- *Electron microscopy:* this can take a number of weeks to perform and allows the identification of glomerular structures in very high magnification (Figure Qc). Thus the fine structure of the glomerular basement membrane and podocytes and endothelial cells can be examined. In addition, any material deposited in the kidneys can be defined more clearly, e.g. amyloid fibrils can be visualised. In minimal change GN, the only histological abnormality present is visualised exclusively at electron microscopy (fusion of podocyte foot processes), therefore it can be extremely useful.

Treatment of renal disease/dysfunction

Treatments can be divided into those aimed at modifying the process or disease causing kidney dysfunction, and

Normal glomerulus (H+E)

Membranous GN (H+E)

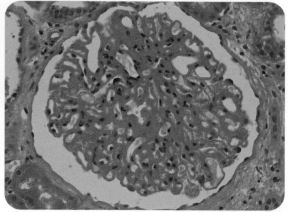

FSGS (PAS staining)

Mesangiocapillary GN (H+E)

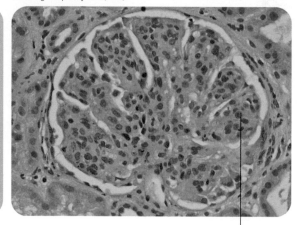

(a)

Sclerosed segment
of the glomerulus

Mesangial proliferation
(>3 cells/lobule)

Figure Q Renal biopsy. (a) Light microscopy. (b) Immunostaining. (c) Electron microscopy.

those aimed at dealing with the consequences of renal dysfunction.

Dealing with the consequences of kidney failure

Hypertension

In addition to general measures such as weight loss and exercise, a number of antihypertensive agents are available. They act to reduce either the total peripheral resistance or the heart rate/venous return (and hence the cardiac output) (see cases of hypertension).

Proteinuria

A number of drugs have been shown to be useful in reducing proteinuria, particularly ACE inhibitors and angiotensin receptor blockers (ARBs). These inhibit the action of angiotensin on the efferent arteriole, causing relaxation of this vessel. This reduces glomerular pressure and associated proteinuria.

Erythropoietin deficiency

Recombinant erythropoietin became available in the 1980s and has revolutionised the treatment of renal anaemia and associated cardiovascular disease in patients

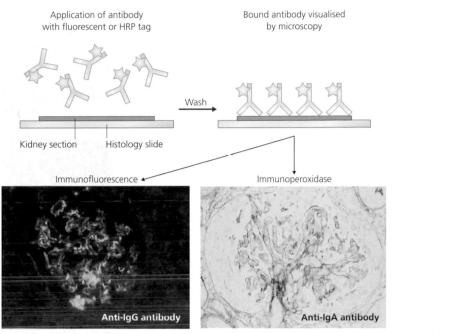

Application of antibody with fluorescent or HRP tag

Bound antibody visualised by microscopy

Wash

Kidney section   Histology slide

Immunofluorescence   Immunoperoxidase

Anti-IgG antibody   **Anti-IgA antibody**

(b)

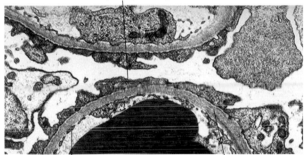

Minimal change GN

Abnormal podocyte foot process

Endothelium   Basement membrane

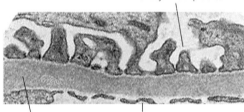

Normal renal biopsy

Podocyte foot process

Basement membrane   Endothelium

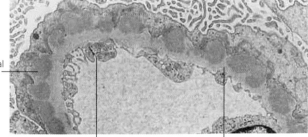

Membranous GN

Subepithelial deposits

Endothelium   Basement membrane forming 'spikes'

(c)

Figure Q *Continued*

with renal dysfunction. It is usually administered once a week as a subcutaneous injection or it can be given intravenously if the patient is receiving haemodialysis.

Vitamin D deficiency and associated hyperparathyroidism

Oral forms of 1α-D3 can be given to prevent the development of tertiary hyperparathyroidism. Patients with CKD are also encouraged to maintain a low-phosphate diet and take oral phosphate binders (for example, calcium carbonate) with food to prevent the absorption of phosphate, which also helps in preventing tertiary hyperparathyroidism. Unfortunately, a number of appetising foods such as cheese, milk, yoghurt and chocolate are high in phosphate.

High potassium levels

Patients with renal failure tend to develop hyperkalaemia, which can lead to serious cardiac arrhythmias. Hence those with CKD are advised to take a low-potassium diet (avoid fruit, nuts, vegetables). In the acute setting, a high potassium level can be treated with a dextrose-insulin infusion to drive potassium back into cells.

Accumulation of waste products such as urea and creatinine, and acid and fluid overload

The filtering and blood-cleaning role of the kidney can be replaced by three treatments, which are collectively termed renal replacement therapy (RRT).

• *Haemodialysis:* blood is taken out of a large vein, pumped around a series of filters and then returned to the patient. This requires a relatively high blood flow, and hence access to a large vein. This can be achieved by placing a large temporary central line containing both an arterial and venous lumen into a sizeable vein such as the femoral or internal jugular vein. This is usually done under ultrasound guidance. These central lines can be tunnelled under the skin to minimise the risk of infection, and allow their use for weeks or even months. If a patient is likely to need long-term haemodialysis then ideally an arteriovenous fistula should be formed. This involves joining a medium-sized artery, such as the radial artery, with a medium-sized vein, usually the cephalic vein. Because the arterial blood flow is no longer subject to decompression at the capillary bed, high pressures and flows of blood occur in the cephalic vein. This enlarges and forms a useful vein into which needles can be easily placed during dialysis (Figure R).

• *Peritoneal dialysis:* a tube is placed into the peritoneal cavity and fluid instilled. This is usually allowed to dwell

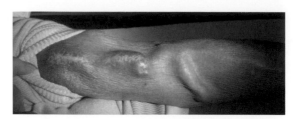

Figure R A well-developed radiocephalic arteriovenous fistula.

for a number of hours and waste products diffuse out from the blood into the peritoneal fluid via the peritoneal membrane. It can be done at home, but requires manual dexterity and an adherence to aseptic technique. Therefore it is often more useful for younger, fitter patients.

• *Renal transplantation:* the treatment of choice for most patients with end-stage renal failure. Physiological renal function is restored, including the production of erythropoietin and vitamin D. The patients are freed from the practical constraints of dialysis and the limiting dietary regimens imposed during end-stage renal failure. On the downside, patients must take lifelong immunosuppressants in order to prevent allograft rejection.

Dealing with the consequences of specific tubular dysfunction

Some specific tubular disorders may lead to abnormalities of electrolytes (typically low potassium) and acid–base balance. In such cases, oral replacement with potassium supplements and bicarbonate is given.

Treating the underlying cause of renal failure

Clearly treatment depends on the underlying cause. Specific treatments will be discussed in the relevant cases in Part 2.

In patients with acute renal failure, treating the underlying cause may be as simple as inserting a urinary catheter to relieve obstruction or giving intravenous fluids in order to restore renal perfusion. An approach to fluid balance in patients with acute renal failure is shown in Box J.

Specific treatments for glomerulonephritides vary, but in the main they are treated with immunosuppressants such as corticosteroids.

In terms of preventing the progression of CKD, patients with recurrent UTI should receive prophylactic antibiotics. Patients with diabetic nephropathy or hypertension should have their glucose or blood pressure optimally controlled.

Box J Fluid balance in ARF

Assessing fluid balance in ARF

- It is important to ensure patients with ARF are well filled in order to optimise the chance of renal recovery. However, an excess of fluid must be avoided to minimise the risk of pulmonary oedema.
- Assessment of fluid balance can be achieved by regular clinical examination including:
  - skin turgor
  - mucous membranes (dry or moist)
  - JVP
  - BP (hypotension or postural drop)
  - lung bases (for crepitations indicative of pulmonary oedema).
- An accurate input–output chart should be established in all patients with ARF.
- The usefulness of input–output charts may be limited by incomplete documentation or in situations where there is an excess of insensible losses (e.g. profuse diarrhoea or persistent fever).
- Measurement of the patient's weight on a daily basis may provide a more accurate day-to-day assessment of net fluid loss or gain in cases where input–output charts are thought to be inaccurate.
- Central venous pressure monitoring is not mandatory for all patients with ARF and is reserved for more complex cases.

Fluid replacement in ARF

- In patients with hypovolaemia (as evidenced by reduced skin turgor, dry mucous membranes, low JVP, hypotension or postural drop in BP), fluid should be given to restore euvolaemia. Normal saline is the fluid of choice and will be distributed in the extracellular compartment (interstitium and intravascular space). In a patient with acute intravascular volume depletion (e.g. following a gastrointestinal bleed), a bolus of colloid (e.g. Gelofusine) may be useful to restore blood pressure as its distribution is limited to the intravascular space. Note: 5% dextrose is distributed throughout the intracellular and extracellular spaces and therefore makes a small contribution to intravascular volume restoration.
- Once euvolaemia has been achieved, fluid replacement in oliguric patients with ARF must be tailored to match the total output (the main elements of which are urine output and insensible losses).
- In an afebrile patient, without vomiting or diarrhoea, insensible losses amount to about 500 mL in 24 hours. Thus a reasonable fluid replacement regimen for a 24-hour period would be the sum of the total urine output for the previous 24 hours plus 500 mL.
- It is important to remember that patients may be taking enough fluid orally to meet their input requirements and may not need additional intravenous (IV) fluids.
- Eu/hypervolaemic, oliguric patients with ARF may need to have their oral intake restricted in order to prevent pulmonary oedema.
- In those patients requiring IV fluid, normal saline (contains 150 mmol/L Na) should be alternated with 5% dextrose. Additional potassium replacement in intravenous fluid is rarely required in patients with ARF, as hyperkalaemia is often an issue. (Note: Hartmann's solution contains 5 mmol/L of potassium and should be avoided in patients with hyperkalaemic ARF.)

PART 2: CASES

Case 1 An 84-year-old man with reduced urine output

Mr Godfrey Griffiths is an 84-year-old man who was admitted to the Care of the Elderly ward 10 days ago with increasing breathlessness. This was felt to be due to a combination of pulmonary oedema and a lower respiratory tract infection. He was treated with intravenous diuretics and antibiotics and rapidly improved. Unfortunately, the occupational therapy and physiotherapy assessment performed on the ward suggested that Mr Griffiths would need some adjustments to his home, as well as a short-term care package to ensure his safe discharge. Whilst waiting for these to be put in place, he has developed severe diarrhoea and vomiting and has been isolated in a side room. You are asked to review him by the nursing staff because they are worried that his urine output is decreasing.

Before taking a history, what basic facts should you establish?

As with any patient who is acutely unwell, before embarking on a prolonged history and examination, you should make sure the patient's ABC are safe.

- **A = Airway** (when patients become drowsy and have a reduced level of consciousness, they may fail to adequately protect their airway)
- **B = Breathing** (make sure the patients respiratory rate (RR) is neither too low (<8 rpm) or too high (>30 rpm)
- **C = Circulation** (does the patient have a normal pulse and blood pressure?) Remember:

$$MAP = CO \times TPR$$
$$CO = SV \times HR$$

Brady- or tachycardias can compromise BP, bradycardia because the reduction in HR leads to a reduction in CO and therefore MAP. Tachycardias compromise BP because the cardiac cycle is so quick that there is inadequate time for the ventricles to fill properly, hence SV falls, leading to a reduction in CO and hence in MAP. Systemic hypotension will also compromise cerebral

circulation. Thus, the patient's pulse and BP may need to be stabilised before tackling the history and examination.

Mr Griffiths is sitting up in bed and answering questions appropriately. His oxygen saturations are 98% on air, his RR 22 rpm, his pulse is 100 bpm and regular and his BP 105/55 mmHg. He has a urinary catheter in situ. You decide that his ABC are stable enough to proceed with the assessment.

His urine output chart is placed at the bottom of the bed and is shown in Figure 1.1.

What does the urine output chart (Figure 1.1) show?

Mr Griffiths' urine output chart shows that he is oliguric. In the last 6 hours (07:00–12:00) he has only passed 70 mL of urine and the main concern is that he may be developing significant renal dysfunction. He was started on an 8-hourly bag (125 mL/h) of intravenous fluid at 06:00 h. The fluid balance given for the morning is +425 mL but this is not likely to be accurate because the chart shows three episodes of diarrhoea which have not been quantified. He is therefore likely to be in a significant *negative* fluid balance. When fluid balance is difficult to assess, for example if losses are difficult to quantify (e.g. profuse diarrhoea, as in this case, or if a non-catheterised patient forgets to keep urine samples for measurement) then daily weights may be a better way of deciding if a patient is in an overall positive or negative balance for the day.

What aspects of his history would you explore?

It is important to ascertain the precise timing and nature of events leading up to this presentation. Although reading the medical notes before approaching the patient can give a useful insight, it should never be a substitute for taking a proper history yourself.

Nephrology: Clinical Cases Uncovered. By M. Clatworthy.
Published 2010 by Blackwell Publishing.

Adult Daily Fluid Balance Chart (simple)

Date: 09/06
Ward: 23
Pump Asset Numbers:
Pump 1
Pump 2

For staff use only:
Surname: GRIFFITHS
First names: GODFREY
Date of birth:
Hospital no: 27/07/24
Male/Female: (Use hospital)

Weight: 69 kg   Fluid Restriction: None

	Previous Days Balance	+	−	N/D

Input in mL

Time	Oral fluid volume	Enteral feed volume	Input 1 IV FLUIDS	Input 2	Running input total
01:00					
02:00					
03:00					
04:00					
05:00					
06:00			125 mL		
07:00			125 mL		
08:00			125 mL		
09:00			125 mL		
10:00			125 mL		
11:00			125 mL		
12:00			125 mL		
Total			825 mL		

Output in mL

Urine	NG drainage/aspiration	NG pH	Diarrhoea	Vomit	Running output total	Balance	Initial
50 mL					60 mL		
			? Volume large!				
100 mL					160+ mL		
20 mL				200 mL	380 mL		
30 mL					410 mL		
			Volume? large				
20 mL					430 mL		
10 mL			+++		440 mL		
10 mL			?		450 mL	+425	
250 mL			?	200	450	+425	

Please record totals from shaded boxes at top of the chart on other side.

Figure 1.1 An example of a simple adult daily fluid balance chart.

PART 2: CASES

Past medical history

Does he have a history of any conditions which cause chronic kidney disease (e.g. DM, hypertension and renovascular disease) which can increase the likelihood of patients developing pre-renal failure if there is volume depletion or hypotension? In men of this age, prostate pathology is common, so he should be asked about urinary stream and hesitancy.

Drug history

Hospitals can be dangerous places for the kidneys, in part because a number of commonly used medications are nephrotoxic and can precipitate renal failure. Examples include ACEI, ARB, NSAID, gentamicin and ciclosporin.

Family history

There are some inherited causes of chronic renal failure, particularly autosomal dominant polycystic kidney disease (ADPKD). Some patients with PKD 2 mutations may present later in life, in their 70s; however, Mr Griffiths is in his 80s, making this less likely.

Smoking history

Is he a smoker? Smoking is a risk factor for atherosclerosis and may point towards some renovascular disease which, as mentioned above, may increase the likelihood of developing pre-renal failure if there is volume depletion or hypotension.

Mr Griffiths was admitted 10 days ago with a 4-day history of increasing breathlessness. This was worse at night when lying flat (although he generally likes to sleep on three pillows). He has also begun coughing up green sputum. Following treatment with antibiotics (amoxicillin and clarithromycin) and furosemide 80 mg IV, he rapidly improved. Unfortunately, just as he was getting back on his feet, he developed severe diarrhoea and vomiting. For the past 2 days, he has had his bowels open up to 10 times/day and has had some accidents. His motions are watery but he has not noticed any blood. He gets intermittent abdominal cramps, and has also been vomiting in the last 2 days, although he is managing to keep his tablets down.

He had a myocardial infarction 5 years ago, and is known to have left ventricular dysfunction. He was also diagnosed with type II diabetes mellitus 10 years ago. This is treated by diet and metformin 500 mg tds. He has not had any documented prostate problems and although he admits his stream is 'not as good as it used to be', he has no major

difficulties passing urine. He is a lifelong smoker (since the age of 14 years) and has no family history of renal disease. His other medications are aspirin 75 mg od, simvastatin 20 mg od, lisinopril 10 mg od.

What are the important aspects of the examination in this case?

The first point is to determine Mr Griffiths' fluid status. Given his admission with pulmonary oedema, he is clearly at risk of volume overload and examination of his chest is essential. However, he is vomiting and has diarrhoea, so he is currently likely to be dehydrated. Examination of pulse, blood pressure (including lying/sitting and standing BP for evidence of a postural drop), skin turgor, dry mucous membranes and the JVP is essential to determine whether he is intravascularly hypovolaemic.

His abdomen should be carefully examined for the presence of an enlarged bladder (in an elderly man with a history of poor stream, prostatic hypertrophy is likely and may cause urinary retention). If present, a rectal examination is mandatory to assess the size of the prostate. He should also be assessed for signs of peritonism (rebound tenderness, guarding). Severe infective diarrhoea (particularly secondary to *Clostridium difficile*) can lead to toxic megacolon and even perforation, both of which are more likely in elderly patients.

What investigations would you perform?

- FBC
- U+E: determine degree of renal impairment
- CRP
- Blood cultures
- Stool culture: this is likely to be a case of hospital-acquired *C.difficile* diarrhoea, commonly associated with the administration of antibiotics. Screening for *C.difficile* toxin can give a rapid diagnosis and allow treatment to be started.
- US renal tract: to rule out obstruction/hydronephrosis and to establish the size and preservation of kidney structure, and therefore the likelihood of pre-existing CKD.

On examination, Mr Griffiths is dehydrated with dry mucous membranes and reduced skin turgor. His temperature is 37.6°C, pulse 100 bpm, BP 105/55 mmHg lying, 90/50 mmHg sitting, JVP not visible. He has a pansystolic murmur audible at the apex, but no pericardial rub. His chest is clear to

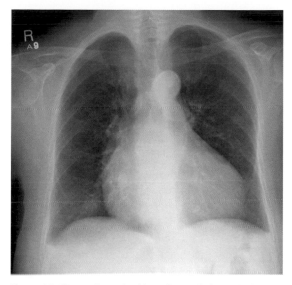

Figure 1.2 Chest radiograph with cardiomegaly (heart shadow is >50% of cardiothoracic diameter) and mildly hyperinflated lungs (consistent with COPD).

auscultation and his abdomen mildly tender, with no rebound or guarding.

His investigations show:

Hb 13.3 g/dL, WBC 11.9 × 10⁹/L, Platelets 455 × 10⁹/L

Na 150 mmol/L, K 4.1 mmol/L, Urea 49 mmol/L, Creatinine 520 μmol/L (185 on admission)

CRP 34 mg/L

CXR: mild cardiomegaly, lungs clear, COPD (Figure 1.2)

US kidneys: 9 cm bilaterally, no obstruction

What is the most likely cause of his renal failure?

The first issue to decide is whether the renal failure is likely to be acute or chronic. Mr Griffiths' kidneys are on the small side and his creatinine was elevated on admission (185 μmol/L, giving an eGFR of 32 mL/min/1.73 m²) indicative of stage 3 CKD. However, although there may be an element of CKD in this case, the current history is of an acute decline in urine output over the last 12 hours and a precipitous rise in creatinine, in keeping with ARF. Therefore this is likely to be acute-on-chronic renal failure.

The causes of ARF are usually classified as pre-renal (e.g. volume depletion), renal (e.g. glomerulonephritis) and postrenal (obstruction). Obstruction is common (5% of cases of ARF, up to 30% of cases of ARF in elderly males) but in this case, the renal ultrasound shows no evidence of hydronephrosis which might indicate

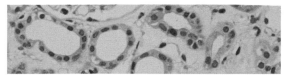

(a) Normal tubules
   (tubular cells are fat and juicy and have nuclei)

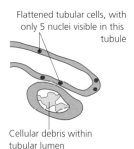

Flattened tubular cells, with only 5 nuclei visible in this tubule

Cellular debris within tubular lumen

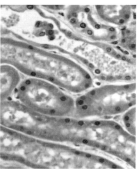

(b) Acute tubular necrosis
   (tubular cells are flattened, many have lost their nuclei)

Figure 1.3 Renal biopsy changes associated with ATN. (a) Normal tubules (tubular cells are fat and juicy and have nuclei). (b) Acute tubular necrosis (tubular cells are flattened, many have lost their nuclei).

obstruction. If obstruction is excluded, then the most likely cause is pre-renal failure, which if left untreated will progress to ATN. ATN occurs if there is persistent hypotension/hypovolaemia +/− exposure to nephrotoxins or sepsis. It is the cause of 70–80% of cases of ARF. Histologically, ATN is manifest as ragged, dying tubular cells which lose their nuclei and begin to slough off into the tubular lumen (Figure 1.3). These dead cells may also fill the tubular lumen and block the flow of any urine. Patients with suspected ATN are not routinely biopsied unless an additional intrarenal pathology is suspected. A number of clinical features in Mr Griffiths' case suggest that the most likely cause of his ARF is pre-renal/ATN, including his obvious dehydration, hypotension and an elevated sodium (due to hypovolaemia).

What immediate management steps would you undertake?

• The most important priority is to restore his intravascular volume with intravenous fluids. There is no evidence that colloids are any better than normal (N) saline in this situation. Therefore he should be given an IV fluid challenge, for example 500 ml N/saline over 30 minutes, followed by a repeat clinical examination to

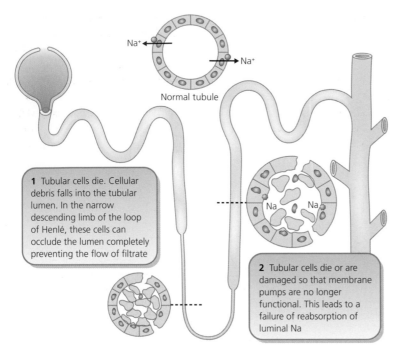

Normal tubule

Na⁺ → Na⁺

1 Tubular cells die. Cellular debris falls into the tubular lumen. In the narrow descending limb of the loop of Henlé, these cells can occlude the lumen completely preventing the flow of filtrate

2 Tubular cells die or are damaged so that membrane pumps are no longer functional. This leads to a failure of reabsorption of luminal Na

Figure 1.4 Tubular dysfunction in ATN.

assess his volume status. If there is no pulmonary oedema, proceed with a further fluid challenge. Mr Griffiths is at risk of developing pulmonary oedema if you fill him up too much (known LV dysfunction with cardiomegaly on CXR). Therefore, he will require frequent clinical examination to determine when his intravascular volume has been restored.

• Any nephrotoxins should be stopped. In this case, he is on an ACEI which should be crossed off his chart.

• Metformin should be stopped, as this can cause lactic acidosis in patients with renal failure. He will probably need an insulin sliding scale in the context of this acute illness.

• Treat underlying cause of volume depletion. Once a stool sample has been sent, it may be wise to empirically start Mr Griffiths on oral metronidazole, given the high likelihood of *C.difficile.*

• Consider gastric protection if the patient is not already on something, since ARF is associated with an increased risk of GI bleeds.

Some textbooks suggest measuring urinary sodium in order to distinguish between pre-renal failure and ATN.

What would you expect the urine sodium to be in a patient with ATN?

In ATN there is dysfunction and death of tubular cells. The normal function of these cells is to pump sodium

Table 1.1 Urine in pre-renal failure and ATN

	Pre-renal	ATN
Urine Na	<20	>80
Urine : plasma creatinine	>50 : 1	<20 : 1
Urine : plasma osmolality	>1.4 : 1	1 : 1

out of the tubular lumen (urine) and into the interstitium (in order to generate an osmotic gradient within the medulla). If the tubular cells are damaged or dead, they cannot move sodium appropriately, so there is an increased concentration of sodium in the urine (Figure 1.4). Typical results for pre-renal failure versus ATN are shown in Table 1.1.

Why is urinary sodium rarely measured in clinical practice in patients with suspected ARF secondary to pre-renal failure or ATN?

Adequate rehydration should correct any pre-renal failure. At this stage the patient should begin to pass urine again. If this does not occur and the patient is intravascularly volume replete with a good blood pressure, then it is likely that the diagnosis is ATN. In practice, this clinical information will be available long before the result of the urine sodium is returned.

Mr Griffiths is given the 500 mL bolus of fluid and still seems dehydrated. He is therefore given a further 2.5 litres of intravenous fluid over the next 6 hours. You come back to review him later in your shift. He is still oliguric but now very well filled with a JVP visible at 7 cm above the manubriosternal angle and some crepitations in both lung bases.

What would you do next?

Mr Griffiths is persistently oliguric but is now volume replete, and indeed is intravascularly volume overloaded. He should therefore be given a bolus of high-dose intravenous furosemide, for example 80 mg IV. If the patient's tubular cells are intact, he should respond to fluid replacement and furosemide. However, if there is established ATN, he may not. It is worth noting that furosemide should not be given to a dehydrated patient with pre-renal failure, as this will only exacerbate the problem. In a man like Mr Griffiths who has high GI fluid losses, it is really important to ensure that he continues to have adequate volume replacement if he responds to diuretics. If he remains oliguric, he will still require some IV fluid to replace insensible losses (normally 500 mL/24 h, in this case likely to be much higher). Care should be taken not to excessively volume overload an oliguric patient as this may lead to pulmonary oedema. If there is pulmonary oedema or the patient has symptomatic uraemia (encephalopathy/pericarditis), resistant hyperkalaemia or severe acidosis then temporary haemodialysis may be required.

Mr Griffiths is given 150 mg of intravenous furosemide in a pump over an hour. His urine output picks up to 100 mL in the following hour and remains at >50 mL/h thereafter.

What would be an appropriate fluid replacement regimen for Mr Griffiths in the next 12 hours?

Mr Griffiths' acute decline in renal function was a result of severe volume depletion secondary to diarrhoea and vomiting. An appropriate replacement regimen should take into account his insensible losses and his urine output. Normally (in a patient without excess GI losses), insensible losses would amount to around 500 mL. Therefore a typical fluid replacement regimen for a 24-hour period would be: urine output + 500 mL. However, in this case insensible losses may be as high as 2 L/24 h. The exact volume of GI losses can be difficult to measure accurately, so these patients need to be examined frequently and weighed daily in order to help assess their fluid balance.

Mr Griffiths' stools are C. difficile toxin positive. His diarrhoea slowly improves over the next few days with metronidazole. He is given intravenous fluids and his fluid status is carefully monitored. By day 5 his creatinine has fallen to 349 μmol/L. Over the next week or so his renal function settles back to a creatinine of around 220 μmol/L. However, he is much weaker than previously and his mobility has declined significantly. On discussion in the multidisciplinary team (MDT) meeting, it is felt that he is unlikely to improve sufficiently to go back to his own home but may now require sheltered accommodation or even a residential home.

Why do so many critically ill patients get ARF secondary to ATN?

The renal tubular blood supply is actually quite precarious, so that any drop in BP (secondary to hypovolaemia or reduced peripheral vascular resistance, as seen in sepsis) can lead to tubular ischaemia. This precarious blood supply is a direct result of the anatomical arrangement of the blood supply, which comes to the tubules only after it has passed through the glomerular capillary bed (see Part 1, Figure B). Thus there is always a relative hypoxia in the renal medulla compared with the cortex. When the MAP falls, there will be a reduced blood flow into the glomerulus via the afferent arteriole and a consequent fall in GFR. In an attempt to maintain GFR, there is an increase in vasoconstriction in the efferent glomerular arteriole. This will further compromise the blood supply to the medulla, leading to increased hypoxia and tubular ischaemia. Tubular cells are also very metabolically active, with a number of energy-requiring electrolyte pumps.

CASE REVIEW

An 84-year-old man with a history of left ventricular dysfunction and type II diabetes becomes oliguric following a 2-day history of diarrhoea and vomiting. On examination, he is severely dehydrated. Investigations show acute-on-chronic renal failure. He is initially treated with intravenous fluid replacement until volume replete and is then given a bolus of intravenous furosemide. He begins to pass urine and his renal function slowly improves over the next few days with careful management of his fluid balance in order to avoid a further episode of pre-renal ARF.

KEY POINTS

- Acute renal failure is relatively common, occurring in about 80/million population/year.
- Urinary obstruction should be excluded (a cause in around 5–10% of cases) because this is readily reversible if diagnosed early. A renal US will be sufficient to identify obstruction in >95% of cases.
- Most cases of ARF are due to pre-renal failure/ATN (70–80%). Risk factors for the development of ATN are:
  - old age
  - drugs (NSAID, ACEI, gentamicin)
  - sepsis
  - CKD (due to any cause).
- If obstruction has been excluded and there is nothing to suggest a more unusual/renal cause of ARF, then ATN is the most likely diagnosis, and patients should be treated with intravenous fluids to restore intravascular volume.

The underlying cause of hypotension should be treated and any nephrotoxins removed. If blood pressure remains low following adequate filling then the patient may require inotropic support which will usually require an ITU bed.
- If intravenous rehydration restores intravascular volume and blood pressure but there is no improvement in oliguria, there is likely to be established ATN and the patient may require a period of renal support (haemodialysis or filtration) whilst tubular cells regenerate. This usually takes days to weeks but can take months.
- ARF in the elderly has a significant mortality, particularly if the patient requires renal replacement therapy (1-year mortality 10–20%).

Case 2 A 74-year-old man with acute renal failure

Mr James Jones is a 74-year-old man who is referred urgently by his GP who saw him this morning and did some blood tests. The results of these tests have been called through to the GP surgery and show:

Na 145 mmol/L, K 6.9 mmol/L, Urea 29.3 mmol/L, Creatinine 686 μmol/L

The GP letter tells you that Mr Jones has had benign prostatic hypertrophy previously but is otherwise usually very fit and uncomplaining. He attended the surgery because he'd been feeling lethargic and under the weather for the past week. Given the blood results, Mr Jones is called by his GP and asked to urgently attend the Medical Admissions Unit. He arrives at 5pm, and his initial observations are unremarkable.

What is your first concern on being asked by the nursing staff to see him?

The morning bloods done at the GP surgery show significant hyperkalaemia. This may be spurious, due to haemolysis of a sample in which there has been delay in processing (potassium is found predominantly within cells, therefore when red blood cells haemolyse, their potassium load is released into the blood). Box 2.1 shows the causes of pseudohyperkalaemia.

However, this degree of hyperkalaemia could be life-threatening, so it should be considered a genuine result until proven otherwise, particularly given the severity of renal impairment present on his blood results. Hyperkalaemia can occur in both acute and chronic renal failure and should be treated as a matter of urgency because it can lead to serious cardiac arrhythmias and even cardiac arrest. Therefore your main concern is: does he have ECG changes associated with hyperkalaemia? If he does have hyperkalaemia, he is at risk of having an arrhythmia and of cardiac arrest.

Nephrology: Clinical Cases Uncovered. By M. Clatworthy. Published 2010 by Blackwell Publishing.

In view of the risk of cardiac arrhythmias associated with hyperkalaemia, what immediate measures would you undertake?

- Establish intravenous access.
- Move the patient to a monitored bed so that any cardiac arrhythmia will be immediately detected.
- Perform an urgent repeat potassium. This is often most quickly achieved by running a venous sample through the arterial blood gas machine (most emergency departments have one).
- Perform a 12-lead ECG looking for signs of hyperkalaemia (Box 2.2).
- If the ECG has significant hyperkalaemia-associated changes, then treat the hyperkalaemia before waiting for the result of the urgent potassium measurement.

The patient's ECG is shown in Figure 2.1.

What does it show and what treatment would you give after viewing it?

The ECG shows broadening of the QRS and early 'sine' waves consistent with hyperkalaemia. Mr Jones is at risk of developing a cardiac arrest. He should be given 10 mL 10% calcium gluconate as soon as possible in order to protect the heart from the development of arrhythmias. He should then be commenced on an insulin-dextrose infusion (preferably through a 18 G+ needle inserted into a large vein; 50% dextrose can be irritant to veins, so it is best to avoid putting into small veins).

Why does insulin-dextrose lower serum potassium?

If 50 mL of 50% dextrose is administered intravenously to a young person with functioning islets of Langerhans, they will rapidly secrete significant quantities of insulin from their β cells. The dextrose infusion is usually given with 10 units of a short-acting insulin, e.g. Actrapid, in case of underlying islet dysfunction, to prevent hyperglycaemia. Insulin stimulates the uptake of potassium from the blood into cells via cell surface sodium-potassium pumps. Thus both the exogenous and endogenous insulin will cause a temporary redistribution of potassium. Patients may need repeated treatments if the underlying cause of the hyperkalaemia is not dealt with. It should be emphasised that insulin-dextrose is only a holding measure because the total body potassium does not fall following its administration, it is merely redistributed.

Box 2.1 Causes of pseudohyperkalaemia

1. Prolonged tourniquet time
2. Test tube haemolysis due to delayed processing of the sample
3. Marked leucocytosis and thrombocytosis: measure plasma (liquid component of unclotted blood) not serum (liquid component of clotted blood) concentration in these disease states
4. Sample taken from a limb infused with IV fluids containing potassium

---

Box 2.2 ECG changes associated with hyperkalaemia

- Tenting of T waves
- Prolonged P-R interval
- Widening of QRS complex
- 'Sine' waves

In Mr Jones' case, the cause of hyperkalaemia is likely to be renal failure given his elevated urea and creatinine.

What other causes of hyperkalaemia do you know?

The causes of hyperkalaemia are summarised in Box 2.3. As mentioned above, 95% of the body's potassium is found within cells. Thus, if there is massive cell lysis (as seen in rhabdomyloysis when muscle is damaged or in tumour lysis syndrome when cancer cells are lysed following the administration of chemotherapeutic agents), potassium will be released into the blood. K+ can also exit cells in exchange for H+ if there is acidosis, in an attempt to buffer the elevated H+ ions in blood. K+ excretion occurs in the kidney and acidosis will lead to a reduced renal excretion of K+ as H+ is preferentially excreted instead.

Renal failure can cause hyperkalaemia because a reduction in GFR will lead to a reduced delivery of Na+ to the distal nephron. This results in reduced Na+ resorption and therefore a lower K+ excretion by the distal convoluted tubule Na/K-ATPase (see Part 1, Figure D). An isolated reduction in function of the Na/K-ATPase pump can also lead to hyperkalaemia, e.g., as seen in Addisons disease, where there is aldosterone deficiency, or following the use of drugs which indirectly block aldosterone production by inhibiting the synthesis or action of angiotensin II, e.g. ACEI or ARB.

In practice, hyperkalaemia is often caused by a combination of factors, e.g. renal failure plus an ACEI.

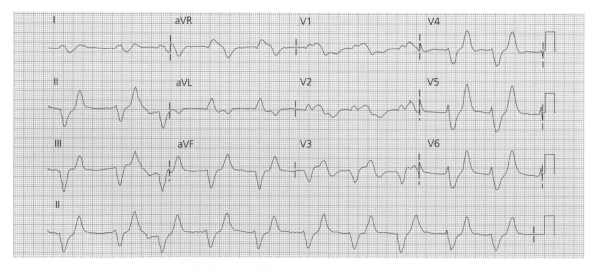

Figure 2.1 An ECG with tented T waves and wide QRS complexes (>3 small squares, i.e. >0.12 seconds).

Box 2.3 Causes of hyperkalaemia

Movement of K+ out of cells
  A. Acidosis: H+ transported into cells at the expense of K+ efflux
  B. Cell death causes release of K+, e.g. rhabdomyolysis, tumour lysis syndrome
Failure of K+ excretion by kidney (distal convoluted tubules)
  C. Renal failure
  D. Aldosterone deficiency
  E. Potassium-sparing diuretics, e.g. spironolactone
  F. ACEI, ARB
Excess intake of K+ from gut

Box 2.4 Treatment of hyperkalaemia

1. 10 mL 10% calcium gluconate (cardioprotectant) intravenously
2. 50 mL 50% dextrose + 10 u Actrapid
3. Consider salbutamol nebulisers if IV access difficult
4. In chronic hyperkalaemia, give advice on low-potassium diet and consider calcium resonium to prevent GI absorption
5. Stop any drugs associated with hyperkalaemia, e.g. ACEI, ARB, postassium-sparing diuretics such as spironolactone or amiloride

---

In the unlikely scenario that IV access cannot be immediately established, what alternative therapy could you use to bring down his potassium?

Salbutamol acts on β2-adrenoreceptors and has the same effect as insulin, in that it stimulates potassium uptake by cells. However, it is only effective if used at relatively high doses, e.g. 2×5 mg salbutamol nebulisers given almost back to back. Patients tend to become rather tremulous and tachycardic and tolerate such high doses poorly.

The treatment of hyperkalaemia is shown in Box 2.4.

Mr Jones' venous blood gas sample showed a potassium of 7.7 mmol/L. Following the calcium gluconate and insulin-dextrose, a repeat measurement shows that his K+ is now 5.9 mmol/L. His ECG changes have resolved. Now that you have tackled the immediate urgent issue of his potassium, you are able to get some more history from the patient.

What questions would you ask?

Mr Jones' bloods show significant renal impairment. The history, examination and investigations should aim to answer three main questions.
• Is this acute or chronic renal failure?
• Why does he have renal failure? A pre-renal (hypotension/hypovolaemia), renal or post-renal (obstruction) cause?
• Does he have any symptoms as a result of his renal impairment?

Is this acute or chronic renal failure, or perhaps acute-on-chronic renal failure?

This is important to establish because many cases of acute renal failure are reversible, if the precipitating/aetiological factors are rapidly remedied. If the patient has no past medical history of renal disease or of diseases which commonly cause chronic kidney disease (e.g. diabetes mellitus, hypertension, prostatic disease), then an acute pathology is more likely. Unfortunately, symptoms such as lethary or vomiting can be associated with both acute and chronic renal impairment. If a patient gives a short history of rapid-onset oligoanuria over a period of days, then an acute cause is more likely. Ultimately, the only definitive demonstration of the acute nature of renal failure is the availability of previous blood test results showing a recent normal creatinine. Chronic kidney disease also tends to be associated with small kidneys on US scan.

Why does he have renal failure?

The GP letter stated that he had a previous history of prostatic disease so a post-renal cause, i.e. obstructive uropathy, is high on the list of possible causes of his renal impairment. Overall, obstruction is the underlying cause in around 5–10% of patients with ARF. In elderly males, up to 30% of cases of ARF may be due to urethral obstruction. It is therefore important to ask about urinary symptoms such as frequency, nocturia, terminal dribbling, hesitancy or poor stream. 'Can you still hit the wall in a public toilet?' is a useful question to assess urinary stream.
• *Pre-renal cause?* Has he had any recent illnesses which might cause volume depletion or hypotension, e.g. vomiting, diarrhoea?
• *Renal cause?* Is there a history of recent pharyngitis or infection which might precipitate a postinfectious GN? Does he have any symptoms suggestive of a systemic inflammatory/autoimmune disease? A past medical

history of MI/CVA/PVD increases the probability of atherosclerotic renovascular disease.

• *Family history.* There are a number of inherited causes of CKD, for example autosomal dominant polycystic kidney disease, Alport's syndrome and familial FSGS, although these are less likely to present for the first time in a patient of this age.

• *Drug history.* Some medications can be associated with CKD including NSAID, ciclosporin, lithium; others can cause ARF due to interstitial nephritis, e.g. PPI and antibiotics.

• *Smoking history.* Smoker? (associated with atherosclerosis and therefore renovascular disease) Alcohol? (chronic liver disease and liver failure can be associated with renal impairment).

Does he have any symptoms associated with the complications of renal failure?

• *Symptomatic uraemia:* nausea, loss of appetite, symptoms associated with uraemic pericarditis (sharp chest pain, worse on lying down, breathlessness) or uraemic encephalopathy (confusion, drowsiness, fitting).

• *Acidosis:* patients may hyperventilate in an attempt to blow off CO_2 and compensate for their metabolic acidosis.

• *Volume overload:* ankle swelling, pulmonary oedema causing shortness of breath.

• *Anaemia:* can be associated with shortness of breath, angina and tiredness.

• *Hyperphosphataemia:* secondary to hyperparathyroidism can cause very troublesome itchiness.

What features of the examination might indicate that Mr Jones needs urgent dialysis?

Dialysis provides a means by which water, K+, urea and H+ can be removed. Whether renal failure is acute or chronic, there are certain features which suggest that urgent dialysis is likely to be required.

• *Pulmonary oedema:* as evidenced by hypoxia, elevated respiratory rate and bibasal coarse inspiratory crackles in the chest.

• *Severe acidosis:* the kidneys are responsible for the excretion of acid. Therefore, in renal failure there is a metabolic acidosis. In an attempt to reduce the H+ ions in the blood, there will be respiratory compensation, i.e. the patient will hyperventilate to blow off CO_2 (which is an acidic gas; Box 2.5) and may have a respiratory rate of 30–40 rpm.

> **Box 2.5 The Henderson – Hasselbach equation demonstrates why CO_2 is an acidic gas**
>
> $$CO_2 + H_2O \leftrightarrow H_2O_2 \leftrightarrow H^+ + HCO_3^-$$

• *Symptomatic uraemia:* evidenced by pericarditis (characterised by a pericardial rub, which classically sounds like feet crunching in the snow, coinciding with each systole). Uraemia can also cause encephalopathy which may cause the patient to be confused (assess this with a mini mental test) or have asterixis (flap).

• In addition, hyperkalaemia refractory to medical treatment should also be treated with dialysis.

On examination, Mr Jones is clinically euvolaemic with a pulse of 90 bpm and a BP of 160/90 mmHg. On auscultation of his chest, there is no pericardial rub but he does have bibasal crackles posteriorly. On examination of his abdomen, his bladder is palpable at 2 cm below the umbilicus. A rectal examination reveals a smooth, significantly enlarged prostate. He has mild peripheral oedema in his ankles.

His admission blood tests show:

Na 145 mmol/L, K 7.7 mmol/L, Urea 34 mmol/L, Creatinine 729 μmol/L, CRP 8 mg/L

Hb 12.7 g/dL, WBC 6.5 × 10⁹/L, Platelets 438 × 10⁹/L.

He has an ultrasound scan performed urgently (Figure 2.2). What does this show?

The ultrasound scan shows a kidney of normal size (10–12 cm) with some preservation of corticomedullary differentiation but gross hydronephrosis (Figure 2.2a) and a full bladder post attempted micturition (Figure 2.2b). The other kidney is also hydronephrotic on US, and both ureters are dilated. This is suggestive of distal obstruction (i.e. at the level of the urethra or beyond). Other causes of obstruction with their typical US patterns are shown in Figure 2.3.

What would you do next for Mr Jones?

Mr Jones has an ultrasound scan which suggests that the most likely cause of ARF is urethral outflow obstruction. Therefore a urinary catheter should be inserted. Given his history of prostatic disease, this may not be easy and may require urology input (Figure 2.4). If a catheter cannot be placed per-urethrally due to the size of the

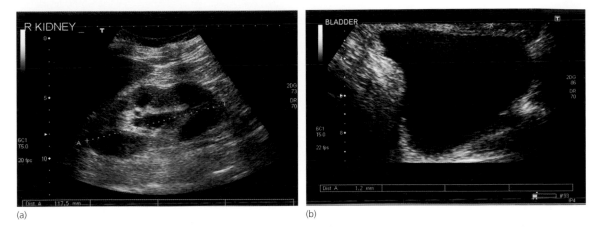

(a)   (b)

Figure 2.2 Ultrasound scan of the renal tract showing (a) pelvicaliceal dilatation of the kidney (dark space centrally in the kidney) and (b) a full bladder.

prostate, then a suprapubic catheter is placed directly into the bladder through the skin.

He will also need repeated U+E measurements to ensure resolution of hyperkalaemia with treatment.

What is the main problem which can develop following resolution of obstruction by insertion of a urinary catheter?

Following treatment of urinary obstruction by insertion of a catheter, patients frequently become polyuric due to temporary tubular dysfunction.

In the 8 hours following catheterisation, Mr Jones passes 6 litres of urine and unless he is placed on an adequate fluid replacement regimen, he will be at risk of developing pre-renal failure due to intravascular volume depletion. Thus his fluid balance should be carefully monitored and he is likely to require intravenous fluids in addition to encouraging increased oral intake.

With the diuresis post catheterisation and adequate fluid replacement, Mr Jones' renal function tests improved rapidly over the next 48 hours. His creatinine plateaus at 150 μmol/L. He is reviewed by the urologists and commenced on tamsulosin (a selective α1a blocker used in the treatment of BPH). His PSA level is unchanged from the last measurement a year previously. He undergoes a successful trial without catheter in the community 2 weeks later.

Two years later Mr Jones is readmitted when he notices a reduction in his urine output and the development of

similar symptoms of lethargy and nausea. His blood tests show Na 135 mmol/L, K 5.8 mmol/L, Urea 36 mmol/L, Creatinine 460 μmol/L. He is clinically euvolaemic and his bladder is not palpable but he does have inguinal lymphadenopathy. His ultrasound does not demonstrate significant hydronephrosis.

What is the most likely cause of his renal failure?

Obstruction is still the most likely cause of his renal failure, given his previous history. Patients with advanced pelvic malignancy may develop functional obstruction in the absence of hydronephrosis because the urinary tract becomes encased in an inflammatory infiltrate or with metastases, thus preventing the development of hydronephrosis. Functional obstruction can be demonstrated using a nuclear medicine scan such as a MAG3 showing delayed tracer excretion to the bladder or encasement of the ureters or other retroperitoneal disease can be visualised on a CT scan.

A MAG3 scan shows obstruction. How should he be treated?

Mr Jones should be treated by insertion of percutaneous nephrostomies. This may lead to a similar polyuric period and thus his fluid balance should be carefully monitored. A nephrostomy will temporarily relieve obstruction but a long-term solution is achieved through the insertion of stents into the ureters, either in an anterograde fashion via the nephrostomy or in a retrograde manner via cystoscopy.

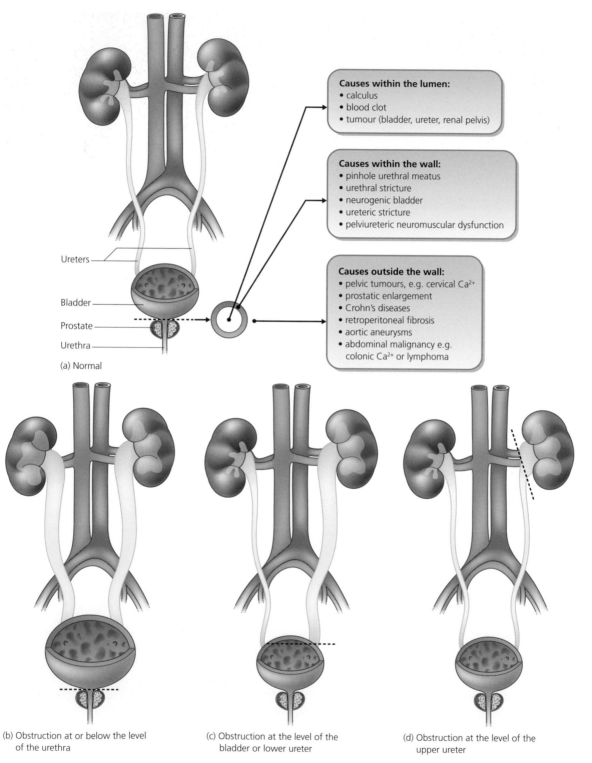

Causes within the lumen:
• calculus
• blood clot
• tumour (bladder, ureter, renal pelvis)

Causes within the wall:
• pinhole urethral meatus
• urethral stricture
• neurogenic bladder
• ureteric stricture
• pelviureteric neuromuscular dysfunction

Causes outside the wall:
• pelvic tumours, e.g. cervical Ca^{2+}
• prostatic enlargement
• Crohn's diseases
• retroperitoneal fibrosis
• aortic aneurysms
• abdominal malignancy e.g. colonic Ca^{2+} or lymphoma

Ureters

Bladder

Prostate

Urethra

(a) Normal

(b) Obstruction at or below the level of the urethra

(c) Obstruction at the level of the bladder or lower ureter

(d) Obstruction at the level of the upper ureter

Figure 2.3 Causes of obstruction (which occur at different sites in the upper and lower urinary tract) and patterns of dilation observed depending on the level of obstruction (b–d).

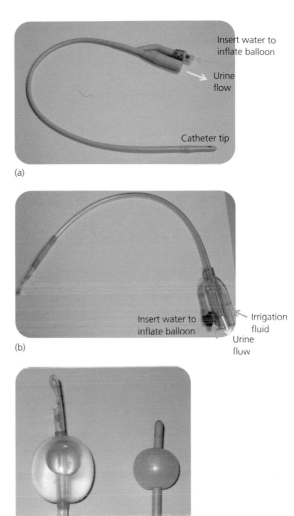

Figure 2.4 Urinary catheter insertion. (a) 14 ch urinary catheter. (b) 18 ch three-way (irrigation) catheter. (c) Catheter tips with balloon inflated in a three-way (irrigation) catheter (left) and a standard catheter (right). The balloon is inflated following the introduction of the catheter into the bladder and prevents it from falling out.

CASE REVIEW

A 74-year-old man with a history of benign prostatic hypertrophy is admitted with acute renal failure. Admission blood tests show significant hyperkalaemia, with ECG changes. This is treated with calcium gluconate and an insulin-dextrose infusion. A renal US shows hydronephrosis and a full bladder post micturition. He is catheterised and has an excellent diuresis and his renal function rapidly improves. He is started on an α-blocker (tamsulosin) and the catheter is successfully removed a week or so later. Two years later, he again presents with ARF. US shows no hydronephrosis but a MAG3 demonstrates functional obstruction. He is therefore treated by nephrostomy placement.

KEY POINTS

- Acute renal failure can be complicated by hyperkalaemia. This is a medical emergency because it can cause significant cardiac arrhythmias and even cardiac arrest.
- The signs of hyperkalaemia seen on ECG are tenting of T waves, prolongation of the QRS complex and the development of sine waves.
- Hyperkalaemia with ECG changes should be treated immediately with calcium gluconate (to stabilise cardiac myocytes) and insulin-dextrose (causes a redistribution of K+ intracellularly).
- Acute renal failure can be caused by pre-renal (e.g. hypovolaemia), renal (e.g. GN) and post-renal (e.g. obstruction) causes.

- Obstruction causes around 5–10% of all ARF and is usually due to prostatic disease. It is usually visible on an US of the renal tract as hydronephrosis. Obstruction should be treated as quickly as possible to prevent long-term damage to the kidneys. In most cases, insertion of a catheter will do the trick. Following relief of the obstruction, patients may develop polyuria and are therefore at risk of developing pre-renal failure unless their fluid balance is managed carefully.

Case 3 · A 64-year-old man with back pain and polydipsia

Mr Gareth Evans is a 64-year-old chartered surveyor who attends A+E after he tripped over a paving stone whilst inspecting a site. He fell with a jolt and has had severe back pain since, prompting his hospital attendance. He also mentions that in recent weeks he has been very thirsty and has been passing urine many times at night, and he is concerned he may have diabetes. He is seen by the A&E F2 who performs an X-ray of the spine and some basic bloods. The results are shown below. He is therefore referred to the medical team on-call.

Na 138 mmol/L, K 5.5 mmol/L, Urea 26 mmol/L, Creatinine 450 μmol/L

Hb 9.0 g/dL, MCV 84, WBC 5.8 × 10⁹/L, Platelets 420 × 10⁹/L

Glucose 4.2 mmol/L, Albumin 30 g/L, LFT NAD, cCalcium 2.98 mmol/L

Why does this man have polydipsia and polyuria?

Polydipsia (increased fluid intake, usually due to increased thirst) often occurs as a result of polyuria. If there is an increased loss of water from the kidneys, the osmolality of blood may increase. This is detected by the hypothalamus which stimulates thirst and the release of ADH in an attempt to restore intravascular volume. Hypovolaemia will also lead to renin release and, via the renin-angiotensin pathway (see Part 1, Figure E), to the generation of angiotensin II. Angiotensin II stimulates thirst, as well as having many other effects, including vasoconstriction. Polyuria occurs if there is an osmotic diuresis, e.g. if there is glycosuria (diabetes mellitus), if there is a deficiency in or insensitivity to ADH (diabetes insipidus) or in the presence of drugs which stimulate diuresis, e.g. alcohol. It can also occur if there is excess water intake, e.g. psychogenic polydipsia.

Nephrology: Clinical Cases Uncovered. By M. Clatworthy.
Published 2010 by Blackwell Publishing.

Given his normal random blood sugar, Mr Evans' symptoms are unlikely to be due to glycosuria. He is hypercalcaemic which can lead to elevated levels of urinary calcium (hypercalciuria), which is associated with an osmotic diuresis and therefore polyuria. An appropriate polydipsia then occurs by the mechanisms described above.

What are the other symptoms of hypercalcaemia?

The classic presenting features of hypercalcaemia are 'bones, abdominal groans, stones, and psychic moans' (Box 3.1). Other features include muscle weakness, hypertension, bradycardia/AV block or short QT interval on ECG.

What are the causes of hypercalcaemia?

The most common causes of hypercalcaemia are primary or tertiary hyperparathyroidism, malignancy and myeloma. A more complete list of causes is given in Box 3.2. Note that a bony fracture does not normally lead to hypercalcaemia.

Parathyroid hormone leads to hypercalcaemia by increasing calcium resorption from bone, gut and kidneys. Hyperparathyroidism is classified as primary, secondary or tertiary. Primary hyperparathyroidism usually occurs because of a parathyroid adenoma (less commonly, carcinoma or hyperplasia). Parathyroid adenomas can occur in isolation or as part of multiple endocrine neoplasia (MEN). Type I MEN is associated with pituitary adenomas and pancreatic islet cell tumours. Type IIa MEN is associated with phaeochromocytoma and medullary carcinoma of the thyroid. Secondary hyperparathyroidism is an appropriate response to a low calcium, and is therefore not a cause of hypercalcaemia. Tertiary hyperparathyroidism occurs in chronic kidney disease, where long-term stimulation of the parathyroids by chronic hypocalcaemia eventually leads to

---

Box 3.1 Presenting features of hypercalcaemia

- 'Bones' – bone pain
- 'Abdominal groans'
  - Nausea/vomiting
  - Anorexia
  - Constipation
  - Pancreatitis
  - Peptic ulceration
- 'Stones' – renal stones
- 'Psychic moans'
  - Malaise/depression
  - Lethargy
  - Confusion

Box 3.2 Causes of hypercalcaemia

- Malignancy
- Myeloma
- Hyperparathyroidism (primary/tertiary)
- Sarcoidosis
- Hyperthyroidism
- Milk – alkali syndrome
- Vitamin D excess
- Thiazide diuretics

parathyroid hyperplasia and autonomous secretion of PTH independent of serum calcium levels (see Part 1, Figure F).

Malignancies cause hypercalcaemia in two ways.

- Through bony metastases, which erode through bone, releasing calcium. The tumours which typically metastasise to bone are lung, prostate, thyroid, kidney and breast (**LPTKB**, easily remembered using the mnemonic 'Lecturers, Professors and Teachers Know Best').
- Through the production of parathyroid hormone related-protein (PTHrP) by the tumour (typically small cell lung cancer), which mimics the actions of PTH on bone, stimulating osteoclasts. It also acts on renal tubules to increase the resorption of Ca from the tubules. There are now assays available which can distinguish PTH and PTHrP.

What are the important points to establish when taking a history from Mr Evans?

History of presenting complaint

When was the last time he was completely well? How long has his polydipsia/polyuria been going on for? Had he had back pain before the fall? Has he had any systemic symptoms associated with solid organ or haematological malignancy, e.g. unintentional weight loss, loss of appetite, fever, night sweats, change in bowel habit, bleeding per rectum, chronic cough or haemoptysis, rashes, jaundice?

Past medical history

Is his renal impairment acute or chronic? Does he have a history of chronic kidney disease or any pathologies that can cause it, e.g. diabetes, hypertension, renovascular disease? Does he have any prostatic symptoms such as hesitancy or poor stream? Has he started on any new medications recently?

Mr Evans has been feeling unwell for 4–5 months with symptoms of lethargy and mild backache. The polyuria and polydipsia have occurred more recently over the last 3–4 weeks. He has previously been very fit and healthy with no history of diabetes or hypertension. His only medications are some multivitamin tablets, which his wife insists he takes on a regular basis.

What are the key points to determine on examination?

As previously emphasised, the central factor to establish in any patient with likely ARF is their intravascular volume status (skin turgor, pulse, BP, JVP). Given his hypercalcaemia and associated polyuria, Mr Evans may well be volume depleted.

Does he have any rashes (can be associated with malignancy and sarcoidosis)? Is there any lymphadenopathy? In a case like this, special attention should be paid to specifically examining for inguinal, axillary, subclavian, cervical and submandibular lymph nodes as well as a careful assessment of the abdomen for any masses or organomegaly. Mr Evans should also have a rectal examination to exclude rectal cancer as well as to assess prostatic bulk.

On examination, Mr Evans has pale palmar creases and mucous membranes. He has no rashes peripherally and no palpable lymphadenopathy. His pulse is 90 bpm, regular, but he has reduced skin turgor, JVP not visible, dry mucous membranes, BP 110/70 mmHg lying, 95/55 mmHg standing. Chest is clear. Abdomen – no masses or organomegaly. Per rectum examination demonstrates no rectal masses and a slightly enlarged, smooth prostate.

Which additional investigations might help to determine the cause of his hypercalcaemia?

Phosphate and alkaline phosphatase (ALP) can help to discriminate between the three most common causes of hypercalcaemia as follows:

$\uparrow$Ca, $\uparrow$PO$_4$, **normal ALP** = myeloma

$\uparrow$Ca, $\downarrow$PO$_4$, $\uparrow$ALP = hyperparathyroidism

$\uparrow$Ca, $\uparrow$PO$_4$, $\uparrow$ALP = malignancy.

ALP is an enzyme released from both liver and bone. These liver and bone isoenzymes can be distinguished if necessary, and it is changes in the bone-derived ALP (released in response to osteoclast activation) which are associated with hypercalcaemia. In the context of hypercalcaemia, ALP is elevated in:

- hyperparathyroidism
- malignancy
- sarcoidosis
- hyperthyroidism.

Does the presence of renal impairment help in determining the underlying cause of hypercalcaemia?

No. Hypercalcaemia can cause renal impairment in and of itself by a number of mechanisms.

- Intravascular volume depletion secondary to polyuria may lead to ATN.
- Hypercalciuria is associated with the development of calcium-containing renal calculi which can cause obstruction and recurrent UTI.
- Chronic hypercalcaemia can lead to the development of nephrocalcinosis, a condition in which there is diffuse deposition of calcium within the medulla, visible on a plain abdominal X ray.

Myeloma can cause renal impairment due to cast nephropathy and direct tubular toxicity with associated TIN. Malignancy is associated with the development of a number of glomerulonephritides, particularly membranous GN.

What other investigations would you perform?

As well as the baseline bloods already performed above, you would also assess ESR, paraprotein levels (elevated in myeloma), PSA (elevated in prostatic cancer). A blood film is useful to check for haematological abnormalities associated with myeloma. A urine specimen for dipstick, microscopy and culture, as well as an early morning specimen for Bence–Jones protein. Imaging should include CXR to exclude a primary lung malignancy, pulmonary metastases or bilateral hilar lymphadenopathy. Ultrasound of the renal tract should be performed to exclude hydronephrosis and to assess the size of the kidneys and corticomedullary differentiation.

Mr Evans' results are returned to you:

ESR 105 mm/h, CRP 20 mg/L, PSA 3 ng/mL
Blood film: rouleaux (red blood cells stuck together)
CXR: clear lung fields, normal-sized heart
Serum IgG is elevated and there is a paraprotein band
   detectable
IgM and IgA levels are normal
Lytic lesions on spine X ray

What is ESR and in what conditions does it become elevated?

ESR is the erythrocyte sedimentation rate. It is estimated by collecting blood and measuring the rate at which erythrocytes (red blood cells) form a sediment in the bottom of the test tube over 1 hour (Figure 3.1). It is a non-specific marker of disease which also rises with age and anaemia. A simple way to calculate the approximate value of a normal ESR for an individual of a particular age is the Westergren method:

- males = age in years/2
- females = age in years + 10/2.

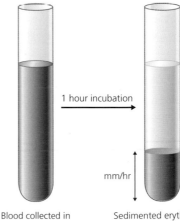

Blood collected in   Sedimented erythrocytes
an EDTA tube to   at the bottom of the upright
prevent coagulation   tube measured in mm

Figure 3.1 Measuring ESR.

Classically ESR becomes elevated in diseases in which there are abnormally high levels of plasma proteins (e.g. immunoglobulins/antibodies) which cover red cells, causing them to stick together in clumps. This is visible on a blood film as rouleaux or stacks of red cells. These clumps of red cells are heavier, so they will fall faster and form a larger sediment within a given time. Diseases classically associated with an elevated ESR include:

- multiple myeloma (raised monoclonal immuno-globulin)
- autoimmune diseases (e.g. SLE and vasculitis, associated with elevated autoantibodies)
- malignancy
- infection.

What is the most likely diagnosis?

The most likely diagnosis is multiple myeloma (MM). MM occurs when a single plasma cell undergoes uncontrolled, malignant proliferation, taking over the bone marrow. Plasma cells are terminally differentiated B cells and are responsible for producing antibodies (immunoglobulins). We normally have plasma cells producing antibodies with many different specificities ($>10^6$). In myeloma, one of these cells clonally expands and is massively over-represented in the overall plasma cell pool. As the clone gets bigger, it eventually squeezes out other cells normally found within the bone marrow (such as erythroid and myeloid precursors), causing anaemia and thrombocytopaenia. The abnormal plasma cell clone also takes up the space occupied by normal plasma cells. Thus, although a patient with an IgG myeloma may have elevated levels of IgG, they may have depressed IgM and IgA levels (immunoparesis) because of loss of the plasma cells producing these antibodies.

In addition, the vast amounts of immunoglobulin produced by the myeloma cells (which form the paraprotein band on serum electrophoresis) all recognise antigen of a single specificity (because they are being produced by a clone derived from a single plasma cell). Hence these antibodies are not particularly useful in defending the body against the vast array of microbes encountered. Patients are therefore at increased risk of developing infections.

Multiple myeloma is usually classified according to the plasma cell product; 55% of patients have an IgG-producing plasma cell clone, 25% an IgA, and 20% a light chain-producing clone. Light chains are also produced by IgG and IgA melomas and can be detected in urine (Bence Jones protein).

To make the diagnosis of myeloma, two out of the following three criteria should be fulfilled:
1. detection of a serum paraprotein band or urine Bence Jones proteins
2. lytic (punched-out) lesions on a skeletal survey
3. >10% plasma cells on bone marrow trephine.
Mr Evans has two of the defining criteria: lytic lesions on X-ray and the paraprotein band.

MM occurs in about 5/100,000 individuals, with a peak age of presentation of 70 years. Clinical features include bone pain, pathological fractures, lethargy (due to anaemia), infections (due to immunoparesis) and symptoms of hyperviscosity due to high immunoglobulin levels (cognitive impairment, visual disturbance).

Why do patients with multiple myeloma develop renal impairment?

Renal impairment in MM is common (50–70%) and is usually multifactorial (Box 3.3). The abnormal protein produced in myeloma can become deposited in the kidneys as casts, crystals or amyloid fibrils, most commonly as casts. Filtration of large quantities of light chain into the tubules leads to the development of cast nephropathy (Figure 3.2). Renal biopsy typically shows large casts in the distal tubule and the collecting duct. They often have a 'hard' and 'fractured' appearance and crystals may be seen within casts, making them angular. Casts are frequently surrounded by mononuclear cells, exfoliated tubular cells and, more characteristically, by multinucleated giant cells. These cells are often seen engulfing the casts and at times actually phagocytosing cast fragments. Light chains can also cause direct tubular toxicity, leading to ATN and TIN.

Patients with myeloma may also develop a degree of nephrocalcinosis secondary to chronic hypercalcaemia or have uric acid stones because of an increased cell turnover (purine catabolism). In addition, patients with myeloma will frequently have a long history of back pain or bony pain, leading them to self-medicate with NSAID which can be nephrotoxic. A renal biopsy will distinguish between these diagnoses, although in many cases biopsy is not undertaken and renal impairment is assumed to be largely due to cast nephropathy.

How would you immediately manage Mr Evans' hypercalcaemia?

Intravenous fluids are the first-line therapy. Once a patient is fully rehydrated, furosemide can be used to encourage diuresis and urinary calcium loss (Box 3.4). If

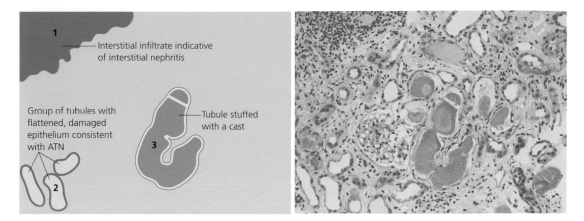

Figure 3.2 Low-power picture of a renal biopsy showing a large cast within a tubule in a patient with multiple myeloma (right panel). A schematic digram of the biopsy is shown in the left panel.

Box 3.3 Causes of renal impairment in multiple myeloma

- Cast nephropathy
- Tubulointerstitial nephritis (TIN)
- Amyloid
- Urate nephropathy
- NSAID
- Hypercalcaemia (associated with calculi/nephrocalcinosis)

Box 3.4 Treatment of hypercalcaemia (if >3 mmol/L)

- N saline infusion (2–4 L/24 h)
- Furosemide 40 mg IV (once rehydrated)
- Bisphosphonates (pamidronate 30–60 mg IV/4 h)
- Steroids (sometimes helpful in malignancy or myeloma-associated hypercalcaemia)
- Calcitonin (rarely used)

---

the patient remains significantly hypercalcaemic following volume replacement and diuretics then intravenous bisphosphonates can be used. However, bisphosphonates are nephrotoxic so should not be used in a dehydrated patient. A urinary catheter would be useful to monitor urine output and would likely be more convenient for Mr Evans whilst intravenous fluids and furosemide are being used to encourage a diuresis.

Mr Evans is rehydrated with intravenous fluids. His calcium falls to 2.68 mmol/L. Renal function also improves (creatinine 212 µmol/l). He is referred to the haematologists for further management of his myeloma, and advised to drink plenty whilst at home.

What is Mr Evans' prognosis?

Overall, the prognosis of MM is poor (50% 2-year survival). Patients with renal failure have a shorter survival than those with normal renal function, particularly if they become dialysis dependent following presentation. In the presence of renal failure, mortality in the first 3 months is about 30% and median survival ranges from 9 to 22 months. Survival time is about 2 years in patients whose serum creatinine returned to normal following treatment, compared to only 5 months in patients with irreversible renal failure.

Current treatment in myeloma is limited. If patients are fit enough, then a combination of melphalan and prednisolone is used. In younger patients, autologous bone marrow transplantation can bring about long-term remission.

In patients with ARF, some nephrologists advocate the use of plasma exchange (PEX), which will remove the monoclonal antibody or light chain. There is an ongoing UK trial (MERIT – MyEloma Renal Impairment Trial) which should provide an answer on whether PEX should be used in all myeloma patients with significant renal impairment.

More recently, a new agent, bortezomib (a proteosome inhibitor), has emerged, which is more efficacious than standard treatment. The proteosome is an organelle found inside cells which is responsible for breaking down misfolded proteins. Plasma cells produce large quantities of proteins (antibodies), so it is inevitable that a proportion will be misfolded and require disposal. If this is not performed properly then misfolded proteins accumulate and the cell will undergo apoptosis. The malignant plasma cell clones in myeloma appear to be highly susceptible to induction of apoptosis following administration of bortezomib.

CASE REVIEW

A 64-year-old man presents with polydipsia, polyuria and back pain. Investigations show hypercalcaemia and acute renal failure. The hypercalcaemia is treated with intravenous fluids. Further work-up shows that he has an IgG paraprotein and lytic lesions on spine X-ray consistent with a diagnosis of multiple myeloma. He is referred to the haematologists, but will likely have a poor outlook (<50% 2-year survival).

KEY POINTS

- Patients with hypercalcaemia classically present with 'bones, (renal) stones, (psychic) moans, and (abdominal) groans'. That is, they have bone pain, renal calculi, depression or psychosis, and intermittent abdominal pain. They will often complain of polydipsia and polyuria and may be dehydrated on examination.
- The most common causes of hypercalcaemia are malignancy, multiple myeloma and hyperparathyroidism (primary and tertiary).
- Treatment of hypercalcaemia is with intravenous normal saline, followed by furosemide once the patient is properly rehydrated. In patients with a persistently elevated serum calcium level (>3.0 mmol/l), then a single dose of pamidronate may also be required.
- Hypercalcaemia can cause renal impairment by a number of mechanisms, for example the development of calcium-containing renal calculi and of nephrocalcinosis.
- Myeloma is a plasma cell dyscrasia which is frequently associated with renal impairment, classically through the development of cast nephropathy (immunoglobulin/light chains aggregate within tubules).

Case 4   A 20-year-old woman with facial swelling and coke-coloured urine

Jane James is a 20-year-old woman who presented to her GP with a 5-day history of increasing facial swelling and right loin pain. Other details noted in the referral letter include a 2-day history of reduced urine output. Her blood pressure is elevated at 150/85 mmHg. In addition, the GP has noted that the urine produced is dark in colour (the patient describes it as 'like coke'). Urine dipstick shows protein+++ and blood++++. She is referred to the on-call renal team for further assessment.

How would you classify or describe this presentation?

This case shows the typical features of nephritic syndrome. This is characterised by:
- acute renal dysfunction
- micro/macroscopic haematuria
- hypertension
- proteinuria
- oedema.

What is the differential diagnosis of a patient with nephritic syndrome?

Nephritic syndrome is generally caused by pathologies which result in glomerular inflammation (glomerulonephritis). This can be primary or occur secondary to other problems such as infection and autoimmune disease. A full differential diagnosis for nephritic syndrome is given in Box 4.1.

What further features of the history would you explore?

Miss James has presented with a nephritic syndrome. Further history should be aimed at identifying the cause, particularly any features suggestive of diseases which can cause GN such as SLE or infection. A reasonable line of questioning would include the following.

Nephrology: Clinical Cases Uncovered. By M. Clatworthy.
Published 2010 by Blackwell Publishing.

- When did she become unwell? Any illness preceding this episode of swelling (particularly pharyngitis or other infection)?
- Any systemic symptoms (fever, joint pain, sweats, rashes, respiratory symptoms /haemoptysis/SOB, nasal crusting discharge, sinusitis, red eyes) which might suggest a systemic autoimmune or inflammatory disease such as SLE or vasculitis?
- Any new medications?
- Any family history of similar disease?
- Any previous similar episodes or any renal or autoimmune past medical history?

Miss James is normally fit and well. She works as a stable hand in the local riding school. She has been unwell for around 3 weeks and things started with a severe tonsillitis. This was so bad that she went along to her GP and was given a 5-day course of penicillin. The tonsillitis cleared but she continued to feel quite tired and lethargic. Five days ago she noticed that her face was a little swollen when she got out of bed in the morning. Since then her legs have become swollen and her urine has darkened and looks 'like coke'. She is also passing much smaller volumes of urine than usual. She has been trying to drink more water to 'make the urine less concentrated' but this has only led to more ankle swelling. Other than the penicillin given by her GP, she has not started any new medicines but does take the oral contraceptive pill. She has no family history of renal or autoimmune disease and no significant past medical history.

Examination shows her to have significant pitting oedema to the knees. There are no obvious rashes. Her pharynx is not erythematous but she does have a couple of palpable cervical lymph nodes bilaterally (1 cm in diameter). Her pulse is 80 bpm, BP 155/85 mmHg, JVP is not elevated and heart sounds are pure. Her chest is clear and oxygen saturations 99% s/v on air. Abdominal examination is unremarkable, with no organomegaly or tenderness.

Box 4.1 Causes of nephritic syndrome

Glomerulonephritis
- Primary
  - ○ IgA nephropathy
  - ○ Mesangiocapillary GN
  - ○ Idiopathic rapidly progressive/crescentic GN
  - ○ Focal segmental glomerulosclerosis (more often presents as nephrotic syndrome)
- Secondary
  - ○ Postinfectious GN
  - ○ Goodpasture's disease (anti-glomerular basement membrane antibody disease)
  - ○ SLE
  - ○ Vasculitides, e.g. ANCA-associated (Wegener's granulomatosis, microscopic polyangiitis), polyarteritis nodosum
  - ○ HSP
  - ○ Systemic sclerosis
  - ○ Cryoglobulinaemia

Acute tubulointerstitial nephritis – may present with acute renal failure and/or nephritic or nephrotic syndrome

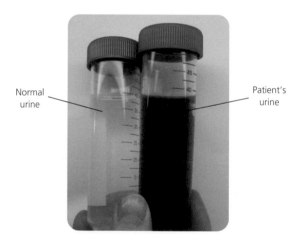

Normal urine

Patient's urine

Figure 4.1 Miss James' urine sample.

She undergoes some investigations in the Medical Admissions Unit including a FBC, U+E, LFT, CXR, ECG, and urine dipstick. The results are shown below.

Hb 11.5 g/dL, WBC 7.7 × 10⁹/L, Platelets 289 × 10⁹/L
Clotting : normal
U+E : Na 134 mmol/L, K 5.6 mmol/L, Urea 22.3 mmol/L,
  Creatinine 213 μmol/L
ESR 46 mm/h, CRP 49 mg/L, LFT normal, Albumin 28 g/L
Coke-coloured urine in pot (Figure 4.1)

Urine dipstick: proteinuria +++ haematuria++++
Urine microscopy: dysmorphic red cells
CXR: NAD
ECG: sinus rhythm

How would you interpret these results?

These results support the initial impression of a nephritic illness. Miss James has significant renal impairment (urea 22.3 mmol/L, creatinine 213 μmol/L). The GP did some routine bloods at the time of the episode of tonsillitis and her creatinine was 68 μmol/L; therefore, this is ARF.

The causes of ARF can be classified as pre-renal (most common), renal and postrenal. The nephritic presentation suggests a renal cause. In particular, Miss James has both haematuria and proteinuria on urine dipstick, dysmorphic red cells on urine microscopy (termed an 'active urinary sediment') and elevated inflammatory markers, all of which are suggestive of glomerular inflammation (glomerulonephritis).

What further investigations would you perform?

Given her ARF and active urinary sediment, a primary or secondary GN is likely (see Box 4.1). The following investigations should be performed.
- Ultrasound of the renal tract (mandatory in any patient with ARF)
- A renal immunology screen, to assess for the presence of systemic autoimmune disease, in particular:
  - ○ SLE – associated with ANA, anti-dsDNA, low complement (C3/C4), high IgG, anti-cardiolipin antibody, anti-Sm antibody
  - ○ vasculitis – associated with ANCA
  - ○ Goodpasture's disease – associated with anti-GBM antibodies
  - ○ cryoglobulinaemia – associated with rheumatoid factor, cryoglobulins and low C3/C4
  - ○ C3 nephritic factor – associated with mesangiocapillary GN and low C3.
- Postinfectious GN typically occurs secondary to group A β-haemolytic streptococci. Throat swabs should be performed, as well as quantification of anti-streptolysin-O (ASO) titres and anti-DNAseB antibody titres, which will allow confirmation of a recent streptococcal infection.
- A US-guided renal biopsy to determine the precise type and cause of glomerular inflammation.

The renal US shows two normal-sized kidneys (left 11.2 cm, right 11.8 cm) with no hydronephrosis or obvious

Wire-loop lesions

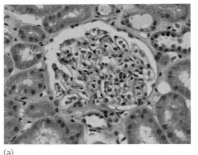
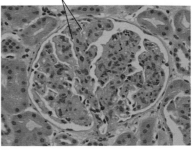

Figure 4.2 Renal biopsy showing diffuse, proliferative glomerulonephritis. (a) Normal renal biopsy (for comparison). (b) Patient's renal biopsy. A representative glomerulus is shown. All glomeruli within the biopsy show similar changes (i.e. diffuse pathology) and there is proliferative change throughout the whole glomerulus (i.e. global pathology).

(a)

(b)

abnormality. This is typical of patients with GN, in which US appearances are often normal or may show some loss of corticomedullary differentiation.

Systemic complement levels are abnormal, with a very low C3 and borderline low C4.

All other immunology is negative (including negative ANA/dsDNA/ANCA/anti-GBM)

What is the most likely diagnosis?

Given the history of pharyngitis with the subsequent development of nephritic syndrome 3 weeks later, and the low complement levels, the most likely diagnosis is a post-infectious GN. The negative immunological investigations make other causes of GN in this age group less likely (e.g. SLE).

The other differential diagnosis of a TIN (secondary to the antibiotic she was given) is unlikely, because this would not lead to complement abnormalities.

Flares of IgA nephropathy can be precipitated by mucosal infection, but these typically occur at the time of pharyngitis or 2–3 days later. Post-infectious GN tends to occur 2–3 weeks after the pharyngitic illness, as an IgG antibody response to the bacteria develops.

Miss James is started on amlodipine 5 mg in order to better control her blood pressure prior to renal biopsy, which is subsequently performed without complication. The H+E staining of the biopsy is shown in Figure 4.2.

What do you think of the glomerular capillary loops? What would you expect the immunostaining to show?

There is global change in all glomeruli in this biopsy. Specifically, there is proliferation of capillaries, with obliteration of capillary loops and so-called 'wire-loop'

lesions. The background tubules and interstitium look relatively normal.

Immunostaining usually shows deposition of IgM and IgG as well as some complement components (particularly C3).

The immunostaining on Miss James' biopsy is positive for IgM, IgG, C3 and C1q. Her ASO titre is 400 iu/mL (normal 0–200) and her anti-DNAse B >1440 iu/mL (0–85), indicative of recent streptococcal infection.

What treatment would you offer this patient?

Post-infectious GN usually resolves spontaneously (provided the associated infection is adequately treated) without any specific immunosuppressive treatment for glomerular inflammation. General management measures include control of hypertension and proteinuria, preferably with an ACEI. Diuretics, e.g. furosemide, are useful in treating oedema.

Miss James is started on furosemide 40 mg and lisinopril 2.5 mg and advised to continue on the OCP whilst on the ACEI.

Why is this advice important?

Angiotensin-converting enzyme inhibitors should be avoided in pregnancy. They are associated with oligohydramnios and developmental abnormalities. If Miss James wants to get pregnant then she should be switched onto a β-blocker or methyldopa.

Miss James' renal function improves rapidly over the next few days but she remains hypertensive. The lisinopril dose is increased to 5 mg prior to discharge. Two weeks later, she is seen in clinic and is feeling very much better. Her oedema has resolved and her creatinine is now 99 μmol/L. However, she is still hypertensive.

She asks about the prognosis of this illness, and whether her kidney function will fully recover.

What do you tell her?

Overall, post-infectious GN is relatively benign, with spontaneous, complete recovery in 95% of children and 80% of adults (the younger, the better the prognosis). Around 5% of patients present with severe hypertension and left ventricular dysfunction. These tend to have a worse prognosis.

On review over the next few months, Miss James' blood pressure and creatinine normalise and her urine dipstick no longer indicates proteinuria.

What do you know about the pathogenesis of post-infectious glomerulonephritis?

Post-infectious GN usually occurs secondary to pharyngitis caused by Lancefield Group A β-haemolytic streptococci. Other causes include staphylococcal osteomyelitis, pneumococcal pneumonia, endocarditis (staphylococcal or streptococcal), and infected atrioventricular shunts (staphylococcal).

Post-streptococcal GN is the most common and widely studied of the post-infectious GNs. Only certain streptococcal strains that contain an M protein within their cell wall can induce glomerular pathology, so-called nephritogenic strains. Three specific streptococcal antigens have been implicated:

- pre-absorbing antigen (PAAg)
- nephritis strain-associated protein (NSAP)
- nephritis plasmin-binding protein (NPBP).

When combined with their respective antibodies, these proteins form immune complexes, which have the right properties to favour glomerular deposition. These deposited immune complexes will activate complement (leading to the low C3/C4 observed) and cause glomerular inflammation.

Other pathogenic mechanisms include the formation of antibodies to bacteria which cross-react with glomerular basement membrane components, and direct activation of the alternative complement pathway by bacterial components deposited subendothelially, leading to C3 consumption.

Host factors also play a role (although these are not well defined), since not all patients infected with nephritogenic strains of streptococcus will develop glomerulonephritis.

In cases of post-streptococcal glomerulonephritis, are there any public health issues which should be addressed?

Post-streptococcal GN can occur in epidemics. Specific strains of β-haemolytic streptococci are nephritogenic and these can be passed around small communities, causing an outbreak of nephritis.

It is therefore useful to enquire whether the patient has any contacts at home or at work with a history of sore throat. Of interest, in Miss James' case, you may also enquire about the horses' health, because animals can pass on nephritogenic strains of streptococcus, for example *Streptococcus equi*. In horses, streptococcal infections are evidenced by 'strangles' (cervical lymphadenopathy) and laminitis.

Final note

Nephritic syndrome was first described in 1827 by English physician Richard Bright. He delineated a patient with oedema (termed 'dropsy' at that time) and appreciated that the symptom was linked to a renal problem, as evidenced by the presence of a reduced quantity of dark, smoky or blood-stained urine. He also demonstrated the presence of large amounts of protein in the urine of such patients by heating it, causing the protein to denature and precipitate in the tube. Nephritic syndrome is therefore sometimes referred to as Bright's disease.

CASE REVIEW

A 20-year-old woman presents with facial swelling and reduced production of abnormally dark urine. She has a history of a severe pharyngitis 3 weeks prior to presentation. She is hypertensive and oedematous and investigations show acute renal failure and blood and protein on dipstick. This presentation shows all the features of a nephritic syndrome. A renal biopsy is performed, which shows appearance typical of post-infectious GN, with diffuse, proliferative changes and deposition of antibody and complement. Her blood pressure and proteinuria are treated with ACEI and her renal function improves over the next few weeks.

KEY POINTS

- Nephritic syndrome is characterised by oliguria due to ARF, micro/macroscopic haematuria, hypertension, proteinuria (1–3.5 g/24 h) and oedema. Urine is typically described as smoky or coke-coloured
- Causes of nephritic syndrome include primary and secondary GN and TIN.
- Secondary GNs presenting with nephritic syndrome include post-infectious GN and lupus nephritis.
- General treatment measures include blood pressure control and inhibition of proteinuria with ACEI. Oedema can be treated with loop diuretics

- The outcome of nephritic syndrome depends on the underlying cause, which should be determined with a renal biopsy
- In post-infectious GN, there is a diffuse, proliferative GN involving the endothelium and mesangium with antibody and complement deposition on immunostaining
- Post-infectious GN usually resolves spontaneously, provided the infection is treated. Some individuals require dialysis for a short period.

Case 5 A 68-year-old man with hearing loss, fatigue and arthralgia

Mr Geoffrey Williams is a 68-year-old man who attends the ENT clinic with increasing hearing difficulties. Mr Williams has a past history of hypertension but has otherwise been fit and well. There is no previous history of ear infections or injury. He is taking bedroflumethazide 2.5 mg for his blood pressure but no other medications. He has run an arable farm for all of his adult life, and does work with noisy machinery from time to time. There is no family history of deafness. His current hearing difficulties started around 5 months ago. They affect both ears but the hearing in his left ear in particular is now very poor with associated discomfort and a feeling of fullness on that side. He has also had night sweats and has noticed some nasal crusting and three episodes of epistaxis in the last 3 weeks. Mr Williams feels lacking in energy and described himself as 'a clapped-out old crock'. In particular, he has noted aches in the muscles of his arms and legs, as well as painful joints.

What are the main differential diagnoses for hearing loss?

Deafness may be conductive (impairment of transmission of sound through the external canal and middle ear to the foot of the stapes, e.g. due to wax, otitis externa, otosclerosis, otitis media) or sensorineural (defects central to oval window of cochlea (sensory) or of cochlear nerve or central connections (neural)).

Given the relatively rapid onset (over months) and the local symptoms of pain and fullness in the left ear, as well as symptoms of nasal crusting, this suggests a conductive cause with pathology in the middle ear.

Mr Williams also gives a history of systemic symptoms including fatigue, lethargy, myalgia and arthralgia which suggest that his problem may not be localised to his ears. The presence of such symptoms should prompt a hunt for systemic infection, inflammation and malignancy.

Nephrology: Clinical Cases Uncovered. By M. Clatworthy.
Published 2010 by Blackwell Publishing.

What features would you seek during clinical examination?

In terms of his hearing loss, the first issue is to confirm that the deafness is indeed conductive. Examine the ear by eye and with an otoscope, assess the external acoustic canal and ear drum. A 512 Hz tuning fork can be used to perform Rinne's test, comparing air conduction with bone conduction. If bone conduction > air conduction, there is conductive hearing loss.

In view of Mr Williams' more widespread symptoms, a careful systemic examination is important.

- *Temperature:* fever can occur in infection, systemic inflammatory disease or malignancy (particularly lymphoma).
- *Weight:* provides a baseline, and may confirm any weight loss objectively.
- *Hands and eyes:* for clinical evidence of anaemia (pallor of skin creases or conjunctiva) which may be associated with chronic infectious or inflammatory disease.
- *Hands/feet/nails:* for splinter haemorrhages, nailfold infarcts, necrotic areas (signs of vasculitis/endocarditis). Leuconychia or Beau's lines (associated with hypoalbuminaemia which may occur with any chronic inflammatory/infectious/autoimmune disease).
- *Rashes:* there are a number of rashes associated with malignancy (e.g. acanthosis nigricans or erythema gyratum repens). Purpuric lesions may indicate vasculitis.
- *Nose:* given the symptoms of epistaxis, it is important to look for nasal crusting or collapse of nasal bridge which may be associated with vasculitis.
- *Facial sinuses:* tenderness can be a feature of vasculitis.
- *Eyes:* red eyes (anterior uveitis) which may be associated with some systemic autoimmune diseases.
- *CVS:* assess intravascular volume status, BP and heart sounds (a new murmur may indicate endocarditis).

• *Chest:* pulmonary malignancy may be associated with a pleural effusion (stony dull percussion note with absent breath sounds). A number of systemic autoimmune diseases (e.g. rheumatoid arthritis and systemic sclerosis) are associated with pulmonary fibrosis (fine inspiratory crepitations).

• *Abdomen:* hepatosplenomegaly may be present in autoimmunity, infection and haematological malignancy. Other abdominal masses should also be sought.

> *Mr Williams' external acoustic canals look normal but there is a fluid level behind his left ear drum which looks bulging and inflamed. Rinne's test confirms conductive deafness on the left. He is febrile with a temperature of 38 °C. He has two splinter haemorrhages in his right hand and one in his left hand but no obvious rashes. He has pale conjunctivae and there is some marked nasal crusting but peripheral examination is otherwise normal. The pulse is 90 bpm and regular. Blood pressure is 150/95 mmHg and there are no audible murmurs. Oxygen saturations are 92% on air, and his respiratory rate 16 rpm. There are some crepitations in both bases. Abdominal examination is unremarkable.*

What blood tests would you request?

• Full blood count: he is clinically anaemic and this should be formally confirmed. In addition, he is febrile and an elevation of both WBC and platelets may occur in infection and inflammation
• Renal function
• LFT
• Albumin — often low if chronic infection/inflammation
• Inflammatory markers (CRP/ESR)
• Blood cultures

> *Investigations show:*
> *Hb 7.5 g/dL, MCV 82, WBC 14.2 × 10⁹/L, Platelets 594 × 10⁹/L*
> *U+E: Na 145 mmol/L, K 3.4 mmol/L, Urea 19.3 mmol/L, Creatinine 346 μmol/L*
> *ESR 118 mm/h, CRP 86 mg/L, LFT, glucose: normal*
> *Albumin 24 g/L*

How would you interpret these results?

The investigations show that the patient is anaemic (normocytic), has significant renal impairment (which may be acute or chronic) and has evidence of systemic inflammation with a grossly elevated ESR.

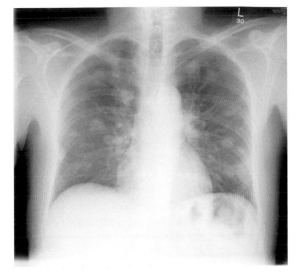

Figure 5.1 Chest radiograph demonstrating multiple opacities in both lung fields. The differential diagnosis for such an appearance includes malignancy (primary or secondary, so-called 'cannon-ball' pulmonary metastases), infection (abscesses/TB/fungal), inflammatory nodules (e.g. vasculitis/rheumatoid arthritis).

> *Mr Williams is referred urgently to the renal physicians who arrange his immediate admission for further investigations and management of his renal impairment.*
> *Further investigations show:*
> *Urine dipstick : blood ++++ protein +++ leucocytes+ negative for nitrites and glucose.*
> *Urine microscopy: red cell casts.*
> *Strongly positive ANCA, specifically a cytoplasmic (c)ANCA, with an anti-proteinase 3 (PR3) titre on ELISA of 130. All other immunological tests are normal.*
> *CXR demonstrates a normal cardiac size and a number of diffuse shadows in both lung fields (Figure 5.1)*
> *ABG: pO₂ 8.8 kPa, pCO₂ 4.5 kPa*
> *A US scan shows a left kidney of 11 cm and a right of 11.6 cm with normal cortical thickness and no hydronephrosis.*

> *The patient undergoes an US-guided renal biopsy which shows a focal necrotising, crescentic GN (Figure 5.2). The immunostaining does not show any antibody or complement deposition, i.e. this is a pauci-immune GN.*

What general treatment measures should you begin?

• The patient is hypoxic and should therefore be placed on supplemental oxygen.

• He has renal failure and therefore his fluid balance should be carefully managed to ensure that he is well hydrated. Daily weights will be helpful for this aspect of his management. His renal function should also be monitored on a daily basis.

• He is also significantly anaemic and will probably need to be transfused.

What is the most likely diagnosis?

The kidneys are of normal size and cortical thickness on US, suggesting that Mr Williams does not have chronic renal damage. The renal biopsy shows a crescentic GN which may be due to a primary GN (idiopathic pauci-immune GN or IgA nephropathy) but more commonly occurs secondary to small vessel vasculitis, Goodpasture's disease or SLE.

Immunostaining (which tests for the presence of immunoglobulin or complement deposition within the

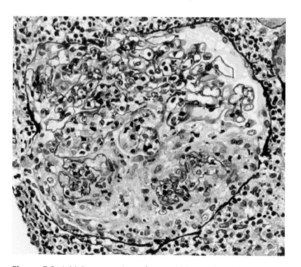

Figure 5.2 A high-power view of a renal biopsy showing a crescentic glomerulonephritis. The cellular crescent occupies the lower part of the glomerulus (silver stain).

glomerulus) is extremely helpful in distinguishing between these diagnoses (Figure 5.3). Pauci-immune staining (no IgG/M/A, no complement) occurs in small vessel vasculitis, linear IgG staining in Goodpasture's disease, strong IgA staining in crescentic IgA nephropathy and full-house staining (positive for IgG/M/A, C1q, C3, C4) in SLE.

In this particular case, immunostaining is negative, making this a pauci-immune, crescentic GN. The underlying diagnosis of a small vessel vasculitis is confirmed by the presence of an ANCA antibody. ANCA are classified into cANCA (c = cytoplasmic) and pANCA (p = perinuclear) according to the pattern of staining observed when the patient's serum is added to neutrophils (Figure 5.4). The precise antigens to which these antibodies bind have been determined: cANCA bind to proteinase 3 (PR3), pANCA bind to myeloperoxidase (MPO). Both are enzymes found within the azurophilic granules of neutrophils. cANCA are classically associated with the clinical syndrome that is Wegener's granulomatosis (WG). pANCA is associated with microscopic polyangiitis. More recently, a further subclass of ANCA has been identified which specifically recognises LAMP-2. This antibody appears to show some cross-reactivity with FimA, a bacterial protein.

Some patients with ANCA-associated vasculitis (AAV) also have pulmonary involvement (particularly those who are cANCA positive, as in this case). This includes pulmonary nodules (which can look like lung tumours), fibrosis and pulmonary haemorrhage. It is important to identify haemorrhage (using CT scan or assessment of gas transfer factor (KCO) on pulmonary function testing) because this should be treated with plasma exchange. One rarer pulmonary involvement is tracheal or bronchial stenosis. Affected patients develop stridor and require repeated bronchoscopy and mechanical stretching of the narrowing.

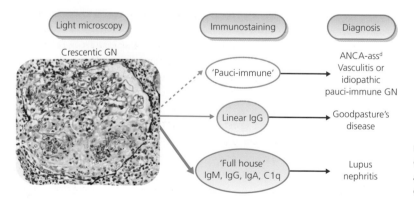

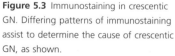

Figure 5.3 Immunostaining in crescentic GN. Differing patterns of immunostaining assist to determine the cause of crescentic GN, as shown.

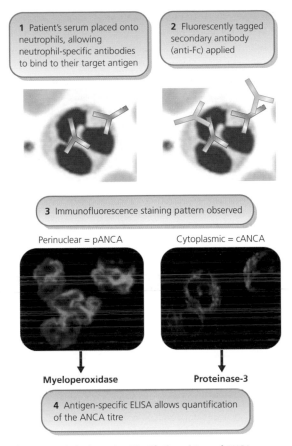

1 Patient's serum placed onto neutrophils, allowing neutrophil-specific antibodies to bind to their target antigen

2 Fluorescently tagged secondary antibody (anti-Fc) applied

3 Immunofluorescence staining pattern observed

Perinuclear = pANCA   Cytoplasmic = cANCA

Myeloperoxidase   Proteinase-3

4 Antigen-specific ELISA allows quantification of the ANCA titre

Figure 5.4 Methods used to identify the subtype of ANCA.

What is vasculitis?

Vasculitis involves inflammation of blood vessels. Vasculitides are classified according to the size of the vessel involved (Table 5.1, Figure 5.5). Clinically, the vasculitic syndromes can have overlapping clinical features, making a precise diagnosis uncertain.

Historically, prior to the identification of ANCA, the small vessel vasculitides were differentially classified according to their clinical presentation. Patients with Wegener's granulomatosis typically have a triad of:
• renal impairment
• upper respiratory tract involvement (sinusitis, nasal crusting, epistaxis, deafness)
• lower respiratory tract involvement (nodules, fibrosis, haemorrhage).
Although clinicians still use the terms Wegener's granulomatosis or microscopic polyangiitis, in general, the small vessel ANCA-associated vasculitides are now grouped together, because their treatment is identical.

The patient's clinical presentation may not include all the classic symptoms outlined in Table 5.1. It is therefore extremely important look for a positive ANCA and to perform a biopsy (often renal or nasal) to confirm the diagnosis of vasculitis. ANCA may be negative in 10–15% of patients with small vessel vasculitis, emphasising the importance of biopsy and history/examination.

Given the diagnosis of an ANCA-associated vasculitis, how would you treat this patient?

Patients with AAV have different degrees of disease severity, ranging from ENT-limited disease through to life-threatening pulmonary haemorrhage and renal failure. The overall treatment is with immunosupressive agents, but the agent, dose and duration depend on disease severity. Mr Williams has severe organ-threatening disease and should therefore receive immunosuppression with corticosteroids and cyclophosphamide. A typical regimen consists of oral steroids (prednisolone 1 mg/kg/day, maximum 60–80mg, tapering to 15 mg od by 3 months, reducing more slowly thereafter) along with oral or intravenous cyclophosphamide. Patients who present with a creatinine of >500 μmol/L or with pulmonary haemorrhage should also receive plasma exchange. At 3 months, the patient should be switched from cyclophosphamide to a less toxic immunosuppressant such as azathioprine or mycophenolate mofetil. Maintenance therapy should be continued for a minimum of 12–18 months after a stable remission has been achieved in order to reduce the risk of relapse.

Immunosuppressive treatments are associated with significant side-effects, particularly cytopaenias and an increased susceptibility to infections. Cyclophosphamide is associated with haemorrhagic cystitis and subsequent increased risk of bladder cancer. Patients are also at increased risk of myeloproliferative disorders later in life and are at risk of infertility (especially with higher cumulative doses of cyclophosphamide). Corticosteroids are associated with osteoporosis, hypertension, glucose intolerance/diabetes mellitus, gastric ulceration, dyslipidaemia, central obesity, thinning of the skin and easy bruising. According to guidelines published by the Royal College of Physicians, in view of his age (>65 years) and his commitment to oral glucocorticoid therapy for a period of greater than 3 months, Mr Williams should commence bone-protective therapy at the time of starting steroids.

More recently, newer treatments for patients with recurrent relapses or resistant disease have been devel-

Table 5.1 Classification of vasculitides

Vessel size	Vasculitis	Clinical features	Investigations
Small	Wegener's granulomatosis	Upper respiratory tract (sinusitis, nasal crusting), Lower respiratory tract (nodules, fibrosis, haemorrhage), renal failure	Elevated ESR, CRP, cANCA Biopsy shows small vessel vasculitis with granulomata
	Microscopic polyangiitis	Vasculitis skin rashes, joint pains, renal failure	Elevated ESR, CRP, classically pANCA (20% cANCA) Histology: arteriolitis
	Churg–Strauss syndrome	Asthma, polyneuropathy, GI involvement, e.g. eosinophilic gastritis	Elevated ESR, CRP, eosinophilia, p or cANCA Histology: eosinophilic vasculitis
Medium	Polyarteritis nodosa	Non-specific symptoms such as malaise, fevers, sweats, weight loss, abdominal pain	Mesenteric angiography demonstrating splenic/renal microaneurysms
Large	Takayasu's arteritis	Often asymptomatic Affects large arteries from heart (e.g. subclavian) Typically affects young women. More common in Far East	MRA or angiography demonstrating large vessel stenosis
	Giant cell arteritis (temporal arteritis)	Headaches, tender scalp, visual disturbance+/– stiffness in shoulders or neck. Age >60 years	Elevated ESR Temporal artery biopsy

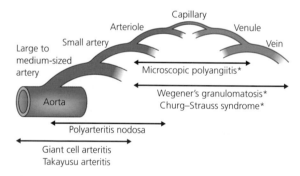

Figure 5.5 Classification of vasculitis. * ANCA associated.

oped. These include the B cell-depleting agent rituximab and the TNF-α neutralising monoclonal antibody inflix-imab. Rituximab is a chimaeric monoclonal anti-CD20 antibody, originally developed as a treatment for B cell lymphomas. CD20 is found on the surface of B cells but not plasma cells, so serum IgG levels tend to remain normal in spite of B cell depletion. Rituximab seems to be useful in the treatment of a number of autoimmune diseases including vasculitis, rheumatoid arthritis, multiple sclerosis and SLE.

The patient asks if the disease is curable. What advice do you give him?

Although most patients will respond to treatment with steroids and cyclophosphamide (90% will achieve remission by 6 months), AAV is a relapsing and remitting disease. Fifty to 60% of patients will have a disease relapse at some stage (more common in Wegener's granulomatosis (60–70% of patients) than in microscopic polyangiitis (30%)).

Most outcome studies now report a 5-year survival rate in AAV of approximately 70%. Untreated, the disease has a mortality rate of 80–90% in the first year, so although immunosuppressant treatments have many side-effects, the risk–benefit balance is in favour of treatment.

Factors associated with a worse outcome include:
- older age
- sepsis
- pulmonary haemorrhage
- creatinine >200 μmol/L at presentation
- presence of end-stage renal failure
- higher % of glomeruli with crescents/prominent interstitial fibrosis/prominent glomerulosclerosis on renal biopsy.

Irreversible dialysis-dependent renal failure essentially halves the 5-year survival rate to 35%. Between 55% and 90% of patients requiring dialysis during the acute phase of disease will become dialysis independent, with between 40% and 70% remaining dialysis independent at 3 years. About 25% of patients with WG eventually reach ESRF.

> *Mr Williams is initially treated with three pulses of intravenous methylprednisolone followed by a pulse of intravenous cyclophosphamide. He is then maintained on oral corticosteroids with further pulses of cyclophosphamide over the next 6 months. His systemic symptoms and renal function improve and his ANCA titres fall. He is switched from cyclophosphamide to azathioprine and remains in remission over the next 6 months.*

What do you know about the aetiopathogenesis of ANCA-associated vasculitis?

The frequency is more common amongst certain occupations (farmers: relative risk (RR) 2.3, livestock: RR 2.9,

silica: RR 3.0), implying that environmental factors may play some role in disease pathogenesis.

There is some evidence that infections may be involved in disease pathogenesis; nasal carriage of *Staphylococcus aureus is* present in 65% of patients with WG versus 20% of controls. Furthermore, in patients with WG, nasal carriage of *Staph. aureus* is strongly associated with disease relapse. The relevance of this observation has been clarified by investigators who have shown that in the presence of TNF-α (which is a cytokine released during infections), PR3 and MPO are translocated to the surface of neutrophils and thus become visible to the immune system. ANCA may then bind to these surface-exposed antigens and cause disease by inducing degranulation of primed neutrophils adherent to, or transmigrating through, the vascular endothelium damaging vessels.

The identification of ANCA which specifically recognises LAMP-2 and which cross-reacts with FimA (a bacterial protein), has led to the suggestion that ANCA may develop due to molecular mimicry. That is, an immune response is mounted against a pathogen which antigenically mimics self-antigen.

CASE REVIEW

A 68-year-old man presents with hearing loss, arthralgia and fatigue. On examination, he was febrile, and had splinter haemorrhages and some crepitations in the lungs. Investigations demonstrated acute renal failure and elevated inflammatory markers. He was cANCA positive with an elevated PR3 antibody titre. Renal biopsy showed a pauci-immune necrotising crescentic GN in keeping with a diagnosis of ANCA-associated vasculitis. He is treated with intravenous corticosteroids and cyclophosphamide.

KEY POINTS

- Vasculitis (inflammation of the blood vessels) can present with a wide variety of systemic symptoms, which are often non-specific. The diagnosis can therefore be difficult and delayed.
- Three different types of small vessel vasculitis have been distinguished, according to their clinical presentation:
  - Wegener's granulomatosis
  - microscopic polyangiitis
  - Churg–Strauss syndrome.
- These small vessel vasculitides are frequently associated with the presence of an autoantibody, antineutrophil cytoplasmic antibody (ANCA), and are therefore grouped together as ANCA-associated vasculitis (AAV).
- AAV occurs in around 20 per million population in the UK. This rate appears to be increasing, although this may

reflect an increased awareness of the diagnosis and an increased availability of one of the diagnostic tests (ANCA). The frequency of AAV increases with increasing age (120 pmp in >65-year age group) and is more common amongst certain occupations such as farmers and those dealing with livestock.

- Treatment depends on severity of disease but severe, organ-threatening disease requires the use of high-dose corticosteroids and cyclophosphamide for the first 3 months followed by azathioprine or mycophenolate mofetil.
- AAV previously had an extremely poor prognosis; untreated, the 1-year mortality rate was between 80% and 90%. With current treatment, the overall 5-year survival rate in AAV is now approximately 70%.

Case 6   A 19-year-old man with macroscopic haematuria

Gary Thomas is 19-year-old man who is referred to the renal services following an episode of macroscopic haematuria.

What questions would you ask the patient?

• Confirm the nature of the haematuria: bright red blood or smoky, 'coke-coloured' urine?
• Duration: when did he first notice blood in his urine?
• Associated symptoms: loin pain, bladder pain, dysuria.
• Any history of previous similar episodes?
• Other systemic symptoms, e.g. fever, rigors, joint pain, red eyes?
• Any history of recent illness, particularly infections?
• Family history of renal disease or renal stones?
• Drug history, including recreational drugs.
• Smoking history and particularly occupational history.

Gary is normally fit and healthy and is an apprentice at the local football club. He has been unwell for the last week with a severe sore throat. He initially attended his family doctor 4 days ago and was started on penicillin but subsequently noticed bright red blood in his urine. He has also had some mild discomfort in both flanks, but no dysuria or frequency. His past medical history includes one episode of right loin pain and macroscopic haematuria at the age of 15 years, which was treated as a urinary tract infection. There was no family history of renal disease and he had taken no medications (including recreational drugs).

What are the main differential diagnoses for macroscopic haematuria?

Haematuria is divided into *macroscopic* (where the urine is obviously discoloured) and *microscopic* (where the blood is found only on dipstick or microscopy examination).

The most common causes of macroscopic haematuria are summarised in Figure 6.1. A full differential for haematuria is as follows (going from proximal to distal in the renal tract).

Renal
Tumours
• *Malignant:* renal cell carcinoma (most common renal tumour) or transitional cell carcinoma.
• *Benign:* angiomyolipoma (hamartomatous lesion, which can grow to great size and be associated with major haemorrhage).

Stones
Stones form within the collecting system. They may cause infection or, if they become large, obstruct the flow of urine. Stones can cause haematuria both during infections and by directly irritating the mucosa.

Infection
Pyelonephritis results from bacteria ascending from the bladder (vesicoureteric reflux). Painless haematuria may occur, but patients will usually also experience loin pain, fever, dysuria and urinary frequency.

Inflammation
• *Glomerulonephritis (GN):* nephritic GN tends to present with microscopic haematuria without renal pain. Macroscopic haematuria is classically associated with two particular forms of GN: IgA nephropathy and postinfectious GN. Very rarely, thin basement membrane disease can present in this way (although this usually presents with asymptomatic microscopic haematuria) and any nephritic GN can present with macroscopic haematuria. The presence of glomerular haematuria is confirmed by the presence of red cell casts on urine microscopy. Urine may look smoky or coke-coloured.
• *Interstitial nephritis:* inflammation affecting the interstitium and sparing the glomeruli. Frequently caused by drugs (more commonly presents with microscopic rather than macroscopic haematuria).

Nephrology: Clinical Cases Uncovered. By M. Clatworthy.
Published 2010 by Blackwell Publishing.

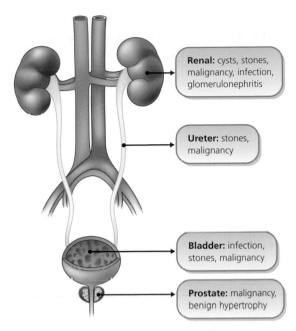

Figure 6.1 Most common causes of macroscopic haematuria.

Cystic disease

A number of genetic diseases (classically autosomal dominant polycystic kidney disease (ADPKD)) can lead to renal cysts which can become very large. Patients can then bleed into the cysts, causing pain and haematuria.

Trauma

This may either occur in the context of external trauma, e.g. post-RTA, or following a renal biopsy. About one in five patients will have haematuria post biopsy.

Vascular

Vasculitis can be associated with haematuria, usually microscopic and with red cell casts in the urine. Arteriovenous malformations can also present with haematuria.

Ureter

• *Stones:* nearly always present with pain which may be severe.
• Malignancy.

Bladder
Infection

Infection-related cystitis is usually associated with pain, dysuria, frequency, and in men is commonly associated with bladder outflow obstruction. Schistosomiasis is a common cause worldwide.

Inflammation

A number of drugs can cause haemorrhagic cystitis, for example cyclophosphamide.

Bladder tumours

These tend to present with painless haematuria. Nearly all are transitional cell cancers, with smoking and aromatic hydrocarbon exposure being risk factors.

Prostate

• Tumours.
• Benign prostatic hyperplasia: can cause haematuria, usually painless.

Spurious

• Eating beetroot.
• Rifampicin treatment.

Non-pathogenic

• Post bladder catheterisation: a trace of blood in the urine is extremely common post catheterisation
• Menstruation

In a young man with macroscopic haematuria, prostatic problems and malignancy are less likely. Infection, stones, cystic disease and glomerular haematuria move to the top of the differential diagnostic list. Gary has had no symptoms typical of pyelonephritis, and his pain is bilateral (therefore unlikely to be stone related). These features do not exclude the diagnoses of infection or stones, but make the clinician alert to the possibility of a GN or polycystic kidney disease. Although he has no positive family history, ADPKD can arise from a new mutation. The patient gives a history of pharyngitis, which can be associated with a post-infectious GN, if caused by a nephritogenic strain of β-haemolytic streptococcus, or with a flare of IgA nephropathy.

What features are important to seek during clinical examination?

Given the patient has had haematuria, you should first assess whether he is haemodynamically stable. The history he gives isn't one of a massive bleed, but any patient who presents with a story of blood loss should be assessed to ensure they are not intravascularly volume depleted, i.e. look for the presence of tachycardia, hypotension (particularly the presence of a postural drop), and whether the patient is peripherally shut down (feel his hands – are they cold and clammy or well perfused?).

Following this assessment, provided the patient is haemodynamically stable or once you have made him stable with fluid resuscitation, important points in the examination include a search for systemic diseases or infections which can lead to glomerular haematuria, (e.g. vasculitis, SLE or pharyngitis, endocarditis, cellulitis).

General

• *Temperature?* Fever can occur in infection or systemic inflammatory disease.
• *Lymph nodes?* Particularly cervical given history of pharyngitis.

Peripheries

• Hands and eyes for clinical evidence of anaemia (pallor of skin creases or conjunctiva).
• Hands/feet/nails for splinter haemorrhages, nailfold infarcts, necrotic areas (signs of vasculitis/endocarditis). Leuconychia or Beau's lines (associated with hypoalbuminaemia which may occur with any chronic inflammatory/autoimmune disease).
• Rashes: particularly purpuric lesions which may be associated with vasculitis, or photosensitivity rashes associated with SLE.
• Other peripheral signs of endocarditis including Osler's nodes (painful erythematous nodules, often in the finger pulps), Janeway lesions (flat, non-tender, erythematous patches, typically on the thenar or hypothenar eminences), Roth spots (focal retinal infarcts). All of these lesions occur because small emboli break off the friable vegetation, circulate around the body and become lodged in the capillaries supplying the skin, retina, etc.

Face

• Inspect the throat in order to confirm pharyngitis and assess its extent. Swabs could be taken for culture at this time. Mouth ulcers are associated with SLE.
• *Nose:* is there collapse of nasal bridge or nasal crusting (associated with vasculitis)?
• *Facial sinuses* (tenderness, can be a feature of vasculitis).
• *Eyes:* red eyes (anterior uveitis) which may be associated with vasculitis.

Cardiovascular system

Intravascular volume status has been assessed above. Heart sound abnormalities and added sounds may indicate endocarditis. Valvular heart disease (typically mitral valve prolapse) also occurs in ADPKD.

Respiratory system

Full examination for signs of infection or fibrosis (the latter can occur in systemic vasculitis).

Abdomen

Organomegaly or masses? Particularly splenomegaly (associated with endocarditis and SLE) or renal enlargement, which may occur if there is polycystic kidney disease or a renal tumour. Large renal AVM may be associated with a bruit.

Gary is febrile with a temperature of 38 °C and is peripherally well perfused. Examination of his throat shows a purulent tonsillitis. His right jugulodiagstric lymph node is enlarged and tender. Peripherally he has no rashes or signs to suggest endocarditis, vasculitis or SLE. His pulse is 62 bpm and regular, and blood pressure is elevated at 150/80 mmHg, with no postural drop. Cardiovascular examination is otherwise normal, with no murmurs. His chest is clear and his abdomen soft, with mild tenderness in both flanks but no masses or renal bruits.

What initial investigations would you request?
Blood tests

• Full blood count
• Clotting tests (occasionally haematuria can occur in a structurally normal urinary tract, if the clotting function is abnormal. This typically occurs in a patient who is anticoagulated with warfarin)
• Renal function
• LFT, including albumin
• Glucose (diabetes is a rare cause of papillary necrosis which can present with microscopic haematuria)
• Calcium and phosphate (many renal stones contain calcium, so you need to ensure that serum calcium and phosphate are normal)
• Inflammatory markers: CRP (raised in infection)

Microbiological tests

Given that he has a fever and an obvious tonsillitis, he should have blood cultures, a throat swab, an ASO titre measured (associated with streptococcal infections), and an MSU sent for culture.

Urine dipstick

To confirm haematuria and provide other clues as to the underlying cause. For example, in a urinary tract infection the dipstick will often be nitrite or leucocyte positive.

In patients with GN, there may be proteinuria as well as haematuria.

Urine microscopy
Specifically looking for red cell casts indicative of glomerular pathology as well as white cells and bacteria (UTI) or crystals (stone disease).

ECG
Useful investigation in any patient with possible renal disease, e.g. may show signs of hyperkalaemia if the patient has acute renal failure.

CXR
To ensure no obvious signs of infection. Again, a useful baseline investigation in a patient who is unwell.

Initial investigations show:

Hb 12.9g/dL, WBC 16.4 × 10⁹/L (neutrophils), Platelets 500 × 10⁹/L

Clotting – normal

U+E: Na 139mmol/L, K 3.8mmol/L, Urea 14.4mmol/L, Creatinine 266µmol/L

CRP 235mg/L

LFT, albumin, glucose, calcium, phosphate: normal

Blood, urine, and throat cultures awaited. ASO titre is within normal limits

Urine dipstick shows protein++, blood++++ negative for leucocytes, nitrites, and glucose

Urine microscopy: red cell casts, white cells, bacteria, crystals not seen

ECG and CXR are normal

How would you interpret these results and how would they help in refining your differential diagnosis?
The investigations show a neutrophil leucocytosis and an elevated CRP, consistent with current infection (probably his tonsillitis). He also has significant renal impairment. For a man of his age, a creatinine of 266µmol/L would give him an eGFR of 28mL/min/1.73m², corresponding to stage 4 CKD. We do not know if this is acute or chronic, given that he has never had his renal function formally assessed previously. In favour of this being acute is his young age and good health prior to this episode. However, the previous history of a similar episode at the age of 15 raises the possibility of a chronic process. In terms of his urine dipstick, the absence of nitrites and

leucocytes in his urine makes a UTI unlikely. The presence of blood and protein in the urine favours a glomerular pathology, renal cystic disease or stones. The absence of red cell casts in the urine does not rule out glomerular inflammation as this investigation is very much dependent on the skill of the technician and is frequently negative in the presence of florid glomerulonephritis. The concurrent pharyngitis and history of a similar episode previously make IgA nephropathy the most likely diagnosis. Stones and cystic disease remain a possibility although the bilateral pain and abnormal renal function make the former unlikely (this would mean the patient would have bilateral stones which are either acutely obstructing the kidneys or have previously obstructed the kidneys or caused UTI, leading to chronic damage).

What further specialist investigation would you undertake?
Given his history of haematuria and loin pain, and the significant renal impairment present, the patient should have a US scan of his renal tract to assess the size of the kidneys and if there is obstruction or any structural abnormalities such as cystic disease. Unless the US scan identifies any obvious non-glomerular cause for his haematuria, he should proceed to a renal biopsy in order to ascertain the cause of his renal impairment and the degree of chronicity.

A renal autoimmune screen should also be performed, including ANA, ANCA, complement (C3/C4), immunoglobulins, anti-GBM antibodies, rheumatoid factor, cryoglobulins, C3 nephritic factor.

He has 2+proteinuria on dipstick which should be quantified.

A US scan shows a right kidney of 12cm and a left kidney of 12.5cm, with normal cortical thickness and no hydronephrosis. A US-guided renal biopsy is performed which on initial H+E shows a crescentic GN (Figure 6.2) with 63% of glomeruli containing crescents. There is also significant ATN. Immunostaining is positive for IgA and C3 (Figure 6.3).

The autoimmune screen is negative, except that he has a polyclonal increase in IgA. Twenty-four hour urine collection contains 2.9g of protein. His renal function has also declined further, with a creatinine of 342µmol/L.

How would you interpret these results?
The kidneys are of normal size and cortical thickness on US, suggesting that he does not have chronic renal

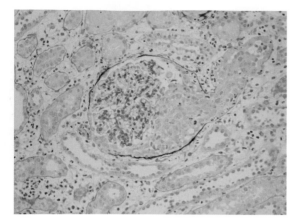

Figure 6.2 Silver stain ×40 showing a glomerulus with a crescent occupying the right half.

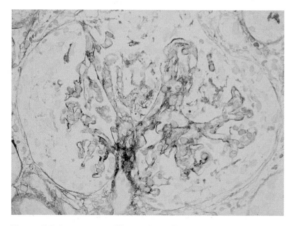

Figure 6.3 Immunoperoxidase staining for IgA shows mainly mesangial positivity.

damage. The biopsy shows a crescentic GN which may be due to a primary GN (idiopathic crescentic GN or IgA nephropathy), but more commonly occurs secondary to small vessel vasculitis, Goodpasture's disease or SLE. The immunostaining is extremely helpful in distinguishing between these diagnoses since pauci-immune staining (no IgG/M/A, no complement) occurs in small vessel vasculitis, linear IgG staining in Goodpasture's disease, strong IgA staining in crescentic IgA nephropathy and full-house staining (positive for IgG/M/A, C1q, C3, C4) in SLE. In this particular case, immunostaining shows IgA deposition, making this a case of crescentic IgA nephropathy. Around 35–50% of patients with IgA nephropathy have a polyclonal elevation of serum IgA (as seen in this case).

Given the result of the biopsy and additional blood tests, how would you treat this patient?

The investigations are consistent with a diagnosis of crescentic IgA nephropathy. He has significant impairment of renal function which has further declined during the admission. Treatments in IgA nephropathy may be divided into those aimed specifically at the disease process and those used to treat associated complications such as proteinuria and hypertension. In terms of the latter, agents such as ACEI and ARB, alone or in combination, can reduce urinary protein excretion and slow the decline in renal function, particularly in those patients with hypertension and IgA nephropathy.

Treatment of IgA nephropathy is controversial and there is a lack of randomised controlled trials to guide clinicians. However, in a patient with acute crescentic IgA nephropathy and declining renal function, most nephrologists agree that a trial of immunosuppressive treatment is warranted. Typically this would be with corticosteroids and cyclophosphamide, although azathioprine and mycophenoate mofetil have also been used. In some patients, recurrent episodes of bacterial tonsillitis precipitate frequent flares of disease. In such individuals tonsillectomy may not only protect from episodic haematuria, but may also have longer term renoprotective effects.

The patient asks you whether his kidney function will continue to deteriorate, requiring dialysis. What advice would you give him?

Acute renal failure, such as that seen in our patient, is a presentation of IgA nephropathy occurring in <5% of cases. In this subgroup of patients, renal biopsy generally demonstrates cellular crescents. A number of studies suggest that patients with crescentic IgA nephropathy tend to present with more severe hypertension, proteinuria and renal impairment.

Prognosis in IgA nephropathy is very variable. However, overall it is estimated that 20–40% of patients with IgA nephropathy progress to ESRF over 10–20 years. Poor prognostic features include heavy proteinuria, renal impairment, hypertension and increasing age. A number of studies suggest that crescentic IgA nephropathy carries a relatively worse prognosis, with some series suggesting that up to 75% of patients had reached ESRF at 10 years. Flares of disease can be precipitated by a number of factors including infections (typically tonsillitis, but also gastroenteritis and pneumonia), vaccinations and exercise.

The patient was treated with three daily 1 g pulses of intravenous methylprednisone followed by a reducing dose of oral prednisolone (40 mg/day initially) and mycophenolate mofetil (MMF) (1 g twice daily) and was commenced on ramipril (5 mg/day) for hypertension and proteinuria. His renal function and urine dipstick abnormalities rapidly normalised over the next few weeks. He remains well on maintenance MMF and has been weaned off oral corticosteroids.

What do you know about the pathogenesis of IgA nephropathy?

The cause of IgA nephropathy is unknown but individuals are likely to possess a number of susceptibility genes and then develop disease following an encounter with specific environmental stimuli. Central to the pathogenesis of IgA nephropathy is thought to be the deposition of IgA within the mesangium. IgA is one of the subclasses of immunoglobulins (antibodies) synthesised in humans, each of which can be distinguished by differences in their heavy chains. It is the most abundant class of immunoglobulin (66 mg/kg body weight versus 34 mg/kg of IgG) and is predominantly found at mucosal surfaces and in secretions, such as saliva and mucus. The pathogenic mechanisms involved in IgA nephropathy are unclear but are thought to involve the production of IgA1 with reduced glycosylation in its hinge region leading to an increased propensity to self-aggregation and aggregation with IgG. Thus if IgA1 aggregates become deposited in the kidney and are not adequately cleared, they may elicit an abnormal inflammatory response in mesangial cells and activate complement.

CASE REVIEW

A 19-year-old man presents with an episode of macroscopic haematuria which was preceded by an episode of tonsillitis. On examination, he was hypertensive and investigations showed blood and protein on urine dipstick as well as significant renal impairment. A renal biopsy was undertaken and demonstrated crescentic IgA nephropathy. He was treated with an ACEI, corticosteroids and mycophenolate mofetil and his renal function significantly improved over the next few months.

KEY POINTS

- IgA nephropathy is one of the most common forms of primary GN. Since the diagnosis can only be made by demonstrating IgA deposition in the glomerular mesangium, its precise prevalence is unknown and estimates vary according to the frequency of renal biopsy. In Europe, IgA nephropathy makes up 15–30% of all primary GN. The prevalence is much higher in Japan where IgA nephropathy is diagnosed in 40–50% of all renal biopsies.
- IgA nephropathy is more common in males and presentation typically occurs in the second and third decades of life.
- A temporal association of disease flare with pharyngitis or tonsillitis is well recognised in IgA nephropathy and generally occurs within days of the infection.
- The clinical presentation of IgA nephropathy is very variable, ranging from asymptomatic microscopic haematuria (30–40% of patients), nephrotic syndrome (<5%) and ARF (5%).

- Patients with IgA nephropathy should be treated with ACEI or ARB to control hypertension and proteinuria. In terms of disease-modifying drugs, many nephrologists would use immunosuppressants if there was a rapid decline in renal function (e.g. a combination of corticosteroids and another immunosuppressant).
- The prognosis of IgA nephropathy is variable. In 10–25% of patients presenting with microscopic haematuria only, there is spontaneous resolution of urine dipstick abnormalities. However, overall it is estimated that 20–40% of patients with IgA nephropathy progress to ESRF over 10–20 years.
- Poor prognostic features include heavy proteinuria, renal impairment, hypertension, increasing age and a crescentic GN on biopsy. The higher the proportion of glomeruli containing crescents, the worse the prognosis.

Case 7 A 27-year-old woman with a rash and renal impairment

Bethan Edwards is a 27-year-old accountant who attends her GP with fever, arthralgia and a rash. On examination, there is an erythematous, macular rash on her forearms. Some blood tests are performed, which show a creatinine of 194 μmol/L. She is therefore referred urgently to the renal services.

What aspects of the history are important to clarify?

Miss Edwards has significant renal impairment (creatinine 194 μmol/L = eGFR 29 mL/min/1.73 m^2). This may be acute or chronic. Some aspects of the history may be helpful in determining which is most likely, e.g. past medical history of diabetes, hypertension, recurrent UTI, renal disease or family history of renal disease such as APKD would be suggestive of CKD. It is also useful to ask if she has ever had her renal function checked prior to this. Previous documentation of normal renal function indicates that this is likely to be ARF.

What is the most likely cause of renal impairment? Causes of renal impairment are classified as pre-renal (e.g. hypotension/hypovolaemia), renal (e.g. GN) or postrenal (e.g. obstruction). If this is ARF, then pre-renal/ ATN is the most likely cause (is there any history suggestive of dehydration/hypotension such as severe diarrhoea and vomiting?). Postrenal causes of ARF are less common in young women (mostly due to prostate problems, therefore more common in older men). If there is nothing to suggest either of the above then think about renal causes. The initial referral from the GP states that she has had fever, arthralgia and a rash. These symptoms make a renal cause (e.g. a GN secondary to a systemic autoimmune disease or TIN) more likely. Further useful history includes the following.

- When did she become unwell? Any illness preceding this episode of swelling (particularly pharyngitis or other infection)?
- Systemic symptoms: precise onset and details of fever, rash, arthralgia plus additional history of night sweats, respiratory symptoms (haemoptysis/SOB), upper respiratory tract symptoms (nasal crusting discharge, sinusitis) or red eyes (anterior uveitis) which might suggest a systemic autoimmune or inflammatory disease such as SLE or vasculitis?
- Any new medications which might cause TIN?
- Any previous similar episodes or past medical history of autoimmune disease?

Miss Edwards has been unwell for around 2 months. Her problems began with symptoms of dyspepsia, which started after taking some ibuprofen for a knee sprain sustained whilst skiing. Initially she had self-medicated with Gaviscon and ranitidine (obtained from her local chemist), but her indigestion became so severe that around 1 month ago she attended her GP. She was prescribed a proton pump inhibitor (PPI; omeprazole), which relieved her symptoms within a few days. About a week later she noticed a faint red rash on her arms. Since then, she has felt increasingly unwell with daily fevers, arthralgia of the small joints of the hand and intermittent loin pain. There is no history of upper or lower respiratory tract symptoms. Her only other regular medication is the OCP, which she has been taking for 7 years. She has no past medical history or family history of renal or autoimmune disease.

On examination, her temperature is 37.4 °C. There is an erythematous, macular rash predominantly over the dorsum of the forearms as well as the legs. BP is 145/90 mmHg. She is mildly tender in both flanks, but examination is otherwise unremarkable.

Miss Edwards' GP is contacted to confirm the date which she started omeprazole and to ask if he has any previous documentation of renal function. Some bloods were performed 5 years ago as part of a routine pre-employment

Nephrology: Clinical Cases Uncovered. By M. Clatworthy.
Published 2010 by Blackwell Publishing.

screen. These showed a creatinine of 68 μmol/L, suggesting that the current decline in renal function is likely to be acute.

What is the most likely underlying cause of her renal impairment?

The features of the case are in keeping with a diagnosis of TIN secondary to one of the drugs which she has been taking (NSAID or PPI). Although it is possible that she has a primary or secondary GN, the documented drug exposure and temporal association of systemic symptoms make this less likely.

The typical clinical presentation of acute TIN includes:

- symptoms of fever, rash, arthralgia, loin pain
- previous history of drug ingestion or infection
- hypertension
- ARF.

A urine dipstick shows +++ protein, ++ blood, +leucocytes and a sample is sent to the lab for microscopy, culture and sensitivity.

What specific feature would you ask the microscopist to look for in the urine sample?

The presence of eosinophils (best visualised with Hansel's stain) in the urine would be suggestive of TIN. A peripheral eosinophilia also occurs in around 70% of patients.

In TIN there is typically microscopic haematuria and non-nephrotic range proteinuria (typically 1.5–2 g/day).

Miss Edwards has an ultrasound of her renal tract performed.

What would you expect this to show?

In ARF secondary to TIN, the kidneys are of a normal size (10–12 cm) or may even be slightly enlarged. There is nothing in her history to suggest CKD (and she has a previously normal creatinine) or obstruction.

A US of Miss Edwards' renal tract is performed, which shows two normal-sized, unobstructed kidneys. An acute renal screen, including ANA, anti-dsDNA, complement (C3/C4), IgG, ANCA, anti-GBM antibodies, RF, cryoglobulins is negative/normal. Other bloods are shown below.

Hb 12.1 g/dL, WBC 11.1 × 10⁹/L (eosinophils 1.2, NR 0.04–0.44), Platelets 534 × 10⁹/L

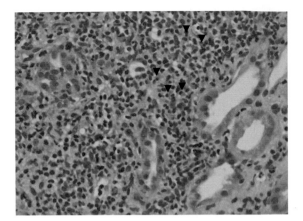

Figure 7.1 Renal biopsy with H+E staining showing an interstitial infiltrate which includes mononuclear cells and eosinophils (stain bright red/pink; arrows).

Clotting : normal

U+Es: Na 139 mmol/L, K 4.4 mmol/L, Uea 14.3 mmol/L, Creatinine 201 μmol/L

ESR 48 mm/h, CRP 36 mg/L, LFT normal, Albumin 34 g/L

A US-guided renal biopsy is performed in order to confirm the cause of ARF (Figure 7.1).

What does the biopsy show?

The biopsy shows typical appearances of acute TIN. These include:

- inflammatory interstitial infiltrate, including eosinophils.
- interstitial oedema and flattening of tubular cells
- necrosis/apoptosis of tubular cells
- tubular atrophy/interstitial fibrosis (indicates chronicity).

Which drugs are associated with acute TIN?

A large number of drugs have been associated with TIN, particularly penicillin-based antibiotics and NSAIDs (see Box 7.1). More recently, UK studies suggest that PPI-associated TIN is not infrequent.

Acute TIN can also be associated with other aetiological factors, particularly infection (Box 7.2). If no obvious cause is demonstrated, then acute TIN is classified as idiopathic.

Box 7.1 Some of the more common drugs associated with acute TIN

- Antibiotics
  - Penicillin based: methicillin, ampicillin, penicillin G
  - Other: cephalexin, tetracycline, erythromycin, gentamicin
- NSAID: particularly fenoprofen and meclofenomate
- Aspirin
- Antacids: PPI and cimetidine
- Diuretics: furosemide, thiazides

Box 7.2 Infections associated with acute TIN

- Bacterial
  - Streptococci, staphylococci
  - Atypicals: *Legionella pneumophilia, Mycoplasma pneumonia*
  - Intracellular: mycobacterial (TB), salmonella
- Viral
  - Measles
  - Mumps
  - Rubella
  - CMV
  - HIV
- Parasitic
  - Toxoplasma
  - Leishmania
  - Schistosoma

What are the pathogenic mechanisms involved in tubulointerstitial nephritis?

It is thought that some medications or pathogens (or bits of pathogens) may bind to tubulointerstitial components, changing their structure so that they become immunogenic. Other drugs/infectious agents may directly damage tubulointerstitial components, again making them immunogenic. The end result of either process is interstitial inflammation (characterised by an inflammatory infiltrate of lymphocytes and eosinophils) and tubular damage. If this is not treated and becomes chronic, then fibrosis and tubular atrophy will result (irreversible changes).

How would you treat Miss Edwards?

- Remove likely causative drug (in this case, it is most likely to be the PPI, but it could be the NSAID or ranitidine. Where possible, all medications should be stopped).
- Treat hypertension and proteinuria (ACEI or ARB).

- Oral steroids (prednisolone 1 mg/kg) to treat the inflammation and prevent progression to fibrosis.

If patients have severe acute renal impairment and oliguria (<20% of patients with TIN) then renal replacement therapy may be temporarily required.

What is the prognosis of acute tubulointerstitial nephritis?

Overall, the prognosis is good. Most patients will gain complete or near complete recovery of renal function once the causative medication is stopped. However, prominent fibrosis and tubular atrophy on renal biopsy indicate irreversible damage, and such patients may not fully regain renal function.

Poor prognostic factors include:
- irreversible biopsy changes (fibrosis + tubular atrophy)
- heavy proteinuria at presentation
- oliguria
- persistent renal failure for >3 weeks
- older age.

The omeprazole is stopped and Miss Edwards is started on lisinopril 5 mg od as well as prednisolone 60 mg od. The steroids are continued at this dose for 2 weeks and then trimmed to 40 mg for 2 weeks before reducing by 10 mg/week until she has weaned off them. Her systemic symptoms improve within 3 days of starting steroids. At follow-up in the renal outpatient clinic 3 months later, her BP is 110/70 mmHg, urine dipstick has 1+protein and creatinine is 110 μmol/L (eGFR = 55 mL/min/1.73 m², i.e. CKD stage 3).

What do you know about chronic tubulointerstitial nephritis?

Chronic TIN is used to describe a renal biopsy which is characterised by significant interstitial fibrosis and tubular atrophy (Figure 7.2). These are rather non-specific findings and can occur as the end result of a variety of aetiological factors (see Box 7.3). If this broad definition of chronic TIN is used, then around 20–30% of patients with ESRF will have chronic TIN on biopsy. However, many nephrologists would consider chronic pyelonephritis, vesicoureteric reflux and obstructive uropathy in a separate diagnostic category. The frequency of chronic TIN of other causes shows great geographic variation, depending on the exposure of different populations to drugs and toxins. Chronic TIN is frequently asymptomatic and thus often remains undiagnosed until the patient reaches ESRF.

Balkan nephropathy is a chronic TIN which is endemic in Bulgaria, Serbia, Montenegro and Romania. The

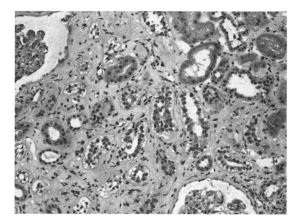

Figure 7.2 Renal biopsy showing an area of tubular atrophy and interstitial scarring. The tubules are not packed tightly, back to back as they should be, but are found infrequently between areas of interstitial fibrosis.

disease begins between the ages of 20 and 30 years, is more frequent in rural populations and is a significant cause of ESRF in these communities. Individuals also develop transitional cell carcinoma (TCC) of the renal pelvis and ureters. Recent research suggests that it is caused by ingestion of *Aristolochia clematitis*, a plant native to the area. This contains aristolochic acid (also found in some Chinese herbal remedies) which has been shown to cause TIN and TCC in animal models.

Box 7.3 Causes of chronic TIN

- Renal infection/obstruction
  - Chronic pyelonephritis
  - Vesicoureteric reflux
  - Obstructive uropathy
- Drugs (chronic exposure)
  - Analgesics
  - Lithium
  - Ciclosporin
  - Gold
- Toxins
  - Lead
  - Aristolochic acid (thought to be the cause of Balkan nephropathy)
- Autoimmune disease
  - Sjögren's syndrome
  - SLE
  - Vasculitis
- Haematological malignancy/dysgammaglobulinaemia
  - Multiple myeloma
  - Amyloidosis
  - Lymphoma
- Metabolic diseases
  - Hyperuricaemic nephropathy
  - Hypercalcaemic nephropathy
  - Cystinosis
  - Fabry's disease
- Radiation

CASE REVIEW

A 27-year-old woman presented with a history of fever, rash and arthralgia after commencing a PPI. Investigations showed acute renal failure, peripheral eosinophilia and eosinophiluria. A renal biopsy was consistent with tubulointerstitial nephritis. The PPI was stopped and the patient was treated with prednisolone and ACEI. Renal function significantly improved, although it did not normalise.

KEY POINTS

- Acute TIN presents typically with fever, rash, arthralgia, loin pain and hypertension. Investigations show ARF, eosinophilia, microscopic haematuria, proteinuria 1.5–2 g/24 h and eosinophils in the urine.
- A renal biopsy is useful, even in cases with a classic presentation, in order to confirm the diagnosis (interstitial infiltrate and oedema, tubular necrosis) and assess for signs of irreversible damage (interstitial fibrosis and tubular atrophy).
- The most common causes of acute TIN are drugs and infections, although some will have no obvious cause (idiopathic). Drugs associated include antibiotics, NSAID and PPI.
- Treatment involves stopping the causative drugs or treating the causative infection, managing hypertension and proteinuria (e.g. with ACE or ARB) and treating inflammation with oral corticosteroids (typically prednisolone 1 mg/kg).
- Overall, prognosis is good, with many patients regaining normal renal function. Poor prognostic factors include older age, oliguric ARF and the presence of significant interstitial fibrosis and tubular atrophy on renal biopsy.

Case 8   A 26-year-old man with haemoptysis and oliguria

Will Roberts is a 26-year-old man who attends his GP complaining that he has coughed up some blood. He doesn't like doctors much so held off visiting his GP until he became really worried because as well as coughing up blood, he also seems to be passing less urine than usual. The GP refers him urgently to the Medical Assessment Unit.

What questions would you ask the patient on arrival?

• *Duration:* how long has he been unwell? When did he first start to cough up blood? How long has there been a reduction in the amount of urine he is passing?

• *Clarification of symptoms:* is he coughing up blood or vomiting blood? Patients sometimes say one when they mean the other. Obviously, the differential diagnosis for haemoptysis is completely different from that for haematemesis, so this is an important point. Occasionally patients with epistaxis (nosebleeds) may also describe coughing up blood, which actually originates from the upper airways.

• *Associated symptoms:* given he has haemoptysis, you should ask about shortness of breath, wheeze, chest pain, fevers/sweats. Painful swelling of calves may indicate a deep vein thrombosis (DVT) with associated pulmonary embolism (PE).

• What is the precise nature of his oliguria? How long has he been oliguric? Are there any other urinary symptoms?

Mr Roberts has had a cough for around a month. This was initially dry but he now brings up small amounts of mucus that contains flecks of bright red blood and he has also been mildly short of breath. He has not had any chest pain. In the last 3 days he has been feeling nauseated and is passing less urine. In fact, now that he comes to think of it, he has passed no urine for 12 hours. He has never had any similar episodes previously.

What are the main differential diagnoses for haemoptysis?

The main differentials are listed in Box 8.1 and include infection, malignancy and autoimmune disease.

What other questions would you ask?

The history so far reveals two major features:
• haemoptysis (causes given in Box 8.1)
• oligoanuria (suggestive of a renal problem, probably ARF).

Further questions should be aimed at determining the underlying cause of these two problems. In particular, pathologies which cause both haemoptysis and ARF (a pulmonary-renal syndrome) should be sought. The differential diagnosis of a pulmonary-renal syndrome is shown in Box 8.2.

In view of these possible underlying diagnoses, the following would be reasonable areas to probe when taking a more detailed history.

• Does the patient have any systemic symptoms (fevers, night sweats, weight loss) which might indicate an infectious or inflammatory process? Duration of such symptoms? It's often useful to ask the patient when they last felt completely well.

• Does the patient have any symptoms specifically associated with the autoimmune diseases listed in Box 8.1? Rash, arthralgia, myalgia, red eyes (anterior uveitis), dry eyes (keratoconjunctivitis sicca), recurrent sinusitis, nasal crusting/discharge, epistaxis, deafness, oral ulceration can all occur in systemic autoimmunity.

• Does he have any significant past medical history? For example, a history of previous DVT or PE may point towards a recurrence and suggest a thrombophilic tendency.

Nephrology: Clinical Cases Uncovered. By M. Clatworthy.
Published 2010 by Blackwell Publishing.

> **Box 8.1 Causes of haemoptysis**
>
> - Malignancy: bronchogenic carcinoma
> - Infection
>   - Pneumonia
>   - Pulmonary tuberculosis
>   - Lung abscess
>   - Aspergilloma
> - Vascular
>   - Pulmonary embolism
> - Autoimmune
>   - ANCA-associated vasculitis (Wegener's granulomatosis)
>   - Goodpasture's disease
>   - Systemic lupus erythematosus
> - Bronchiectasis
> - Pulmonary oedema
>   - Patients will usually describe coughing up frothy pink sputum, but occasionally it can appear more bloodstained

---

> **Box 8.2 Causes of pulmonary-renal syndrome**
>
> **Non-immune mediated**
> - ARF with volume overload/pulmonary oedema
> - Severe pneumonia with ATN, e.g. legionella
> - Infections with respiratory involvement and acute interstitial nephritis, e.g. leptospirosis
> - Thrombosis of renal vein/IVC with PE
>
> **Immune-mediated**
> - ANCA-associated vasculitis
> - Goodpasture's disease
> - SLE
> - Henoch–Schönlein purpura (HSP)/crescentic IgA nephropathy
> - Cryoglobulinaemia

- Has he noticed any other urinary symptoms? Other important points in the history include the presence of frank haematuria, frothy urine, fluid retention (swelling of face or ankles) and loin pain.
- Does he have any past medical history of any of the diseases listed in Boxes 8.1 and 8.2? Vasculitis, SLE and IgA are all diseases characterised by recurrent relapses and so the patient may have had similar presentations previously.
- Smoking history? Is the patient a smoker? Smoking is a major risk factor for pulmonary haemorrhage in Goodpasture's disease. What is the patient's job? Exposure to

hydrocarbons can also predispose to pulmonary haemorrhage in Goodpasture's disease.

The patient has previously been very fit and healthy and has never had any medical problems prior to this. He was last completely well around 2 months ago. Initially he felt generally tired, lethargic and washed out before developing the respiratory symptoms described above 1 month ago. He takes no medications and has never travelled abroad. He has smoked 20 cigarettes/day for the past 10 years and works as a car mechanic, and has done so since he left school at the age of 16 years.

What features are important to seek during clinical examination?

- *Temperature?* Fever can occur in infection or in systemic inflammatory diseases.
- *Hands/feet/nails* for splinter haemorrhages, nailfold infarcts, necrotic areas (signs of vasculitis). Leuconychia or Beau's lines (associated with hypoalbuminaemia which may occur with any chronic inflammatory/ autoimmune disease).
- *Rashes:* purpuric lesions (vasculitis), butterfly rash, photosensitivity rash on arms, neck, face or discoid lesions (SLE).
- *Mouth:* mouth ulcers (SLE).
- *Nose/sinuses:* nasal crusting, sinusitis (vasculitis).
- *Ears:* deafness (vasculitis).
- *Eyes:* red eyes (anterior uveitis) which may be associated with vasculitis.
- *CVS:* assess intravascular volume status (tachycardia may indicate volume depletion or systematic infection/ inflammation. A low BP or postural drop suggests hypovolaemia). Auscultate heart sounds: murmurs occur in endocarditis (infection-associated or aseptic in SLE). Pericardial rub may occur secondary be uraemic pericarditis or in lupus-associated serositis.
- *Chest:* oxygen saturations will be reduced if there is pulmonary haemorrhage, fibrosis or infection. Crepitations may occur if there is bronchiectasis, pulmonary haemorrhage, fibrosis/nodules which can be associated with vasculitis. A pleural rub may be heard if there is PE or serositis associated with SLE.
- *Abdomen:* splenomegaly (associated with SLE and some infections).
- *Legs:* rashes, particularly vasculitic lesions.

Mr Roberts is febrile with a temperature of 39.2 °C. He has one splinter haemorrhage in the first finger of his right hand but no obvious rashes. He has pale conjunctivae but

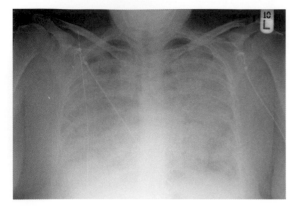

Figure 8.1 Chest radiograph demonstrating diffuse, extensive bilateral alveolar infiltrates, consistent with pulmonary oedema, haemorrhage or inflammation/infiltration.

peripheral examination is otherwise normal. The pulse is 105 bpm and regular. Blood pressure is 100/60 mmHg and there are no audible murmurs. Oxygen saturations are 90% on air, and his respiratory rate 26 rpm. There are coarse crepitations bilaterally in all lung zones. Abdominal examination is unremarkable.

Investigations show:

Hb 7.1 g/dL, WBC 11.2 × 10⁹/L, Platelets 567 × 10⁹/L

Clotting: normal

U+E: Na 145 mmol/L, K 5.4 mmol/L, Urea 29.3 mmol/L, Creatinine 546 µmol/L

ESR 98 mm/h, CRP 46 mg/L, LFT calcium: normal, Albumin 24 g/L

Urine dipstick : blood ++++ protein ++ leucocytes+ negative for nitrites, and glucose

Urine microscopy: red cell casts

ECG normal,

CXR: see Figure 8.1

ABGs: pH 7.29, pO₂ 7.9 kPa, pCO₂ 3.5 kPa

How would you interpret these results?

The investigations show anaemia and evidence of systemic infection or inflammation (WBC, CRP and ESR are elevated). In addition, the urea and creatinine are grossly abnormal, consistent with a diagnosis of ARF/acute kidney injury. There is an active urinary sediment, and red cell casts indicate glomerular inflammation. The patient is hypoxic and the CXR demonstrates shadowing in both lung fields indicative of fluid. This could be water (pulmonary oedema) or blood (pulmonary haemorrhage).

What general treatment measures could you begin?

Mr Roberts is hypoxic and should therefore be placed on high-flow oxygen. He is tachycardic and hypotensive, so intravenous fluid replacement should be commenced to restore intravascular volume. He is anaemic, and it would be prudent to ensure he has some blood cross-matched for transfusion. A urinary catheter should also be inserted to monitor urine output more accurately.

What further specialist investigations would you undertake?

The patient's blood tests indicate renal failure. He has no past medical history of renal disease, so this is likely to be ARF. In all patients with acute kidney injury, an ultrasound of the renal tract is required to ensure that the patient has two kidneys, of a normal size with no obstruction. This patient should then undergo a renal biopsy as a matter of some urgency to determine the underlying problem.

Other useful immunological investigations include a screen for autoimmune diseases which can be associated with a pulmonary-renal syndrome. These include:

- *SLE:* ANA, anti-dsDNA, complement (C3/C4), IgG
- *Vasculitis:* Anti-neutrophil cytoplasmic antibody (ANCA)
- *Goodpasture's disease:* anti-GBM antibodies
- *RF, cryoglobulins:* cryoglobulinaemia.

Mr Roberts' pulmonary problem also needs to be investigated further with:

- *lung function tests:* gas transfer factor (KCO) (increased if there is pulmonary haemorrhage)
- CT chest.

The patient has a US scan which shows two 12 cm kidneys with normal cortical thickness and no hydronephrosis. The patient undergoes a US-guided renal biopsy which on initial H+E shows a crescentic GN (Figure 8.2). The immunostaining shows linear deposition of IgG (Figure 8.3). The immunology results are awaited.

How would you interpret these results?

The kidneys are of normal size and cortical thickness on US, suggesting that Mr Roberts does not have chronic renal damage. Crescentic GN may be due to a primary GN, idiopathic crescentic GN, but more commonly occurs secondary to small vessel vasculitis, Goodpasture's disease or SLE. In a case of crescentic GN, the immunostaining is extremely helpful in making the diagnosis.

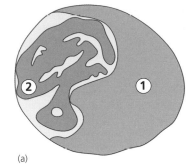
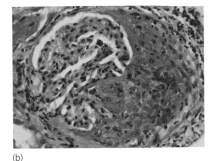

Figure 8.2 Schematic diagram (a) and H+E stained renal biopsy (b) showing a crescentic GN. A large cellular crescent (1) occupies the right-hand side of the glomerulus, and compresses the normal glomerular capillary loops (2).

(a)   (b)

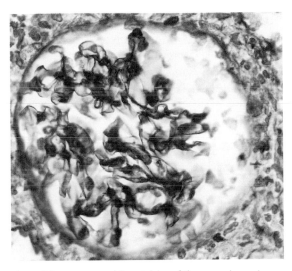

Figure 8.3 Immunoperoxidase staining of the same glomerulus, showing linear IgG deposition (dark brown) in the glomerular capillaries.

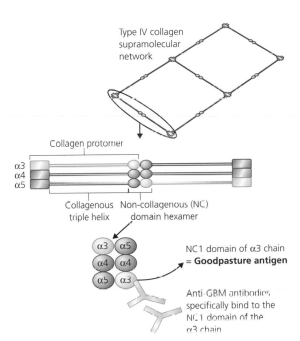

Figure 8.4 The Goodpasture antigen.

• Pauci-immune (no IgG/M/A, no complement): ANCA-associated vasculitis or idiopathic focal necrotising GN
• Linear IgG staining: Goodpasture's disease (anti-glomerular basement membrane disease)
• Linear IgA staining: crescentic IgA nephropathy
• Full-house staining (+ve for IgG/M/A, C1q, C3, C4): SLE

In this case, immunostaining shows linear staining with IgG, making Goodpasture's disease (anti-glomerular basement membrane disease) the most likely diagnosis.

Given the biopsy result, what would you expect the immunology tests to show?

In Goodpasture's disease (anti-GBM disease), patients develop an autoantibody which binds to type IV collagen.

Type IV collagen is found in both glomerular and pulmonary basement membranes. This IgG antibody is detectable in the blood of all patients with Goodpasture's disease and is usually termed an 'anti-glomerular basement membrane' (GBM) antibody. The precise antigen specificity of anti-GBM antibodies has been determined as the non-collagenous domain of the α3 chain of type IV collagen (Figure 8.4). This is also present in the pulmonary basement membrane, so haemoptysis can develop. However, pulmonary haemorrhage is not a universal feature (present in 50–70% of cases). This is because the alveolar endothelium is not fenestrated (in contrast to glomerular capillary endothelium), so in normal lungs anti-GBM antibody has no access to the alveolar basement membrane. If the patient is a smoker or there is damage of endothelium secondary to other toxins (e.g. hydrocarbons, fluid overload, infection) then pulmonary haemorrhage can occur. The most sensitive test for diagnosis of pulmonary haemorrhage is an increased gas transfer factor (KCO) on lung function testing. Rarer clinical manifestations of Goodpasture's disease include retinal detachment (due to antibody binding to the Brusch membrane in the eye) and epileptic fits (due to the binding of antibody to the choroid plexus).

In patients with Goodpasture's disease, all other immunological tests, including ANA, anti-dsDNA, ANCA and complement, are usually normal.

Occasionally, some patients with vasculitis (pANCA positive) also have anti-GBM antibodies (usually of a low titre). These patients tend to have a better renal prognosis than those with 'pure' Goodpasture's disease. The anti-GBM antibodies in such cases are thought to arise because the vasculitis-associated inflammation in the glomerulus acts to unveil the Goodpasture's antigen to the immune system, thus facilitating an immune response to type IV collagen.

Mr Roberts' anti-GBM antibody titre is markedly elevated at 230 iu. All other immunological tests are normal.

Given the result of the biopsy and additional blood tests, how would you treat this patient?

The investigations are consistent with a diagnosis of Goodpasture's disease (anti-GBM disease). Anti-GBM disease is one of the most extensively investigated glomerulonephritides and the archetypal example of an antibody-mediated disease. The pathogenicity of the antibody has been cleverly proven by demonstrating that the serum from humans with Goodpasture's disease can transfer disease to other primates and that antibody titre correlates with disease severity. Thus antibody removal is the principal acute treatment.

Mr Roberts should receive plasma exchange as quickly as possible in order to remove pathogenic antibody from the blood. Corticosteroids (to suppress active inflammation) and cyclophosphamide (kills by actively dividing lymphocytes and prevents an ongoing immune response to the Goodpasture's antigen) should also be commenced.

The patient asks whether the treatment has any side-effects

Immunosuppressive therapy has a number of generic side-effects.

- An increased risk of infection; for example, *Pneumocystis carinii*, CMV and candida.
- An increased risk of malignancy; in particular, patients are at increased risk of myeloproliferative disorders later in life.

Specific side-effects related to corticosteroids include osteoporosis, hypertension, glucose intolerance, gastric ulceration, dyslipidaemia, central obesity, thinning of the skin and easy bruising. Oral cyclophosphamide treatment is associated with haemorrhagic cystitis and a subsequent increased risk of bladder cancer. Higher cumulative doses are also associated with infertility.

In order to prevent some of these adverse events, patients are routinely given prophylactic treatment: co-trimoxazole (Septrin) to prevent pneumocystis; Calcichew D3 +/− bisphosphonates to prevent osteoporosis; proton pump inhibitor, e.g. omeprazole, to prevent peptic ulceration.

The patient asks you whether this disease is curable. What advice would you give him?

If treatment with plasma exchange is started before the patient has established renal failure, then he may recover renal function. However, this is not the case for most patients, including Mr Roberts. Unfortunately, those who are oligoanuric at presentation will usually become dialysis dependent. Hence it is important to recognise Goodpasture's disease as quickly as possible and to start treatment if irreversible renal failure is to be avoided.

Treatment with plasma exchange and immunosuppression is useful in preventing pulmonary haemorrhage, which can become severe and life-threatening without intervention. Plasma exchange usually results in a measurable fall in anti-GBM titre. Unlike small vessel vasculitis, Goodpasture's disease does not tend to relapse.

Overall, the 1-year mortality in patients with Goodpasture's disease is between 10% and 20%. At this stage, 60% of survivors will be dialysis dependent. For those patients who do not recover renal function, transplantation is an option, provided anti-GBM antibodies have been undetectable for a sustained period (this may take a number of months or even years).

Mr Roberts is started on plasma exchange. He is also given three pulses of intravenous methyl prednisolone, followed by oral prednisolone and a pulse of intravenous cyclophosphamide. After six exchange sessions, the anti-GBM titre falls to 34. The haemoptysis improves but his renal function continues to decline. Unfortunately, he becomes dialysis dependent and there is no recovery of renal function.

What do you know of the aetiology of Goodpasture's disease?

The aetiology of Goodpasture's disease appears to involve a genetic susceptibility (Goodpasture's is more common in patients with the HLA-DR15 genotype) and an environmental trigger (as evidenced by the many reported clustering of cases, including its occurrence in genetically unrelated next-door neighbours!). There are now some data suggesting that microbial peptides can act as 'molecular mimics' if they possess a similar molecular structure to the GBM antigen. Thus a cross-reactive immune response is triggered following infection.

Ernest Goodpasture (1886–1960) was a pathologist and assistant professor at Harvard University. He trained under George Whipple and in fact, his first publication was on haemorrhagic pancreatitis. He was interested in the pathological processes occurring in influenza infection, and in 1919 described the autopsy findings of an 18-year-old man who died at the height of the 1918 influenza pandemic with the clinical features of pulmonary haemorrhage and ARF secondary to a crescentic GN.

Final note

Interestingly, Goodpasture's disease can occur for the first time following transplantation in patients with Alport's syndrome. This is a rare genetic condition in which patients have mutations in the genes encoding type IV collagen. This leads to defective or deficient type IV collagen which manifests as deafness and a nephritis, progressing to end-stage renal failure in some patients. Following transplantation, the recipient's immune system mounts a response to the normal type IV collagen found within the allograft because they have never developed self-tolerance to it in the usual way. Thus, Goodpasture's disease can develop *de novo* post-transplant in patients with Alport's syndrome.

CASE REVIEW

A 26-year-old man presents with haemoptysis and oliguria. Investigations demonstrate acute renal failure, anti-GBM antibodies and a crescentic GN with linear IgG staining consistent with a diagnosis of Goodpasture's disease. He is treated with plasma exchange, corticosteroids and cyclophosphamide. The pulmonary haemorrhage improves, but he develops irreversible, dialysis-dependent renal failure.

KEY POINTS

- The combination of pulmonary haemorrhage and acute renal failure is known as pulmonary-renal syndrome. This clinical presentation is also sometimes referred to as Goodpasture's syndrome (note, this is different from Goodpasture's *disease*, which is specifically due to anti-GBM antibodies). The two main differential diagnoses to consider in a case of pulmonary-renal syndrome or Goodpasture's syndrome are ANCA-associated vasculitis (AAV) and Goodpasture's disease (now often termed anti-GBM disease to avoid confusion).
- Renal biopsy and immunological investigations allow AAV and anti-GBM disease to be distinguished.
- Both AAV and anti-GBM disease result in a crescentic GN. However, in AAV, there is circulating ANCA and a pauci-immune GN. In anti-GBM disease there are circulating anti-GBM antibodies and linear IgG deposition on renal biopsy.
- Anti-GBM disease is rare (1 pmp) but makes up 1–5% of all biopsy-proven GN and 10–20% of crescentic GN. It is more common in caucasians than in other racial groups. It is slightly more common in men (M:F 1.5)
- Unfortunately, many patients present with established renal failure (particularly if they are non-smokers and do not get pulmonary haemorrhage which often prompts patients to seek medical attention at an earlier stage). In these cases, renal failure is usually irreversible and patients will become dialysis dependent.
- Treatment is with plasma exchange and immunosuppression with corticosteroids and cyclophosphamide.

A 25-year-old secretary, Miss Tracy Peel, presents with joint pains, lethargy and a rash. She has no significant past medical history. Investigations show renal impairment (creatinine 120 μmol/L, eGFR 50 mL/min/1.73 m²) prompting referral to the nephrology services.

What additional questions would you ask the patient?

Miss Peel has renal impairment (eGFR 50 mL/min/1.73 m²) which may be acute or chronic. The absence of any past medical history (e.g. diabetes, hypertension, recurrent UTI or renal disease) makes CKD less likely, but still possible, in this case.

The causes of renal impairment can be divided into pre-renal/ATN, renal or post-renal. There is nothing in the referral to suggest hypovolaemia/hypotension (e.g. history of diarrhoea/vomiting) and post-renal causes of renal failure are less common in young women (mostly due to prostate problems, therefore more common in older men).

The referral mentions a rash and arthralgia. The presence of such systemic symptoms make a renal cause (e.g. a GN secondary to a systemic autoimmune disease, infection or TIN) more likely. Further useful history includes the following.
- Duration of illness: acute or chronic? Any infection preceding this episode (particularly pharyngitis or GI infection)?
- Systemic symptoms: precise onset and details of rash (e.g. exacerbating factors such as sunlight or trauma (Koebner phenomenon)), mouth ulcers (multiple? Presence of genital ulceration which is seen in Behçet's disease), arthralgia (which joints are involved, is there associated back pain indicative of sacroiliitis?), plus additional history of night sweats, respiratory symptoms (haemoptysis/SOB), chest pain (pleuritic or pericardial,

associated with serosis), upper respiratory tract symptoms (nasal crusting discharge, sinusitis) or red eyes (anterior uveitis) which might suggest a systemic autoimmune or inflammatory disease such as SLE or vasculitis?
- Any new medications which might cause TIN?
- Any previous similar episodes or past medical history of autoimmune disease?

What are the possible causes of her rash?

Rashes can occur as part of a primary dermatological problem, e.g. psoriasis, contact dermatitis, or may occur in association with a number of other conditions, particularly systemic autoimmune diseases, infections and malignancy. These are classified in Box 9.1. In this particular case, the patient also has documented renal impairment and arthralgia. It is most likely that her rash is caused by a disease which is also associated with these two features (Occam's razor – if possible, seek a diagnosis that will account for all symptoms). Thus autoimmunity and infection rise to the top of the list.

Occam's razor

Occam's razor is a concept said to originate with the 14th-century English logician and Franciscan friar William of Okham. He advocated the law of parsimony ('less is better', from the latin *parcere*, 'to spare'), that the simplest hypotheses, with fewest assumptions, should be favoured. In medicine, Occams's razor is usually used to refer to diagnostic parsimony. Thus, a physician should, if possible, seek a single diagnosis which accounts for all symptoms and signs, however disparate.

Further history is obtained from Miss Peel. She has been unwell for around 6 months. During this time she has had aches in her finger joints and has been finding typing increasingly difficult. She has also noticed some stiffness and has been feeling increasingly tired and lacking in energy.

Nephrology: Clinical Cases Uncovered. By M. Clatworthy.
Published 2010 by Blackwell Publishing.

Box 9.1 Causes of a rash

- Primary dermatological diagnosis, e.g. eczema, psoriasis
- Irritant or contact dermatitis
- Drug-induced
- Autoimmune-associated (a number of systemic autoimmune diseases are associated with a rash, as described in Table 9.1)
- Infection-associated
  - Purpuric rash (meningococcal septicaemia)
  - Erythema nodosum (β-haemolytic streptococci, mycobacterium (TB and leprosy), chlamydia, leptospirosis)
  - Erythema marginatum (rheumatic fever)
  - Erythema chronicum migrans (Lyme disease)
- Malignancy-associated: acanthosis nigricans, erythema gyratumm repens
- Associated with diseases of other systems
  - Insulin resistance/DM (acanthosis nigricans, necrobiosis lipoidica diabeticorum)
  - Inflammatory bowel disease (pyoderma gangrenosum)

Table 9.1 Dermatological manifestations of autoimmune diseases

Autoimmune disease	Rash
SLE	Photosensitivity rash Butterfly rash Discoid lupus Mouth ulcers
Dermatomyositis	Photosensitivity rash, Gottron's papules
Vasculitis	Purpuric rash, digital gangrene
Cryoglobulinaemia	Livedo reticularis
Sarcoidosis	Lupus pernio
Systemic sclerosis	Digital gangrene, finger pulp infarcts, telangiectasia, sclerodactyly, calcinosis

She first noticed the rash 1 month ago. It appeared following a day at the seaside, and at first she thought it was sunburn. This rash has persisted since then, mainly on her arms, neck, upper chest and cheeks. She has also had four or five mouth ulcers in this period, which is unusual for her. There is no history of genital ulceration. Miss Peel is normally very fit and healthy and has never had any similar episodes previously. Her only medication is the OCP which she has been taking for the past 6 years and she has never been pregnant or had a miscarriage. She is a non-smoker and denies the use of any recreational drugs. She does have a family history of autoimmune disease in that her maternal grandmother had rheumatoid arthritis.

What features are important to seek during clinical examination?

The history so far is suggestive of an autoimmune disease. Less likely is the possibility of a chronic infection. Examination features which might confirm the presence of a systemic autoimmune disease include the following.

- The presence of fever, cachexia, palor (anaemia).
- *Rash:* distribution, characteristic features (macules, papules, etc.), involvement of mucous membranes, presence of rheumatoid nodules.
- Hands/feet/nails for splinter haemorrhages, nailfold infarcts, necrotic areas (signs of vasculitis/endocarditis).

- Leuconychia or Beau's lines (associated with hypoalbuminaemia which may occur with any chronic inflammatory/autoimmune disease).
- *Joints:* hands in particular given symptoms. Are there signs of inflammation? The classic features of inflammation were defined by Celsus (30 BC) as calor (heat), dolor (pain), rubor (redness), tumor (swelling). Functio laesa (reduced function) was added as an additional feature by Virchov in 1870. Therefore assess range of movement and functional limitation.
- *Mouth:* mouth ulcers (SLE, Behçet's).
- *Nose:* nasal crusting (vasculitis).
- *Eyes:* red eyes (anterior uveitis, which may be associated with vasculitis), scleritis, episcleritis, keratoconjunctivitis sicca, scleromalacia perforans (associated with rheumatoid arthritis).
- *Abdomen:* splenomegaly is associated with a number of infections and autoimmune diseases.

Miss Peel has pale conjunctivae and palmar creases. Her temperature is 37.2 °C and pulse is 72 bpm and regular. Blood pressure is elevated at 150/85 mmHg, cardiovascular examination is otherwise normal. Chest is clear with no signs of a pleural effusion. There is an erythematous macular rash on the dorsum of her forearms, around her neckline in the sun-exposed areas and on her cheeks and over the bridge of her nose (Figure 9.1). She also has two mouth ulcers on her right buccal mucosa. The proximal interphalangeal joints in her right hand look slightly swollen but they are not

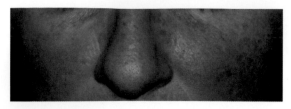

Figure 9.1 Butterfly rash over the cheeks and bridge of the nose.

erythematous and there is no obvious involvement of any other joints. Abdominal examination is unremarkable; in particular, there is no obvious splenomegaly.

Investigations show:

Hb 9.1 g/dL, MCV 79, WBC 11.2 × 10⁹/L, Platelets
567 × 10⁹/L
Clotting: PT normal, APTT prolonged
U+E: Na 138 mmol/L, K 5 mmol/L, Urea 12.3 mmol/L,
Creatinine 155 μmol/L
ESR 98 mm/h, CRP 26 mg/L, LFT normal, Calcium normal
Albumin 26 g/L
Urine dipstick: blood ++++ protein +++ leucocytes+ negative
for nitrites and glucose
Urine microscopy: red cell casts
ECG normal
CXR demonstrates a normal cardiac size and no pleural
effusion

What do the urine findings suggest about the cause of Miss Peel's renal impairment?

The presence of blood, protein and leucocytes on dipstick with red cell casts on microscopy points towards a renal pathology, more specifically glomerular inflammation (GN).

What is the most likely underlying diagnosis?

The features of this case are most in keeping with a diagnosis of SLE (see Box 9.2 for diagnostic criteria). In particular she is the right age and sex (young female) and has evidence of inflammation in a number of systems, specifically skin, joints and kidneys. The prolonged APTT suggests the presence of lupus anticoagulant.

Cutaneous manifestations occur in 85% of patients with SLE and range from the classic butterfly rash through to alopecia, discoid lupus and mouth ulceration. Ninety-five percent of patients will have musculoskeletal symptoms including arthralgia and myalgia; the arthritis

> **Box 9.2 American College of Rheumatology (ACR) diagnostic criteria for SLE (4/11 features required)**
>
> - Malar rash
> - Discoid rash
> - Photosensitivity
> - Oral ulcers
> - Arthritis
>   - Non-erosive
>   - Two or more joints
> - Serositis
>   - Pleuritis or pericarditis
> - Renal disorder
>   - Proteinuria or casts (glomerular haematuria)
> - Neurologic disorder
>   - Fits or psychosis
> - Haematologic disorder
>   - Haemolytic anaemia or lymphopaenia or leucopaenia or thrombocytopaenia
> - Immunological disorder
>   - Anti-dsDNA or anti-Sm abs
> - ANA

seen in SLE is usually non-erosive. Seventy-five percent will have a fever.

Inflammatory markers (ESR and CRP) are also raised. In SLE, the ESR is typically significantly elevated, whilst CRP may be within the normal range or only mildly elevated, unless there is intercurrent infection. This is said to be a useful guide to distinguish when patients with SLE have infection once they are on immunosuppressive medications.

The ECG does not show any evidence of pericarditis (saddle-shaped, elevated ST segments), although SLE can be associated with serositis (pleurisy or pericarditis, found in 60% of patients). On CXR there may be a small pleural effusion if there is active pleurisy or an enlarged heart if there is a pericardial effusion associated with pericarditis. Occasionally SLE is associated with an aseptic endocarditis (Leibmann–Sachs endocarditis). Other manifestations include neuropsychiatric symptoms (seizures, psychosis, depression 55%), renal involvement (50%) and haematological features (70% including haemolytic anaemia, thrombocytopenia and lymphopenia).

Clearly, the clinical manifestations of SLE are extremely variable, so the diagnosis can sometimes be difficult and delayed. Diagnosis is based on a combina-

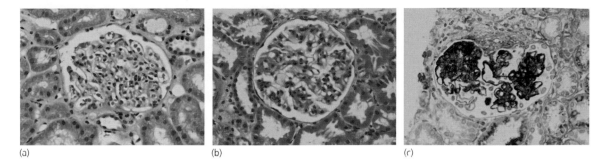

(a) (b) (c)

Figure 9.2 Renal biopsy with lupus nephritis. (a) Normal glomerulus (for comparison). (b) Patient's biopsy (H+E). The glomerulus is hypercellular and lobulated, with thickening of capillary basement membrane to form 'wire loops'. If >50% of the glomeruli are involved, then this is class IV lupus nephritis. (c) Patient's biopsy (immunostaining for IgG).

tion of clinical features and the results of laboratory investigations.

What further specialist investigations would you undertake?

Given the clinical features, a diagnosis of SLE is most likely. An acute renal immunological screen should be undertaken including:

- screen for SLE: ANA, anti-dsDNA antibodies, anti-Sm, anti-cardiolipin antibodies, complement (C3/C4) and Ig
- screen for other autoimmune diseases: ANCA, anti-GBM, cryoglobulins, RF.

As with all patients with ARF, an ultrasound of the renal tract is required to ensure that the patient has two kidneys, of a normal size with no obstruction. Miss Peel has ARF with evidence of glomerular inflammation. She should therefore undergo a renal biopsy to identify the precise pathological pattern and likely cause.

> A US scan shows two 11.0 cm kidneys with normal cortical thickness and no hydronephrosis. Miss Peel undergoes a US-guided renal biopsy (Figure 9.2) which on initial H+E shows a diffuse, proliferative GN with thickened glomerular capillary loops (so-called 'wire-loop' lesions) and with 'full house' immunostaining (i.e. positive for IgM, IgG, IgA, C1q, C3, C4). Immunology investigations show that she has ANA, anti-dsDNA, anti-Sm and anticardiolipin. C3 low normal, whilst C4 very low. There is also a polyclonal elevation of IgM and IgG.

How would you interpret these results?

The kidneys are of normal size and cortical thickness on US, suggesting that she does not have chronic renal damage. The biopsy findings are typical of lupus nephri-

tis. Lupus nephritis is classified (class I–V) depending on the extent and severity of the lesions. Class V lupus nephritis shows a membranous GN on biopsy.

The immunological investigations confirm this diagnosis. Patients with SLE have a breakdown in self-tolerance, particularly to nuclear components, and therefore have antibodies which bind a variety of self-antigens normally found within the nucleus. Ninety-five percent of patients with lupus are ANA positive, 80% are anti-dsDNA positive, and 40% are anti-Sm (Smith, named after the first patient in which it was described) positive. The latter is highly specific for lupus. Anti-phospholipid antibodies are associated with a prolonged APTT and an increased frequency of venous and arterial thrombosis. These antibodies are also associated with recurrent miscarriages. Other autoantibodies identified in patients with SLE are shown in Table 9.2.

C4 is typically low in patients with lupus due to activation of the classic complement pathway by deposited immune complexes (Figure 9.3).

How would you manage Miss Peel?
General management measures

She is hypertensive, so it would be prudent to commence an anti-hypertensive to ensure her blood pressure is well enough controlled to perform a renal biopsy. Given she has proteinuria on dipstick, an ACEI or ARB would be a reasonable choice.

Specific management measures

Lupus nephritis is caused by the deposition of immune complexes within the glomerulus, which initiates inflammation. Similarly if the rash is biopsied, linear IgG deposition will be demonstrated, indicating immune complex

Table 9.2 Autoantibodies in SLE

Self-antigen recognized by autoantibody	Prevalence in SLE
ssDNA	70–90%
Ubiquitin (DNA/chromatin-binding protein)	60–80%
dsDNA	50–70%
Histones (nuclear)	60–80%
Sm (soluble nuclear RNA protein)	20–30%
SS-A/Ro (cytoplasmic antigen)	30–40%
SS-B/La (cytoplasmic antigen)	15–25%
Phospholipid (associated with thrombosis and foetal loss)	20–30%
Red cell antigens (causing haemolytic anaemia)	20–30%
Lymphocyte antigens (including CD24, TCR, CD4, IL-2R, which can lead to autoimmune lymphopaenia)	30–50%
Platelet antigens (causing immune thombocytopenic purpura)	10–25%

deposition within the skin. Treatments are therefore aimed at suppressing the immune system, in order to reduce the production of immune complexes and inhibit inflammation generated in response to immune complex deposition. The agents of choice for lupus nephritis are corticosteroids and mycophenolate mofetil (associated with diarrhoea and bone marrow suppression). Other immunosuppressants used in SLE include hydroxychloroquine (mainly if disease limited to skin and joints), azathioprine and cyclophosphamide. The latter was often used in the treatment of lupus nephritis but this has significant implications for fertility and therefore is a difficult drug to use in young women.

Miss Peel is also lupus anticoagulant positive and is therefore at increased risk of developing both arterial and venous thromboses; a careful search should be made in the history for evidence of previously clinically unrecognised thromboses. In the absence of these, some physicians would start her on prophylactic aspirin. If there is any suggestion that she has had previous thromboses then she should be formally anti-coagulated with warfarin.

Given that she is on a number of potentially teratogenic medications (mycophenolate, ACEI), then she should use some form of contraception, although oestrogen-containing preparations may add to the thrombotic risk.

> *Miss Peel is started on ramipril 1.25 mg, pulsed with intravenous methylprednisolone and then maintained on oral prednisolone and mycophenolate mofetil (1 g tds). She is also placed on omeprazole, to protect against gastric ulceration, and Calcichew D3 to prevent osteoporosis. On review in clinic 2 weeks later, she feels much better in herself. Creatinine is now 156 µmol/L.*

Miss Peel asks you whether this disease is curable. What advice would you give her?

Systemic lupus erythematosus is a relapsing, remitting disease. Patients may respond to immunosuppression and remain in remission for a number of years on maintenance immunosuppression, but subsequently experience a relapse. Therefore they need to be monitored frequently (every 3–6 months). A rise in dsDNA titre frequently precedes renal relapse. Relapses do not necessarily affect the same organ as the primary presentation, e.g. a patient may present with nephritis and skin disease but subsequently relapse with an episode of serositis or a cytopaenia. Other possible future complications include venous or arterial thrombosis (given that she is lupus anticoagulant positive).

Overall, ESRF develops in approximately 20% of patients with lupus nephritis. This is more likely in patients with proliferative changes on biopsy (class III/IV).

What do you know about the aetiopathogenesis of systemic lupus erythematosus?

Systemic lupus erythematosus occurs in about 30/100,000 individuals and is more common in young women (F:M 9:1; mean age 30 years, range 15–65). It is also more common, and more severe, in certain racial groups, for example Afro-Caribbeans and South-East Asians.

The aetiology of SLE is thought to have both genetic and environmental influences.

Genetic factors

A genetic influence on pathogenesis is suggested by:
• 15x increased risk in siblings of patients with SLE
• 3% of dizygotic twins will get disease if their twin has it (concordance), compared with a 30% concordance rate in monozygotic twins

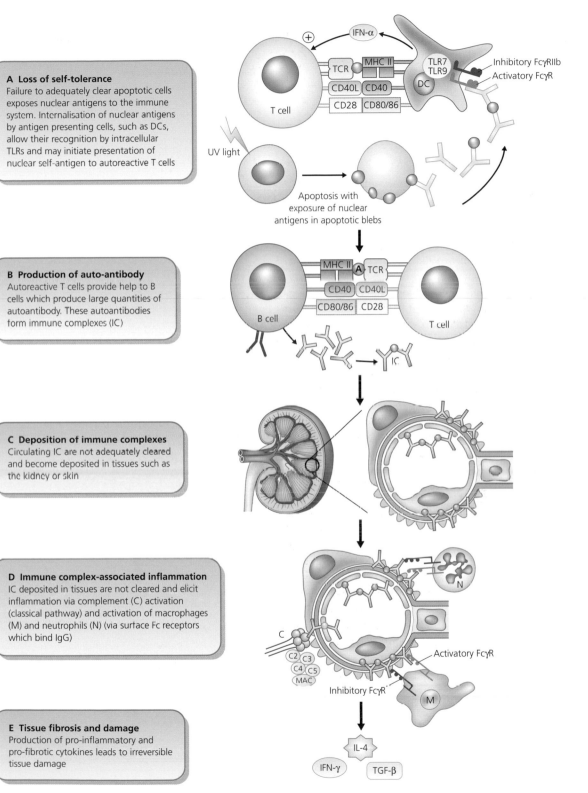

A Loss of self-tolerance
Failure to adequately clear apoptotic cells exposes nuclear antigens to the immune system. Internalisation of nuclear antigens by antigen presenting cells, such as DCs, allow their recognition by intracellular TLRs and may initiate presentation of nuclear self-antigen to autoreactive T cells

B Production of auto-antibody
Autoreactive T cells provide help to B cells which produce large quantities of autoantibody. These autoantibodies form immune complexes (IC)

C Deposition of immune complexes
Circulating IC are not adequately cleared and become deposited in tissues such as the kidney or skin

D Immune complex-associated inflammation
IC deposited in tissues are not cleared and elicit inflammation via complement (C) activation (classical pathway) and activation of macrophages (M) and neutrophils (N) (via surface Fc receptors which bind IgG)

E Tissue fibrosis and damage
Production of pro-inflammatory and pro-fibrotic cytokines leads to irreversible tissue damage

Figure 9.3 Pathogenesis of SLE.

• variation in susceptibility between different racial groups.

Systemic lupus erythematosus is a polygenic disease; that is, a number of genes confer disease susceptibility. Genes implicated in the pathogenesis of SLE include those encoding HLA molecules, complement components, Fc receptors and Toll-like receptors (TLR).

Environmental factors

A number of environmental influences have been identified which can precipitate disease in individuals with a susceptible genotype. SLE is more common in women than men, suggesting that hormonal factors may influence pathogenesis. Disease flares can also be triggered by environmental stimuli such as ultraviolet light or certain drugs (Box 9.3). Thus an individual may be genetically predisposed to the development of SLE but will only develop the disease if they encounter the correct environmental triggers. Once initiated, other genetic, environmental and hormonal factors act to modify the spectrum and severity of clinical manifestations.

Interaction of factors

The way in which genetic and environmental factors interact to produce disease is a subject of intense research. The discovery of TLRs has provided an explanation of some of the observed associations between environmental stimuli and disease. TLRs are innate immune receptors which have evolved to facilitate a rapid immune response to invading micro-organisms by recognition of pathogen-associated molecular patterns (PAMP). TLR7 and TLR9 detect microbial RNA and DNA respectively, and are located within intracellular compartments. Exposure to sunlight is a well-known trigger of both

---

> **Box 9.3 Environmental factors which may contribute to the pathogenesis of SLE**
>
> **Chemical/physical factors:**
> • Aromatic amines
> • Drugs: hydralazine, procainamide, chlorpromazine, isoniazid, penicillamine
> • Tobacco
> • Hair dyes
> • Ultraviolet light
>
> **Dietary factors:**
> • L-canavanin (alfafa sprouts)
>
> **Infectious agents:**
> • Bacterial DNA
> • Endotoxin
> • Viruses

---

cutaneous (photosensitivity rash) and systemic manifestations of lupus. It is thought that skin exposure to UV light alters the location of DNA and other nuclear antigens, by inducing apoptosis in keratinocytes. Previously inaccessible nuclear self-antigens are then internalized by immune cells (e.g. B cells and dendritic cells) and are recognised by TLR 7 or 9, triggering an immune response to these antigens.

Some drugs, including hydralazine and procainamide, can cause SLE. This is thought to be because they can alter DNA methylation or RNA structure which subsequently enhances TLR activation.

A summary of the pathogenesis of SLE is shown in Figure 9.3.

CASE REVIEW

A 25-year-old woman presents with rash, mouth ulcers, arthralgia and renal impairment. Investigations demonstrate elevated inflammatory markers and a range of auto-antibodies, including ANA, anti-dsDNA, anti-Sm, and anti-phospholipid antibodies, indicating a diagnosis of SLE. A renal biopsy confirms lupus nephritis. Blood pressure is controlled with an ACEI and she is treated with steroids and mycophenolate mofetil.

KEY POINTS

- Systemic lupus erythematosus is a multisystem autoimmune disease. Clinical features include rashes, arthralgia, GN, pleurisy, pericarditis, cytopaenias and neurological involvement.
- Immunological abnormalities include the presence of autoantibodies (particularly ANA and anti-dsDNA), hypergammaglobulinaemia and hypocomplementaemia (particularly C4).
- Histopathological examination of affected tissues (typically skin or kidneys) demonstrates IgG immune complexes

which activate complement and phagocytes via Fc receptors.
- Treatment of lupus nephritis is with immunosuppression, typically corticosteroids and mycophenolate mofetil.
- Patients with SLE should be monitored every 3–6 months to screen for renal involvement (active urinary sediment) and a rise in anti-dsDNA titres which often precede flares of nephritis.

Case 10 An 18-year-old girl with lethargy and headache

Pauline Thorburn is an 18-year-old girl who presents with a 2-week history of lethargy and headache. In the last 24 hours she has also noticed a rash on her arms and feet. On examination, she is febrile with a temperature of 38°C and looks mildly jaundiced. There is a petechial rash on both forearms and feet (Figure 10.1). Pulse 95 bpm, BP 150/90 mmHg, JVP not visible, normal heart sounds. Chest clear. Abdominal examination showed diffuse tenderness, but no rebound or guarding and no organomegaly.

What does a petechial rash indicate?

Petechiae are small (1–2 mm) red or purple spots, caused by haemorrhage from skin capillaries. The most common cause is physical trauma of the capillaries. This may occur if the patient has a vigorous bout of coughing or vomiting (typically leads to periorbital petechiae) or when a tight tourniquet is applied for a prolonged period. Petechiae can also occur if there is thrombocytopaenia or platelet dysfunction. Occasionally, petechiae occur if blood vessels are more fragile than usual, e.g. vasculitis, although in such cases the amount of haemorrhage is usually greater, leading to purpura (non-blanching, purple lesions >2 mm) rather than petechiae.

The results of Pauline's investigations are shown below. How would you interpret these?

Hb 7.9 g/dL, MCV 100, WBC 14.4 × 10⁹/L (neutrophils),
    Platelets 57 × 10⁹/L
Clotting: PT 13.9 s, APTT 31 s
U+E: Na 139 mmol/L, K 4.7 mmol/L, Urea 14.4 mmol/L,
    Creatinine 268 μmol/L
CRP 155 mg/L, albumin 27 g/L
Urine dipstick shows protein++, blood+++ negative for
    leucocytes, nitrites, and glucose
ECG and CXR are normal

Nephrology: Clinical Cases Uncovered. By M. Clatworthy.
Published 2010 by Blackwell Publishing.

She has significant anaemia, an elevated white cell count and low platelets. The elevated white cell count and CRP are in keeping with systemic infection or inflammation. There is also renal impairment (eGFR 21 mL/min/1.73 m²).

What are the causes of thrombocytopaenia?

Broadly speaking, this can be divided into pathologies which cause a reduced production of platelets, those which cause an increased consumption and conditions in which there is platelet aggregation (summarised in Box 10.1).

What does the MCV suggest about the cause of her anaemia?

The MCV, i.e. size of red cells, is useful and can distinguish between different causes of anaemia, as shown in Table 10.1. In this particular case, the MCV is elevated, therefore it is a macrocytic anaemia.

What tests should you do to investigate the cause of anaemia?

Given that Pauline also has low platelets, one would be concerned about B12/folate deficiency (associated with megaloblasts in the bone marrow and pancytopaenia) so these levels should be measured. However, in megaloblastic anaemia the MCV is often very elevated, i.e. >110 fl.

The presence of jaundice would be consistent with liver disease or haemolysis as a possible cause of macrocytic anaemia. Therefore her LFT should be measured and a haemolysis screen performed. This includes the following.

• Bilirubin: a breakdown product of haem and will be **HIGH** and in its unconjugated form if there is haemolysis and will therefore not be found in urine, although urinobilinogen may be.

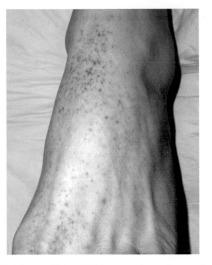

Figure 10.1 A petechial rash. This occurs due to haemorrhage from capillaries, and can be associated with thrombocytopaenia.

Table 10.1 MCV and causes of anaemia

Low MCV (MCV <80 fl) Microcytic anaemia	Normal MCV (MCV 80–95 fl) Normocytic anaemia	High MCV (MCV >95 fl) Macrocytic anaemia
Iron deficiency	Anaemia of chronic disease	B12/folate deficiency
Thalassaemia		Liver disease
Sideroblastic anaemia	Mixed iron and B12/folate deficiency	Alcohol
Aluminium toxicity	Some cases of haemolysis	Hypothyroidism
	Marrow failure, e.g. post chemotherapy	Reticulocytosis, e.g. secondary to haemolysis or haemorrhage

Box 10.1 Causes of thrombocytopaenia

- Reduced production
  - Marrow infiltration, e.g. leukaemia, myelodysplasia/fibrosis
  - Marrow destruction: irradiation
  - B12/folate deficiency (required to synthesise purine bases, which are needed if the DNA for new cells is to be made). This usually leads to a pancytopaenia and a megaloblastic anaemia
  - Drugs: cytotoxins inhibit or kill dividing cells
- Increased destruction
  - Splenomegaly with hypersplenism, e.g. cirrhosis with portal hypertension
  - Antibody-mediated immune destruction, e.g. immune thrombocytopaenic purpura (ITP) or SLE
  - Excess consumption due to inappropriate aggregation, e.g. disseminated intravascular coagulopathy (DIC), HUS, TTP
- Abnormal aggregation

• Reticulocytes: these are immature red cells and are larger than mature erythrocytes. They are called reticulocytes because they have a reticular (lace-like) network of ribosomal RNA within their cytoplasm. They are released from the marrow if there is an excess turnover of RBCs (normal lifespan 120 days). The presence of **HIGH** numbers of reticulocytes (>2%) contributes to the high MCV, although in fact the MCV tends to be biphasic, i.e. there are two populations of cells, some normal-sized mature erythrocytes and then the large reticulocytes.

• Haptoglobin level: this is a plasma protein which binds free haemoglobin released from erythrocytes, for example during intravascular haemolysis. The haptoglobin-haemoglobin complex is then removed by the reticuloendothelial system of the liver and spleen. In cases of haemolytic anaemia, the constant formation and removal of the haptoglobin-haemoglobin lead to **LOW** haptoglobin levels.

• Blood film: damaged red cells may be abnormal in shape or even fragmented.

• Coombs test: this assesses for the presence of an antibody which binds to red cells and causes their destruction. It is positive in cases of autoimmune haemolytic anaemia and negative in cases of microangiopathic haemolytic anaemia.

The results show a bilirubin of 57 μmol/L but otherwise normal LFT.
Reticulocytes 5% (elevated)
Haptoglobin: low
Blood film: fragmented red cells
Coombs test: negative

These features are in keeping with a microangiopathic haemolytic anaemia (MAHA). The differential diagnosis for MAHA is shown in Box 10.2.

Pauline also has a US of her renal tract which shows two normal-sized kidneys with no hydronephrosis or thinning of the cortices. This is in keeping with acute rather than chronic renal failure.

What is the most likely diagnosis?

This patient has the classic features of haemolytic uraemic syndrome (HUS), i.e. the triad of MAHA, thrombocytopaenia and acute renal failure.

What feature of the history is important to go back and clarify?

Haemolytic uraemic syndrome can be associated with diarrhoeal illnesses (D+ HUS), particularly those secondary to verocytotoxin/shigatoxin(Stx)-producing *Escherichia coli* (typically *E.coli* 0157:H7, also known as STEC). This can occur in epidemics, e.g. if food contaminated with bacteria is eaten by a number of individuals. The vero- or shigatoxin is thought to bind to leucocytes and is transported to the kidney where it mediates damage to glomerular endothelial cells via its cellular receptor globotriaosylceramide (Gb3). This promotes the formation of platelet and fibrin microthombi at sites of damage. The turbulent blood flow through these narrowed areas produces sufficient shear stress to cause damage and hae-

Box 10.2 Causes of a microangiopathic haemolytic anaemia (MAHA)

- Disseminated intravascular coagulopathy (DIC): abnormal clotting and low fibrinogen are usually prominent features. Erythrocytes fragment as they pass through strands of deposited fibrin
- Haemolytic uraemic syndrome
- Thrombotic thrombocytopaenic purpura
- Malignant hypertension
- Mechanical destruction of erythrocytes, e.g. associated with prosthetic valves or aortic grafts

molysis of red cells (Figure 10.2). Overall, D+ HUS (also known as Stx-HUS) is more common in children than in adults, and mainly occurs in those under 5 years old. In some circumstances HUS can occur in the absence of diarrhoea – so-called D– or atypical HUS (aHUS).

The history is clarified with Pauline. She did have slightly loose motions in the 2 days prior to presentation, but stools were not watery and she did not pass blood or mucus. She has not eaten anything unusual and is not aware of any friends or relatives with diarrhoea. Her stool culture did not indicate the presence of any pathogenic micro-organisms, including STEC PCR, and her STEC serology is negative.

What other tests should be performed?

D– or atypical HUS is about 10 times less common than D+ HUS and may be familial. Around half of the aHUS cases have a defect in the regulation of the complement cascade, leading to inappropriate activation of the alternative complement pathway, particularly within renal glomerular and arteriolar endothelial cells. Excessive complement activation is due either to loss of function mutations in complement regulatory genes such as factor H, factor I or membrane co-factor protein (MCP, also known as CD46) or gain of function mutations in complement-activating genes such as factor B and C3 (Table 10.2). The mechanisms by which regulator proteins control complement activation is shown in Figure 10.3.

More recently, autoantibodies to factor H and factor I have been demonstrated in some patients with aHUS. These are thought to bind and inhibit normal function, producing a similar phenotype to patients with mutated proteins. The common endpoint is persistent deposition

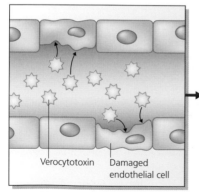
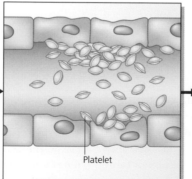
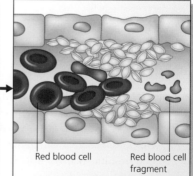

Verocytotoxin | Damaged endothelial cell | Platelet | Red blood cell | Red blood cell fragment

Verocytotoxin or shigatoxin damages endothelial cells

Platelet and fibrin thrombi form at sites of endothelial damage

Red blood cells are destroyed due to turbulent flow through narrowed vessels

Figure 10.2 Pathogenesis of D+ HUS.

Table 10.2 Mutated proteins in aHUS

Complement protein	Normal function of protein	Location of protein	Mutation frequency in aHUS
Factor H	Inhibitor	Plasma	25%
MCP (CD46)	Inhibitor	Endothelial cell surface	10%
Factor I	Inhibitor	Plasma	7.5%
Factor B	Activator	Plasma	5%
C3	Activator	Plasma	10%

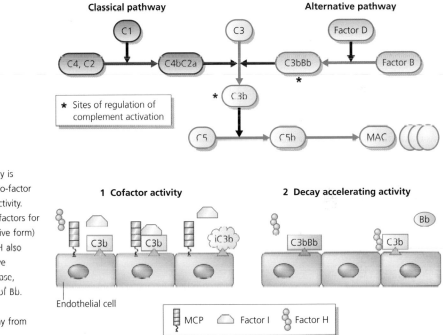

Figure 10.3 The activity of the alternative complement pathway is regulated by two methods: 1. co-factor activity; 2. decay accelerating activity. Both factor H and MCP are co-factors for factor I, which cleaves C3b (active form) to iC3b (inactive form). Factor H also facilitates the decay of the active alternative pathway C3 convertase, C3bBb by causing dissociation of Bb. These mechanisms prevent the alternative complement pathway from being excessively activated.

of activated C3 on endothelium which attracts and activates phagocytes as well as activating the terminal complement components to produce a membrane attack complex (MAC) (Figure 10.4). Both activated phagocytes and MAC can damage endothelium and lead to platelet consumption and haemolysis as described for D+ HUS.

These conditions lead to low C3 levels and normal C4 levels (C4 normal because the classic complement pathway is not activated).

A screen for mutations associated with aHUS is requested and the results are awaited. Complement studies show C3 low, C4 normal. Pauline's renal function continues to decline; the creatinine is now 480 μmol/L.

How should she be managed?

- Supportive treatment
  - Blood and platelet transfusions
  - BP control
  - Haemodialysis if renal function continues to decline
- Plasma exchange: this will require the insertion of a large central line, such as those used for haemodialysis.

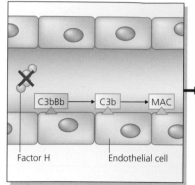
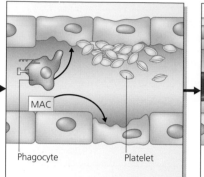
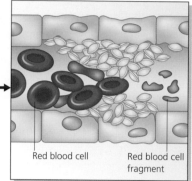

(a) Factor H deficiency or dysfunction leads to inappropriate activation of alternative complement pathway on glomerular endothelial cells

(b) Activated phagocytes and complement membrane attack complex (MAC) mediate endothelial damage, which results in the formation of platelet thrombi

(c) Red blood cells are destroyed due to turbulent flow through narrowed vessels

Figure 10.4 Pathogenesis of D– HUS.

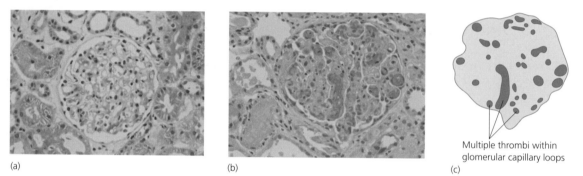

(a)   (b)   (c)

Multiple thrombi within glomerular capillary loops

Figure 10.5 (a) H+E stain of a normal glomerulus. (b) Renal biopsy from a patient with HUS, showing thrombotic microangiopathy. (c) Schematic diagram of the glomerulus shown in (b).

This can be difficult in patients with HUS who may need multiple platelet transfusions before and during line insertion. Fresh frozen plasma (FFP) must be given with the exchange (rather than albumin, which is sometimes used). It is thought that the FFP may help to replenish some plasma complement regulatory proteins. In some refractory cases steroids and intravenous immunoglobulin have been used. Plasma exchange with FFP replacement is also the standard treatment for D+ HUS. In cases where a factor H-binding autoantibody is identified, B cell depletion with the anti-CD20 monoclonal antibody rituximab may prevent relapses.

Pauline undergoes a renal biopsy (Figure 10.5b). What does this show?

The biopsy shows thickening of the glomerular capillary walls. The glomerular capillaries are distended by thrombi, i.e. a thrombotic microangiopathy.

What is the prognosis of her condition?

This depends on the underlying cause. Patients with aHUS and factor H or I mutations have a poor prognosis, with around 70% developing renal failure or dying. Patients with MCP mutations do slightly better, with only 20–30% progressing to ESRF. These patients often run a relapsing/remitting course, but do relatively well nonetheless. Those with autoantibodies to factor H tend to respond well to plasma exchange. In aHUS patients in whom no mutations have been identified, the outcome is probably somewhere between the two, with around 60% alive and dialysis-free at 1 year.

In D+ HUS the prognosis is better, with around 3% mortality and 10–20% progression to ESRF.

The aHUS screen showed a mutation in factor H. Although Pauline's platelet and Hb levels stabilised following a prolonged course of plasma exchange, she remained dialysis dependent.

> **Box 10.3 Clinical features of TTP**
>
> - MAHA
> - Thrombocytopaenia
> - Neurological abnormalities
> - Fever
> - Acute renal failure

What is the difference between haemolytic uraemic syndrome and thrombotic thrombocytopaenic purpura?

Haemolytic uraemic syndrome and TTP have overlapping clinical features, which has often led to difficulties in assigning patients to one diagnosis or another. However, as the pathological mechanisms underlying the two conditions have been better worked out, the distinction is now easier.

Clinically, TTP is characterised by a pentad of features (Box 10.3). Patients with HUS usually have three of these five features but as mentioned above, there is often overlap. In general, HUS is considered to be primarily a renal disease with limited systemic complications whilst TTP is a systemic disease with a relatively low frequency of renal complications.

Thrombotic thrombocytopaenic purpura is now known to be due to an inherited or acquired deficiency of the metalloproteinase enzyme ADAMTS13. This defective function of ADAMTS13 can also be caused by anti-ADAMTS13 autoantibodies in some cases. This protein normally cleaves unusually large multimers of von Willebrand factor oligomers secreted by endothelial cells. In the absence of normal ADAMTS13 activity, uncleaved multimers lead to platelet aggregation and the occlusion or partial occlusion of vessels (Figure 10.6), which in turn causes haemolysis, by the same mechanism as described in Figure 10.3.

Recent research has identified links between HUS and TTP and may explain some of the overlapping clinical features. Platelets activated by shigatoxin may adhere to unusually large multimers of von Willebrand factor that are secreted from toxin-stimulated renal endothelial cells. In addition, shigatoxin has also been shown to impair ADAMTS13 function.

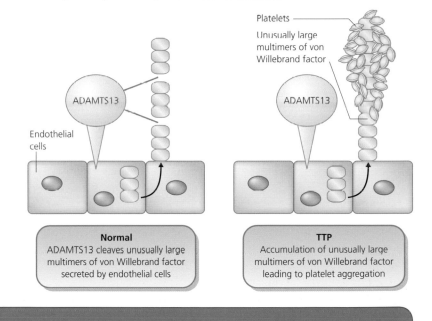

Figure 10.6 Pathogenesis of TTP.

CASE REVIEW

An 18-year-old girl presents with lethargy and headache and is found to have a petechial rash and hypertension. Investigations show haemolysis with fragmented red blood cells on film, thrombocytopaenia and renal failure, features typical of HUS. There is no history of diarrhoea and no evidence of shigatoxin-producing *E. coli* (STEC). A genetic screening reveals a mutation in factor H, one of the complement regulator proteins which can be abnormal in some patients with D− or atypical HUS. She received supportive therapy and plasma exchange but remained dialysis dependent in the long term.

KEY POINTS

- Haemolytic uraemic syndrome is characterised by a triad of microangiopathic haemolytic anaemia (MAHA), thrombocytopaenia and renal failure.
- The most common type of HUS is diarrhoea-associated (D+ HUS/Stx-HUS) which occurs because shigatoxin produced by some bacteria can directly or indirectly damage renal endothelial cells. It mainly occurs in children under the age of 5 years. It is treated supportively and does not require plasma exchange.
- Non-diarrhoeal associated (D– or atypical HUS) is 10 times less common than D+ HUS. More than half of cases are caused because of deficiency or dysfunction of proteins which regulate the alternative complement pathway. Inappropriate activation of complement on glomerular endothelial cells leads to endothelial damage.

- In both D+ HUS and D– HUS the final common pathway of damage is platelet aggregation and consumption at sites of endothelial damage. This causes narrowing of the lumen of blood vessels and red cells are destroyed as they squeeze through.
- Haemolytic uraemic syndrome is treated by supportive therapy (transfusions and dialysis) and plasma exchange, with FFP replacement.
- D+ HUS has a better prognosis than D– HUS.
- Thrombotic thrombocytopaenic purpura and HUS have overlapping features, although patients with TTP are much less likely to have renal involvement.
- The predominant pathology in TTP is deficiency or dysfunction of the metalloproteinase ADAMTS13.

Case 11 A 56-year-old man with ankle swelling

Mr Ieuan Davies, a 56-year-old man, is referred by his GP to the medical team on call with increasing swelling of the legs. In the referral letter the GP states that both legs are swollen to the mid-thighs and the patient is having difficulty walking.

What additional questions would you ask the patient?
• *Duration:* when did the leg swelling first appear?
• *Onset:* sudden or gradual?
• *Extent/distribution:* one leg or both legs involved? Did the swelling start proximally or distally?
• *Swelling elsewhere:* hands/arms? Abdomen? Face?
• Previous similar episodes?

Mr Davies tells you that he first noticed the swelling in both legs around 6 weeks ago. This was initially confined to his ankles but gradually extended upwards to his thighs. His hands have also been slightly puffy, as has his face. He has never had any similar episodes previously.

What are the main differential diagnoses for bilateral leg oedema?
Increased hydrostatic pressure
Swelling can occur because of increased hydrostatic pressure forcing fluid out of vessels. Pathology causing increased hydrostatic pressure includes:
• right heart failure (RHF)/congestive cardiac failure (CCF)
• cirrhosis with portal hypertension
• bilateral venous obstruction due to pelvic mass
• bilateral deep vein thrombosis
• bilateral lymphatic obstruction – previous radiotherapy, filariasis.

Reduced oncotic pressure
Peripheral oedema can also occur if there is a reduction in oncotic pressure within blood vessels, so that fluid is not retained within the vasculature. Intravascular oncotic pressure is maintained by circulating proteins, principally albumin. Hence any pathology in which there is a failure to produce albumin or an abnormal loss of albumin will lead to oedema. Examples include:
• chronic liver disease with reduced protein/albumin synthesis
• nephrotic syndrome with renal loss of protein
• malabsorption with inadequate absorption of protein
• protein-losing enteropathy with GI loss of protein (rare).

What other questions would you ask?
• Does the patient have any other symptoms consistent with RHF or CCF, e.g. orthopnoea, paroxysmal nocturnal dyspnoea (PND)?
• Does he have any significant cardiac past medical history? CCF is likely to occur in a patient with a previous history of cardiac disease, e.g. previous MI.
• Does he have any symptoms of liver disease, e.g. jaundice, symptoms consistent with synthetic failure, e.g. bruising?
• Does he have any significant past medical history of liver disease, e.g. cirrhosis of any cause (alcoholic liver disease, hepatitis B/C, autoimmune liver disease)?
• What is his current alcohol intake? Is this sufficient to cause liver disease?
• Has he noticed any urinary symptoms, particularly frothy urine which is characteristic of heavy proteinuria?
• Does he have any past medical history of renal disease, particularly glomerulonephritides which are known to be associated with nephrotic syndrome, e.g. minimal change, membranous, FSGS?
• Any GI symptoms consistent with malabsorption, e.g. diarrhoea, floating stools?

Nephrology: Clinical Cases Uncovered. By M. Clatworthy.
Published 2010 by Blackwell Publishing.

• Past medical history of pelvic malignancy, e.g. bladder or prostatic cancer?
• Drug history? Some medications are associated with peripheral oedema, e.g. amlodipine.
• Travel history? Filariasis caused by *Wuchereria bancrofti* found in tropics and subtropics, e.g. northern Australia, Pacific Islands, South America, India, West and Central Africa.

> Mr Davies has previously been very fit and healthy. He has not had any heart, liver or kidney problems previously. He has not been short of breath on exertion, nor does he give any history of orthopnoea/PND. He has not noticed any bruising or jaundice, nor has he had any GI symptoms but has noticed that his urine has been frothy in recent weeks. He takes no medications and has never travelled abroad.

What features are important to seek during clinical examination?

Examination should attempt to ensure that there are no signs of cardiovascular disease, particularly CCF, e.g. atrial fibrillation (AF), raised JVP, displaced apex beat, left parasternal heave (right ventricular hypertrophy – RVH), murmurs, bibasal crepitations (pulmonary oedema). Leuconychia indicates hypoalbuminaemia. The presence of jaundice, hepatomegaly, ascites, intra-abdominal masses and lymphadenopathy (inguinal in particular) should be sought. Pleural effusions can occur in patients with nephrotic syndrome. The extent of peripheral oedema should be assessed, as sometimes this can extend up onto the abdominal wall.

> Mr Davies' pulse is 72 bpm and regular. Blood pressure is elevated at 150/85 mmHg, cardiovascular examination is otherwise normal. His chest is clear, with no signs of a pleural effusion. His abdomen is distended with shifting dullness. There is no liver or spleen palpable and no signs of chronic liver disease in the peripheries. He has pitting oedema to his upper thighs and extending onto his anterior abdominal wall. There are no palpable inguinal lymph nodes. He also has mild oedema in his hands.

Given the history and examination so far, what is the most likely cause for his oedema?

There are no symptoms or signs to suggest underlying RHF/CCF or liver disease. The presence of oedema in upper and lower limbs makes venous or lymphatic obstruction unlikely. Given the history of frothy urine together with the widespread oedema and ascites, he is most likely to have nephrotic syndrome.

What investigations would you request in the emergency room?

• Blood tests
  ○ Full blood count
  ○ Renal function (abnormal in some causes of nephrotic syndrome)
  ○ LFT
  ○ Albumin (usually part of LFT)
  ○ Glucose (diabetes can cause proteinuria)
  ○ Cholesterol (frequently elevated in nephrotic syndrome)
• Urine dipstick
• 24-hour urine collection for protein or an albumin/creatinine ratio (ACR) or protein/creatinine ratio (PCR)
• *ECG:* to assess for signs of cardiac disease, e.g. Q waves indicative of previous MI, signs of LVH or RVH
• *CXR:* to assess heart size (looking for cardiomegaly), small pleural effusions (blunting of costophrenic angles), pulmonary masses, e.g. metastases

> Investigations show normal FBC, renal function, LFT and glucose but an albumin of 16 g/dL. Urine dipstick shows protein++++, blood+, negative for leucocytes, nitrites and glucose. ECG is normal, CXR demonstrates a normal cardiac size but a blunted left costophrenic angle (Figure 11.1).

How would you interpret these results?

The investigations are consistent with a diagnosis of nephrotic syndrome with a very low albumin and heavy proteinuria on urine dipstick. His 24-hour urine collection has 12 g of protein in it, confirming this diagnosis (see Part 1, Box C).

What general treatment measures could you begin?

Patients with nephrotic syndrome are treated with diuretics in an attempt to reduce the oedema and bring symptomatic relief. Typically loop diuretics are used, e.g. furosemide, and often high doses will be needed, e.g. 80–150 mg. If the patient has established oedema this may include gut mucosal oedema, making oral diuretics ineffective and necessitating the use of intravenous diuretics. While using diuretics, the patient should be fluid restricted, e.g. 1 L/day.

Regardless of the cause of proteinuria, ACEI or ARB should be started in an attempt to reduce proteinuria.

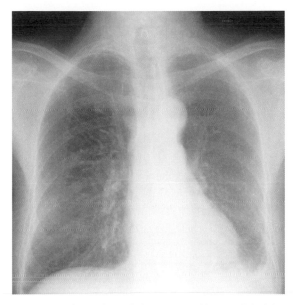

Figure 11.1 Chest radiograph demonstrating blunting of the left costophrenic angle, indicative of a small pleural effusion.

Once the patient has been started on diuretics and antiproteinurics, renal function should be carefully monitored since the patient may be at risk of developing pre-renal failure.

What further specialist investigation would you undertake?

All adults with nephrotic syndrome should proceed to a renal biopsy in order to ascertain the underlying cause. In order to perform a biopsy, patients must undergo an ultrasound scan of the renal tract to ensure they have two kidneys, of a normal size with no obstruction. The patient's clotting should also be assessed prior to biopsy.

A US scan shows two 12 cm kidneys with normal cortical thickness and no hydronephrosis. The patient undergoes a US-guided renal biopsy which on initial H+E shows thickened glomerular capillary loops (Figure 11.2), with IgG deposition on immunostaining and subepithelial deposits on electron microscopy (EM).

How would you interpret these results?

The kidneys are of normal size and cortical thickness on US, suggesting that the patient does not have chronic renal damage. Primary GN likely to cause nephrotic syndrome include minimal change GN, membranous GN

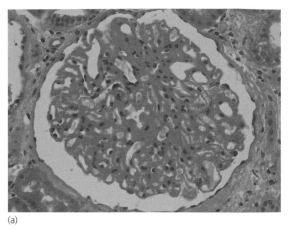

(a)

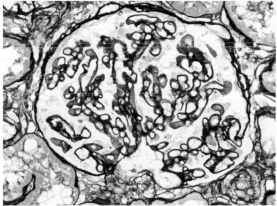

(b)

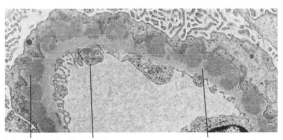

| Sub-epithelial deposits | Endothelium | Basement membrane forming 'spikes' |

(c)

Figure 11.2 Renal biopsy findings in membranous GN. Both H+E (a) and silver staining (b) show thickening of the basement membrane (BM). (c) EM demonstrates sub-epithelial immune deposits and 'spikes' extended from the BM.

and FSGS. In minimal change GN, light microscopy and immunostaining are normal. The findings of thickened glomerular capillary loops and subepithelial deposits are consistent with membranous GN.

> **Box 11.1 Secondary causes of membranous nephropathy**
>
> - Autoimmunity
>   - SLE (Class V lupus nephritis)
>   - Rheumatoid arthritis
>   - Dermatomyositis
> - Infections
>   - Hepatitis B, C
>   - HIV
>   - Leprosy
> - Drugs
>   - Captopril
>   - Penacillamine
>   - Gold
>   - NSAID
> - Malignancy
>   - Carcinomas
>   - Hodgkin's disease
>   - Melanoma
>   - Mesothelioma

Given the biopsy result, are there any additional investigations that you would perform?

Membranous GN is primary (idiopathic) in two-thirds of cases but can occur secondary to a number of other pathologies (Box 11.1) including some malignancies, infection (e.g. hepatitis B) and autoimmune disease (e.g. SLE). Therefore these diagnoses should be excluded by performing the following investigations.

- Investigations for occult malignancy as symptoms dictate, e.g. faecal occult blood (FOB)/endoscopy, PSA if enlarged prostate on examination
- Hepatitis B/C serology
- Autoimmune screen (ANA, anti-dsDNA antibody, anti-Sm antibody, complement (C3/C4), immunoglobulins, rheumatoid factor)

The patient has no symptoms suggestive of an underlying malignancy. Hepatitis serology and autoimmune screen are all negative.

Given the result of the biopsy and additional blood tests, how would you treat this patient?

The investigations are consistent with a diagnosis of primary/idiopathic membranous GN. As well as diuretics

and anti-proteinuric agents, this patient should be anti-coagulated. Given the degree of proteinuria and his albumin of <20 g/dL, most nephrologists would formally anticoagulate with warfarin, aiming for an INR of 2–3 since he is at significantly increased risk of thromboembolic disease. Patients with an underlying cause of membranous GN are particularly prone to thromboembolism, with some series suggesting a rate of 15–20% renal vein thrombosis.

Specific treatments for membranous GN include oral corticosteroids alternating with chlorambucil on a monthly basis (known as the Ponticelli regime). Other immunosuppressants used include cyclophosphamide, ciclosporin and tacrolimus. However, given that some patients undergo a spontaneous remission, many nephrologists would advocate a 6-month period of observation along with the general treatment measures outlined.

The patient asks you whether this disease is curable. What advice would you give him?

Roughly speaking, membranous GN is a disease of thirds: 25–30% get better spontaneously, 25–30% continue to have some proteinuria but stable renal function, 40–50% will develop progressive renal impairment and may eventually require renal replacement therapy.

What are the complications of nephrotic syndrome?

Nephrotic syndrome of any cause is associated with a number of complications, particularly thromboembolism, due to urinary loss of antithrombin III as well as intravascular volume depletion. Studies show that around 10% of patients have PEs detectable on VQ scan, 25% of patients have DVT if Doppler scanned and renal vein thrombosis may occur in 15–20% of nephrotics. Membranous GN is associated with a particularly heightened risk of thromboembolism.

Patients are also at increased risk of infection, e.g. pneumococcal peritonitis, due to urinary loss of immunoglobulins.

CASE REVIEW

A 56-year-old man presents with a gradual onset of worsening oedema. Investigations confirm a low serum albumin and nephrotic range proteinuria. A renal biopsy demonstrates membranous glomerulonephritis. He is treated with diuretics and ACEI and is anticoagulated with warfarin to prevent thromboembolic complications.

KEY POINTS

- Nephrotic syndrome is characterised by a triad of oedema, proteinuria (>3.5 g/24 h) and hypoalbuminaemia. Additional features include hypercholesterolaemia
- All adults with nephrotic syndrome should undergo renal biopsy which assists in identifying the underlying pattern of glomerular damage. Three patterns are commonly seen in adults with nephrotic syndrome.
  1. Minimal change: where light microscopy and immunostaining are normal but podocyte fusion is seen on EM. This pattern is most commonly seen in children and young adults.
  2. Membranous GN is the most common cause of nephrotic syndrome in adults and is characterised by thickening of the glomerular basement membrane.
  3. FSGS: focal (some but not all glomeruli) and segmental (some but not all of a glomerulus) sclerosis/fibrosis.
- Membranous GN is idiopathic in two-thirds of cases. Associations include drugs, SLE, hepatitis B and malignancy.
- Prognosis is variable: 25% of patients with membranous GN go into complete remission spontaneously and around 50% develop progressive renal impairment of varying severity
- Poor prognostic factors include male sex, heavier proteinuria, renal impairment at presentation and tubulointerstitial fibrosis on biopsy.

PART 2: CASES

An 80-year-old man with abdominal discomfort and ankle swelling

Mr John Popham is an 80-year-old man who attends his GP complaining of indigestion and upper abdominal discomfort. His GP diagnoses gastritis and prescribes omeprazole. Two weeks later Mr Popham returns, having had little improvement in his abdominal pain and he has now noted increasing swelling of his legs.

What questions would you ask the patient?

• Duration, nature, onset, site, exacerbating and relieving factors of the abdominal pain.

• Are there any associated abdominal symptoms? For example, loss of appetite, weight loss, nausea, vomiting, haematemesis, jaundice, change in bowel habit, blood PR.

• Is the swelling limited to his legs or is it elsewhere? For example, hands/arms, abdomen, face? Does it involve one or both legs?

The patient has had epigastric and occasionally a more general upper abdominal discomfort for around 2 months. He describes the pain as burning; it sometimes radiates up into his chest and is worse when he lies down and after a large meal. He has also noticed a generalised increase in his abdominal girth, such that his trousers no longer fit. In spite of this increased girth, his weight is actually decreasing and he has lost more than a stone in weight in the last month. He has not noticed any change in bowel habit or other abdominal symptoms. The swelling of his legs began around 2 weeks ago, although he's not quite sure if it predates the omeprazole. It is bilateral and although initially confined to his ankles, it now extends up to his mid shins.

What possible causes would you consider for his upper abdominal pain?

The list of differential diagnoses for abdominal pain is vast. However, this patient's pain is localised to the upper

abdomen. Hence, the main diagnoses to consider are as follows.

• Oesophageal (pain usually retrosternal or epigastric)
  ○ Oesophagitis secondary to acid reflux or infection (e.g. candida)
  ○ Perforation/tear
  ○ Oesophageal cancer
• Gastric
  ○ Gastritis
  ○ Peptic ulceration
  ○ Perforation
  ○ Gastric carcinoma
• Pancreas
  ○ Pancreatitis – pain is worse on lying down, boring through to the back. Vomiting is often prominent
  ○ Pancreatic cancer
• Gallbladder
  ○ Cholecystitis
  ○ Biliary colic
• Liver
  ○ Hepatitis
  ○ Congestive hepatomegaly
• Duodenum
  ○ Duodenal ulcer
  ○ Duodenal malignancy
  ○ Perforation
  ○ Obstruction – pain is colicky in nature
• Non-abdominal
  ○ Myocardial infarction
  ○ Basal pneumonia
  ○ Basal pulmonary embolus

Patients with perforation will have acute peritonitis and are therefore acutely unwell, and generally do not walk into the consulting room. They tend to lie still and do not like being prodded.

The patient's pain sounds very much like gastro-oesophageal reflux, in that it is brought on by eating, radiates retrosternally and is worse if he lies flat. However, he also has a number of worrying features including

Nephrology: Clinical Cases Uncovered. By M. Clatworthy. Published 2010 by Blackwell Publishing.

weight loss and swelling of his abdomen. Abdominal swelling/distension can be caused by the 5 Fs: Fluid, Flatus, Fat, Faeces, Foetus. Specific causes include the following.

• *Flatus (air):* classically gastrointestinal obstruction. This patient's abdominal pain does not have the typical features of obstruction-associated pain (i.e. colicky and cramping in nature, and associated with vomiting).

• *Fluid (ascitic fluid):* ascites can be caused by any pathology in which there is a failure to produce albumin or an abnormal loss of albumin, for example, chronic liver disease with reduced protein synthesis and nephrotic syndrome with renal loss of protein. Ascites can also occur if there is right heart failure or portal hypertension. Ascitic fluid with a high protein content occurs in malignancy and infection.

• *Organomegaly:* hepatosplenomegaly, or massively enlarged polycystic kidneys can give rise to abdominal distension.

> Further history reveals that the patient has previously been very fit and healthy. He has not had any heart, liver or kidney problems and has always 'steered clear of hospitals and doctors' until now. He was an extremely fit 80 year old, living independently and taking daily 1-mile walks until about a month ago. He had not been short of breath on exertion until that time, but now finds exercise increasingly difficult. He has not noticed any bruising or jaundice, but has thought that his urine has been frothy in recent weeks. He takes no medications other than the omeprazole. He is a lifelong non smoker and drinks a bottle of Newcastle Brown ale on most evenings, but never drinks wine or spirits.

What features are important to seek during clinical examination?

The abdominal pain and swelling mean that a careful search should be made for signs of abdominal disease, including liver disease. Weight loss in a man of this age is a worrying feature, and in the absence of signs indicative of hyperthyroidism raises the possibility of internal malignancy. The frothy urine suggests proteinuria (which occurs in a number of glomerulonephritides, some of which can be associated with malignancy, e.g. membranous GN).

Bearing these facts in mind, examination should attempt to confirm or exclude the presence of the following.

• *Hands:* leuconychia (indicating hypoalbuminaemia). Pale palmar creases (anaemia) or koilonychia (iron deficiency).

• Rashes associated with internal malignancy including:
   ○ acanthosis nigricans (dark, slightly raised, velvety eruptions in the inguinal area, sides of the neck, abdomen and mouth)
   ○ erythema gyratum repens (associated with lung, breast, gastric carcinoma)
   ○ Superficial migratory thrombophlebitis, or Trousseau's syndrome, occurs as a cancer-associated coagulopathy. Classically associated with pancreatic or gastric carcinoma.

• Peripheral signs associated with chronic liver disease including jaundice, excoriations, tattoos, xanthelasma, clubbing, telangiectasia, palmar erythema, Dupuytren's contracture and a paucity of body hair.

• Lymphadenopathy, particularly in the left supraclavicular fossa (Virchow's node, Troissier's sign), associated with gastric carcinoma.

• *Cardiovascular system:* raised JVP (RHF), displaced apex beat (LV dilation), left parasternal heave (RVH), murmurs, bibasal crepitations (pulmonary oedema).

• *Respiratory system:* pleural effusions can occur in patients with hypoalbuminaemia or in those with lung cancer.

• *Abdominal system:* hepatosplenomegaly, intra-abdominal masses, ascites (as evidenced by the presence of shifting dullness +/ a fluid thrill. The latter is elicited by getting the patient to place their hand vertically on the midline of the abdomen, whilst the examiner places the palm of their left hand on the left side of the abdomen and flicks the right side of the abdomen with their right hand. If there is a large ascites, a fluid thrill will be transmitted from the right to the left side of the abdomen).

• The extent of peripheral oedema should also be assessed.

> In the peripheries, he has leuconychia (Figure 12.1) but no other signs suggestive of chronic liver disease. His pulse is 82 bpm and regular. Blood pressure is 140/80 mmHg, cardiovascular examination is otherwise normal. Chest is clear with no signs of a pleural effusion. His abdomen is distended with shifting dullness. Both liver and spleen are enlarged (Figure 12.2). He has pitting oedema to his knees. There are no palpable lymph nodes.

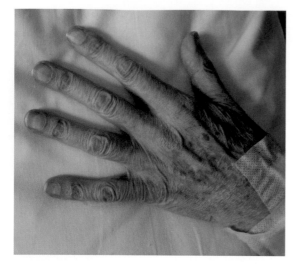

Figure 12.1 Examination of hands showing leuconychia with Beau's lines.

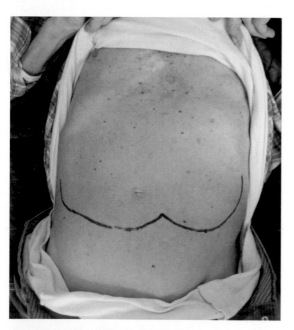

Figure 12.2 Examination of abdomen – massive hepatosplenomegaly.

As the reviewing GP, what initial investigations would you request?

- Blood tests
  - Full blood count
  - Renal function
  - LFT
  - Albumin (usually part of LFT)

> **Box 12.1 Most common causes of nephrotic syndrome**
>
> - Primary GN
>   - Minimal change GN
>   - Membranous GN
>   - FSGS
> - Secondary causes
>   - Diabetes mellitus
>   - SLE
>   - Amyloidosis

  - Glucose
  - Bone function tests (BFT)/calcium (often elevated in malignancy)
- Urine dipstick (given history of frothy urine)
- 24-hour urine collection for protein or ACR if urine dipstick positive for protein
- ECG
- CXR: to assess heart size (looking for cardiomegaly), small pleural effusions (blunting of costophrenic angles), pulmonary masses, e.g. metastases

Investigations show:

Hb 10.1 g/dL, WBC 9.2 × 10⁹/L, Platelets 467 × 10⁹/L
Clotting normal
U+E: Na 138 mmol/L, K 4.4 mmol/L, Urea 18.3 mmol/L,
*   Creatinine 374 μmol/L*
LFT: Bilirubin 7 μmol/L, ALT 27 iu/L, Alk phos 274 iu/L, γGT
*   159 iu/L, Amylase 96 iu/L*
Albumin 24 g/dL
Glucose 5.2 mmol/L
cCa normal
Urine dipstick shows protein++++, blood+ negative for
*   leucocytes, nitrites and glucose*
24-hour protein collection 7.6 g
CXR demonstrates a normal cardiac size but a blunted right
*   costophrenic angle*
His ECG shows first-degree heart block

How would you interpret these results?

The history, examination and investigations show two major features.

- Heavy proteinuria (3.5 g/24 h, i.e. nephrotic range), with a low albumin and oedema (i.e. nephrotic syndrome) in association with significant renal impairment. The most common causes of nephrotic syndrome are shown in Box 12.1.

- Abnormal LFT with massive hepatomegaly. The causes of hepatomegaly are:
  - malignancy (primary or secondary)
  - cirrhosis (early)
  - congestion secondary to right heart failure
  - infection (e.g. hepatitis B, C, EBV, CMV, visceral leishmaniasis)
  - myelo- and lymphoproliferative disorders
  - infiltration (amyloid or sarcoid)

He has no signs indicative of chronic liver disease or right heart failure. Neither does he have any lymphadenopathy or signs of bone marrow failure on FBC which may indicate a myelo- or lymphoproliferative disorder.

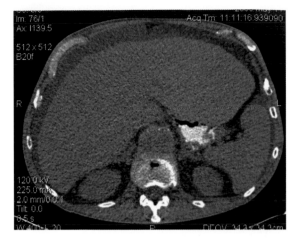

Figure 12.3 CT abdomen showing hepatosplenomegaly with some ascites.

Based on the above, Mr Popham is immediately admitted for further investigation and management under the care of the nephrologists.

What further specialist investigation would you undertake?

All adults with nephrotic syndrome should proceed to a renal biopsy in order to ascertain the underlying cause. In addition, Mr Popham also has significant associated renal impairment of unknown cause. He will need an US scan prior to this to confirm the presence of two normal-sized kidneys and to exclude obstruction. An US scan will also allow confirmation of the presence and size of an enlarged liver and spleen and ascites.

He has abnormal LFT so a hepatic screen should also be undertaken including hepatitis A/B/C, EBV and CMV serology, an autoimmune liver screen (antimitochondrial antibodies and ANA are associated with primary biliary cirrhosis (PBC), and anti-smooth muscle antibodies and anti-liver kidney microsomal (LKM) antibody are associated with chronic active autoimmune hepatitis (CAH)). Immunoglobulin levels can also be useful (polyclonal elevation of IgA in ALD, IgG in CAH and IgM in PBC). Other useful immunological investigations (given that SLE is in the differential diagnosis of nephrotic syndrome) are anti-dsDNA antibody, anti-Sm antibody and complement (C3/C4).

The ECG shows a conduction abnormality, so one might proceed to a 24-hour tape to exclude any significant pauses. In addition, an echocardiogram would be useful to assess whether he has any focal wall abnormalities suggesting ischaemic heart disease or a more generalised myocardial pathology suggesting infiltration or restrictive/hypertrophic cardiomyopathy. Thyroid function tests would also be performed.

Mr Popham has a number of these investigations over the next few days, including US abdomen, which showed a massively enlarged liver, particularly the left lobe. No focal lesions in liver. The spleen also mildly enlarged. The kidneys are both 12.5 cm in size and unobstructed. He also goes on to have a CT scan of his abdomen to screen for intra-abdominal malignancy. This confirms massive hepatomegaly (Figure 12.3), an enlarged spleen and some ascites but does not demonstrate any obvious neoplasm. Other results include:

Autoimmune screen negative (including ANA, dsDNA, ANCA, LKM, mitochondrial, smooth muscle antibodies)
Immunoglobulins: polyclonal IgA increase, no paraprotein band
Hepatitis virology negative (including Hep A, B, C, CMV, EBV)
Echocardiogram:
  Normal LV function, moderate global hypertrophy
  Thickened pericardium
  No restrictive defect

The patient undergoes a US-guided renal biopsy following which he has significant macroscopic haematuria. This lasts for around 3 hours post biopsy and settles spontaneously. However, his repeat haemoglobin has dropped to 7.9 g/dL and he is therefore given a 2 unit transfusion.

What general treatment measures could you begin whilst awaiting the results of the renal biopsy?

Patients with nephrotic syndrome are treated with diuretics in an attempt to reduce the oedema and bring symptomatic relief. Typically loop diuretics are used, e.g. furosemide, and often high doses will be needed, e.g. 80–150 mg. If the patient has established oedema this may include gut mucosal oedema, making oral diuretics ineffective due to reduced absorption and necessitating the use of intravenous diuretics. Whilst using diuretics, the patient should be fluid restricted, e.g. 1 L/day. Daily weights and an accurate fluid balance chart will be useful in the overall management of his oedema.

Normally an ACEI or ARB would be started in an attempt to reduce the proteinuria. However, this patient already has significant renal impairment and given his blood loss post biopsy and your introduction of a diuretic and fluid restriction, his renal function is already at high risk of declining. Therefore in this case, you would hold off an ACEI or ARB and carefully monitor renal function.

> The patient is commenced on furosemide 80 mg intravenously and is placed on a fluid restriction, aiming for a 0.5 kg weight/fluid loss each day. His oedema begins to improve in response to this regimen, but his renal function continues to decline. His creatinine is now 440 µmol/L.
>
> His renal biopsy result returns, showing extensive deposition of an amorphous pink hyaline material on H+E staining, filling much of the mesangium (Figure 12.4). After

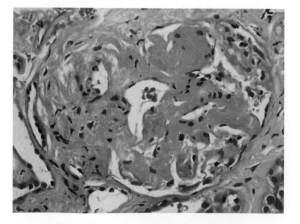

Figure 12.4 Renal biopsy. Deposition of an amorphous pink hyaline material on H+E staining, filling much of the mesangium of this glomerulus.

> Congo red staining, the deposits appear red under normal conditions of light microscopy but show characteristic apple-green birefringence under polarised light. At EM, randomly deposited bundles of non-branching fibrils of 8–10 nm are seen.

How would you interpret these results?

The kidneys are on the large side for a man of 80 years of age (12.5 cm). This immediately suggests the possibility of an infiltrative process. The biopsy changes are typical of renal amyloidosis.

Amyloid is defined as an extracellular substance composed of non-branching, 8–10 nm diameter fibrils which stain apple-green with Congo red when viewed by birefringent light. Fibrils are insoluble and arranged in β-pleated sheets when studied by X-ray diffraction. Each fibril is made from a complex of glycoproteins and proteins, which individually are normally soluble.

Amyloid can be classified as localised (e.g. as seen in Alzheimer's plaques in which Aβ protein precursor forms part of the fibrils) or systemic, as seen in this case. Systemic amyloidosis was traditionally classified into primary (AL) or secondary (AA) forms. AL amyloidosis is considered to be a plasma cell dyscrasia, in which there are plasma cells producing abnormal light chain (quantity and quality usually abnormal). In AL amyloid, these immunoglobulin light chains combine with serum amyloid P (SAP) and glycosaminoglycans (GAG) to form insoluble fibrils. In AA amyloid, fibrils are composed of the acute phase protein serum amyloid A (SAA) together with SAP and GAG (Figure 12.5). SAP and GAG are found in all amyloid fibrils. SAP is a glycoprotein produced in the liver and is a member of the pentraxin family (which includes CRP).

As a variety of constituent proteins in amyloid fibrils have now been identified, the classification system has

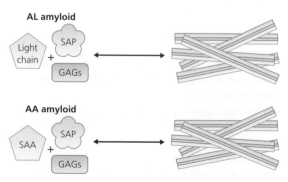

Figure 12.5 Primary (AL) and secondary (AA) amyloid.

Table 12.1 Classification of amyloidoses

Type	Protein	Clinical features
Acquired		
AA	Serum amyloid A	Chronic infection or inflammatory disease (amyloid in liver, kidney and spleen)
AL	Light chain	Plasma cell dyscrasia leading to deposition of amyloid in liver, kidney, heart, nerves, tongue
AβM	β2-microglobulin	Associated with long-term dialysis, fibrils found in joints and ligaments
Inherited		
AA	Serum amyloid A	Periodic fever syndromes, e.g. familial Mediterranean fever (amyloid in liver, kidney and spleen)
ATTR	Transthyretin	Familial amyloid polyneuropathy (amyloid in nerves and heart)
AFib	Fibrinogen Aα	Hereditary non-neuropathic amyloidosis (amyloid in kidneys and liver)
Alys	Lysozyme	As above
AApoAl	Apolipoprotein Al	Hereditary non-neuropathic and neuropathic amyloidosis (amyloid in kidneys, liver and nerves)

evolved so that amyloidoses are now classified according to the protein involved (Table 12.1). Indeed, reinvestigation of patients previously given a label of AL amyloid has led to around 10% being reclassified as having one of the inherited forms.

Given the biopsy result, are there any additional investigations which you would perform?

Biopsies should be stained for SAA to differentiate AA and AL amyloid. Staining for light chains is much less reliable, so the diagnosis of AL amyloid is given if the AA stain is negative. Eighty percent of patients with AL amyloid have a detectable paraprotein in blood or detectable serum or urinary free light chain. They will usually

undergo a bone marrow biopsy which shows <10% plasma cells (i.e. does not reach formal diagnostic criteria for myeloma).

Serum amyloid A is an acute phase protein produced in response to infection or inflammation. Therefore patients with AA amyloid will usually have a source of chronic infection or inflammation, e.g. long-standing rheumatoid arthritis, chronic osteomyelitis or bronchiectasis, which should be sought.

Overall, investigation of a patient with amyloid can be divided into four areas.

• Confirm the diagnosis by biopsy (in this case a renal biopsy), showing typical amyloid fibril deposition and apple-green birefringence of Congo red-stained fibrils under polarised light.

• Find the protein
  ○ Evidence of infection/inflammation
  ○ Family history (FH)
  ○ Serum electrophoresis
  ○ Serum and urine free light chains

• Assess organ involvement. Clinical examination for organomegaly, neurological features, urine dipstick for protein, ECHO for cardiac involvement. The National Amyloid Centre also uses SAP scintigraphy to assess the total amyloid load and the organs involved. This test involves the administration of radiolabelled ^{123}I-SAP which becomes incorporated into amyloid fibrils and can then be viewed radiologically.

• Genetic testing. There are a number of genetic mutations which lead to amyloidosis. For example, mutations in the genes encoding apolipoprotien A-I, lysozyme, transthyretin, fibrinogen Aα have been identified, which lead to the production of abnormal proteins which have an increased tendency to form fibrils. In the UK, all amyloid patients are referred to a specialised centre in which genetic testing occurs.

Mr Popham's renal biopsy is stained for SAA. This is negative, as are stains for light chains. The patient has no serum paraprotein band but does have detectable urinary free light chains. His bone marrow biopsy shows 7% plasma cells, which are polyclonal.

Given the result of the biopsy and additional blood tests, how would you treat this patient?

The investigations are consistent with a diagnosis of primary AL amyloid. The patient has involvement of kidneys, liver, spleen and heart. UK patients with amyloid

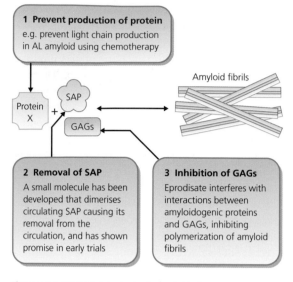

1 Prevent production of protein
e.g. prevent light chain production
in AL amyloid using chemotherapy

Amyloid fibrils

Protein X + SAP

GAGs

2 Removal of SAP
A small molecule has been
developed that dimerises
circulating SAP causing its
removal from the
circulation, and has shown
promise in early trials

3 Inhibition of GAGs
Eprodisate interferes with
interactions between
amyloidogenic proteins
and GAGs, inhibiting
polymerization of amyloid
fibrils

Figure 12.6 Treatment strategies in amyloidosis.

are usually referred to the National Amyloid Centre which is based at the Royal Free Hospital in London.

The treatment depends on the type of amyloid, but generally most strategies involve preventing the production of the excessive or abnormal protein (Figure 12.6). For example, in AL amyloid, chemotherapy+/− bone marrow transplant is used to prevent the production of light chains. In AA amyloid chronic infections are treated

aggressively to prevent the production of SAA and chronic inflammatory conditions can be targeted with anti-TNF-α therapies. In familial cases where the abnormal protein is produced by the liver, e.g. transthyretin mutations, liver transplantation can dramatically improve disease. Newer treatments are being developed which target other components of the fibril, namely SAP and GAG.

The patient asks you whether this disease is curable. What advice would you give him?

AL amyloid has a pretty dismal prognosis, particularly if there is extensive cardiac involvement. In early studies, the median survival was about 1 year while more recent studies suggest a 2–3 year median survival. There are a number of groups actively researching new treatments, and this is facilitated by the presence of a national centre in the UK which can co-ordinate trials.

Mr Popham's renal function continues to decline and he becomes dialysis dependent. He is referred to the National Amyloid Centre and offered treatment with melphalan and prednisolone. After hearing about the side-effects of treatment and the likely limited extension to his lifespan, he decides that he has had 'a good innings' and will opt for palliative treatment only. He dies at home with his family 6 months later.

CASE REVIEW

An 80-year-old man presents with abdominal discomfort and swelling. On examination, he has hepatosplenomegaly, ascites and peripheral oedema. Investigations show that he has nephrotic range proteinuria and renal impairment. A renal biopsy demonstrates changes consistent with AL amyloidosis. His oedema is treated with diuretics and he is offered chemotherapy for the amyloid, but declines. He is managed conservatively and dies comfortable at home 6 months later.

KEY POINTS

- This is a complex case, which illustrates that the kidneys may be involved in a multisystem disease (such as amyloid). The key in such cases is to think about the underlying causes of each problem separately, and then look at where there are overlapping pathologies which account for all features.
- Mr Popham's clinical presentation was typical of amyloidosis, with massive organomegaly, cardiac

conduction disturbances and renal involvement with nephrotic syndrome. Other presenting features include periorbital ecchymoses and prominent bruising. This occurs due to blood vessel fragility, resulting from amyloid fibril deposition in blood vessel walls and in skin. Hence patients with amyloid will sometimes have a significant bleed following a renal biopsy (as in this case).

- As well as enlargement of internal organs such as the liver, spleen and kidneys, some patients will also have an enlarged tongue (macroglossia). Neurological involvement can also occur, including sensorimotor peripheral neuropathy (often with enlarged, palpable peripheral nerves), as well as autonomic neuropathy and compression neuropathies such as carpal tunnel syndrome.
- Some patients present with cardiac problems, particularly cardiac failure due to a restrictive cardiomyopathy or conduction defects (as seen in this patient). Echocardiogram can demonstrate a typical 'bright speckled pattern' or merely thickening of atria and ventricles.
- Amyloid is defined as an extracellular substance composed of non-branching, 8–10 nm diameter fibrils which stain apple-green with Congo red when viewed by birefringent light, are insoluble and arranged in β-pleated sheets.
- Systemic amyloidosis is mainly an acquired disorder cause by dysgammaglobulinaemia, chronic infection or inflammation. It is classified according to the type of protein found in the fibril, e.g. AL (light chain) or AA (serum amyloid A). There are also a number of familial forms of amyloidosis.
- The overall prognosis is still relatively poor. With current treatments, the median survival in a patient with AL amyloid is now up to 50 months in some series using more aggressive therapeutic regimens, while for AA amyloid it is around 130 months.

Case 13 A 23-year-old obese woman with ankle swelling

Miss Bronwen Price is a 23-year-old woman who is referred to the renal services with ankle swelling and proteinuria. The referral letter states:

'Thank you for assessing this 23-year-old female who came up to the surgery today complaining of increasing ankle swelling and shortness of breath. Her BP was elevated at 145/90 mmHg and she has pitting oedema to the knees. Her urine dipstick showed 4+ protein. The other main point to mention is that she is currently seeing the practice dietician, because she has a significantly elevated BMI'.

What is the most likely cause of her ankle swelling?

A reduction in oncotic pressure in circulating blood.

Peripheral oedema can occur because of an increased hydrostatic pressure which drives fluid out of the vessels into the interstitium (as occurs in right heart failure, cirrhosis with portal hypertension or venous obstruction) or a reduced oncotic pressure – that is, fluid seeps out of the vessels because there is inadequate circulating protein to exert an osmotic pressure sufficient to keep it there. A reduction in oncotic pressure occurs in any condition which leads to low levels of plasma protein, the most important of which is albumin. Plasma protein levels can be low in hepatic failure with inadequate protein synthesis or malabsorption of protein from the gut, as can an excessive loss of protein from the urine. In this case, the presence of heavy proteinuria on dipstick points towards renal loss of protein with subsequent hypoalbuminaemia and a reduction in oncotic pressure as the likely cause of oedema.

Examination shows an overweight young lady (105 kg) who is 1.63 m tall. She is afebrile and has no obvious rashes. Pulse is 90 bpm and regular. BP is 150/90 mmHg. Her JVP is

not elevated. Her heart sounds (HS) are quiet, but there are no obvious additional sounds. Respiratory examination demonstrates reduced expansion bilaterally and a stony dull percussion note at the right base with reduced breath sounds. Abdominal examination is unremarkable, other than that there is a large apron of fat. She has pitting oedema to the mid thighs.

What are the causes of quiet or inaudible heart sounds?

Assuming there are likely to be HS (i.e. the patient is alive and has a pulse!) then they can be quiet because fluid (pericardial effusion), air (COPD with hyperinflated lungs or bullae) or fat (obesity) lies between the heart and the stethoscope. In this case, it is likely to be the latter. Pericardial effusions are associated with quiet heart sounds, hypotension and an elevated JVP, which make up Beck's triad. She does not have the other features of pericardial effusion, and there is no history or examination features which makes COPD likely (e.g. hyperinflated chest).

What is her Body Mass Index, based on the clinic examination?

$$BMI = weight\,(kg)/(height\,(m))^2$$

In this case, $105/1.63^2 = 39.5\,kg/m^2$. A BMI of $>30\,kg/m^2$ is classified as obese, $>40\,kg/m^2$ is classified as extreme/morbid obesity.

What are the critical investigations which should be performed in clinic?

• *Pregnancy test:* pregnancy can be associated with proteinuria and hypertension (pre-eclampsia). Although the presentation is not typical, pregnancy should always be excluded in any young woman presenting with hypertension.

• *Quantification of proteinuria:* the clinical presentation is suggestive of nephrotic syndrome, with peripheral oedema and proteinuria on dipstick. This should be

Nephrology: Clinical Cases Uncovered. By M. Clatworthy.
Published 2010 by Blackwell Publishing.

quantified, by either a 24-hour urine collection and ACR or PCR. If proteinuria exceeds 3.5 g/24 hours then this is nephrotic range proteinuria.

• *Quantification of serum albumin:* the diagnosis of nephrotic syndrome requires the triad of oedema, hypo-albuminaemia (30 g/L) and >3.5 g proteinuria/24 hours. Therefore, serum albumin should be assessed.

• *U+E:* she has significant hypertension. Hypertension can be both a cause and an effect of renal disease. Hypertension can cause end-organ damage in the kidney with thickening of vessel walls. In addition, both acute and chronic kidney disease (of any cause) can be associated with hypertension so it is important to determine renal function.

• *CXR.*

What would you expect her chest X-ray to show?

The examination findings (stony dull percussion note at the right base with reduced breath sounds) are consistent with a small right-sided pleural effusion. Other causes of a dull percussion note include an elevated right hemidiaphragm, pleural plaques/thickening and consolidation.

Investigations show:

Na 140 mmol/L, K 3.5 mmol/L, Urea 8.2 mmol/L, Creatinine 123 µmol/L

Albumin 22 g/L, cholesterol 7 mmol/L, glucose 6.8 mmol/L

24 hour urine collection – 7 g protein

CXR – blunting of right costophrenic angle

Comment on these results

Miss Price has renal impairment. Although a creatinine of 123 µmol/L does not seem greatly elevated, this value gives an eGFR of 50 mL/min/1.73 m^2 (normal GFR is around 100 mL/min/1.73 m^2). The low albumin, nephrotic range proteinuria and elevated cholesterol are all consistent with nephrotic syndrome.

The random glucose is high, so she may have impaired glucose tolerance (IGT) or even frank diabetes. IGT is a pre-diabetic state that is associated with insulin resistance. IGT is formally defined by the patient having two random glucose levels of between 6 and 7.8 mmol/L or a 2-hour glucose level of 7.8–11.0 mmol/L following a 75 g oral glucose tolerance test.

Blunting of the right costophrenic angle on CXR is consistent with a small right-sided pleural effusion.

A renal US scan is undertaken. Although views are suboptimal, she appears to have two normal-sized, unobstructed kidneys.

What conditions (for which Miss Price should be screened) can cause nephrotic syndrome?

She should be screened for secondary causes of nephrotic syndrome, including SLE (ANA, dsDNA, IgG, C3/C4), infections such as hepatitis B/C and HIV, and plasma cell dyscrasias such as AL amyloidosis (serum paraprotein, serum/urine free light chains).

In Miss Price's case, the above investigations are all normal/ negative.

What investigation should be performed next?

The general rule is that all adults with nephrotic syndrome should undergo renal biopsy in order to determine the underlying cause, unless there is a clear contraindication, e.g. single kidney.

Her blood pressure is optimised (by starting an ACEI; see later) and she undergoes a US-guided renal biopsy. This is a difficult procedure because of Miss Price's body habitus and requires three passes before renal tissue is obtained. She is placed on bed rest and standard 'biopsy obs'. Her post-biopsy observation chart is shown in Figure 13.1.

What does this show and what is the likely cause?

The chart shows a tachycardia and drop in BP post biopsy. This is most likely to be due to significant haemorrhage. Other causes of haemodynamic instability such as pulmonary embolism or myocardial infarction are less likely, although the former should be borne in mind because nephrotic syndrome is a major risk factor for venous thromboembolism.

Within 15 minutes of the biopsy, Miss Price feels that she is desperate to pass urine. Given the instruction that she should be maintained on bed rest, a bed pan is provided. She promptly passes 500 mL of bright red, heavily blood-stained urine.

How would you mange this lady?

Given the haemodynamic instability, intravenous access should be obtained as quickly as possible (preferably two

Renal Biopsy Care Plan

Name	Miss Bronwen Price
No.	

Problem	Date & Sign	Plan	Date & Sign	
Potential haemorrhage, pain and/or infection following renal biopsy.		Explain reason for biopsy and details of procedure and post-biopsy care to patient.		
Reason for biopsy: DIAGNOSIS OF RENAL IMPAIRMENT		Ensure patient has the following:		
		Hb, clotting, group & save 2 units	✓	AB
		Consent	✓	AB
Aim		Baseline BP, temperature & pulse	✓	AB
To prevent or detect and treat any pain,		Urinalysis	✓	AB
haemorrhage and/or infection following biopsy		Check need for FFP/platelets	✓	AB
		Prepare trolley and assist with procedure		
		Post-Biopsy care:		
Evaluation		Bedrest for 6 hours (unless doctor specifies longer)		
Time of biopsy:	10:00 AB	BP, pulse and wound check:		
		1/4 hrly for 2 hours		
		1/2 hrly for 2 hours		
		hourly for 2 hours		
		Then 6 hourly		
		Check patient has pased urine -note any haematuria		
		Monitor pain, note type & severity-use pain scale		
		Give analgesia if required as prescribed		
		Assist with hygiene/elimination needs		
		Inform patient of result and intended treatment		

Time	10:00	10:15	10:30	10:45	11:00	11:15	11:30	11:45	12:00	12:30	13:00	13:30	14:00	15:00	16:00							
Pain score	8	9	10	7	7	6	6	5	4	4	3	3	1	1	1							
Site	✓	✓	Bleed		✓	✓	✓	✓	✓	✓	✓	✓	✓	✓								

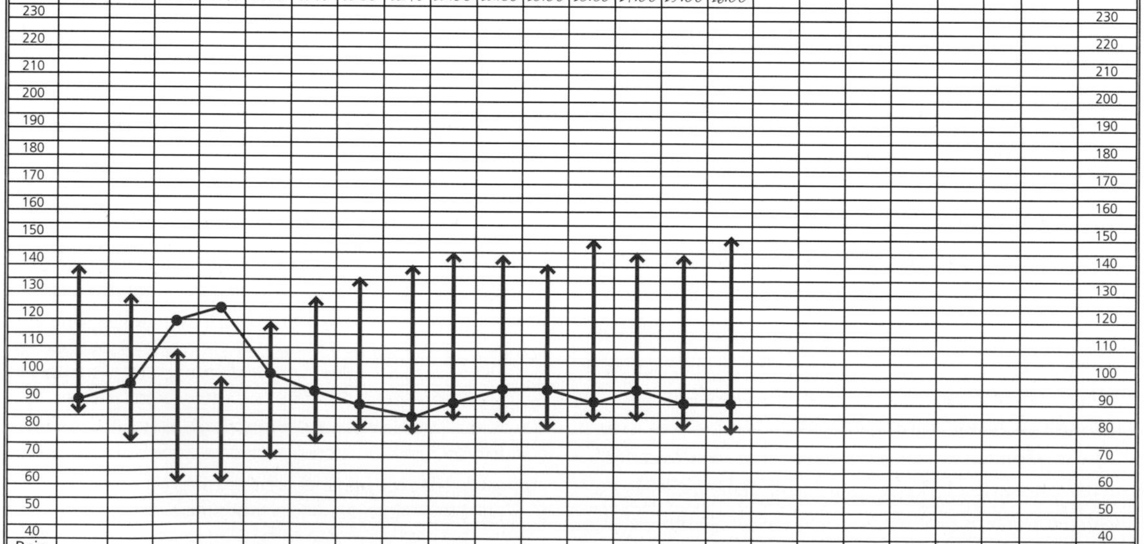

Please date, time and sign all entries

Figure 13.1 The patient's observation chart post-renal biopsy.

large cannulae in reasonable sized veins), and any fluid (colloid or crystalloid) given in an attempt to restore her intravascular volume.

On inserting the cannula, blood should be withdrawn and sent for a FBC, U+E, clotting and urgent cross-match of four units of blood.

A three-way urinary catheter should be inserted to allow flushing of the bladder with saline to prevent the formation of clot. If clot forms in the bladder, this is extremely uncomfortable for the patient and may require removal by cystoscopy.

The patient is given 500 mL of Gelofusine. Her pulse drops to 95 bpm and her BP comes up (see chart). A three-way urinary catheter is inserted (Figure 13.2). The fluid flushing the bladder continues to be heavily blood-stained and a repeat Hb shows that her Hb has dropped from 13 g/dL pre-biopsy to 9 g/dL. In view of the ongoing bleeding, she is given a two-unit transfusion. Unfortunately, over the next 12 hours the bleeding fails to settle, and she requires an additional two units of blood.

What further management would be appropriate at this stage?

Renal angiography should be undertaken so that a coil or glue can be deployed at the bleeding point.

Miss Price undergoes renal angiography with coil insertion. This procedure is successful, and the haemorrhages stops.

The primary glomerulonephritides causing nephrotic syndrome are:
- minimal change
- membranous
- FSGS
- membranoproliferative glomerulonephritis (MPGN).

What is her biopsy likely to show?

Overall, membranous GN is the most common cause of nephrotic syndrome in adults but in younger adults, minimal change is more likely. However, in Miss Price's case, her increased BMI is potentially a significant aetiological factor. Obesity is well known to be associated with FSGS, so-called 'obesity-related glomerulopathy' (ORG).

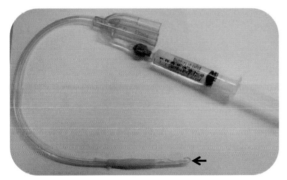

(a) The tip of the catheter (arrow) is introduced into the bladder. Note: a three way catheter is much larger than a regular urinary catheter.

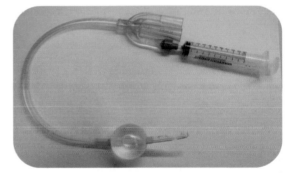

(b) Once in the bladder, the balloon is inflated with 10 mL of sterile water. This prevents the catheter from slipping out of the bladder.

(c) Urine+/−debris/blood clots drain through a large opening at the tip of the catheter — A second tube/port allows the delivery of irrigation fluid into the bladder

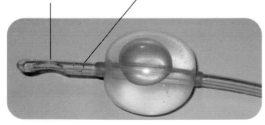

(d) Irrigation fluid is delivered though one port (blue arrow), urine/blood clots are drained via a second port (yellow arrow), whilst the third port is used to deliver fluid to the balloon.

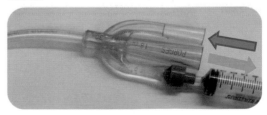

Figure 13.2 A three-way catheter is used to flush the bladder.

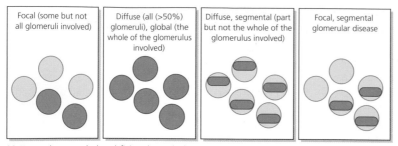

(a) Nomenclature used when defining glomerular lesions

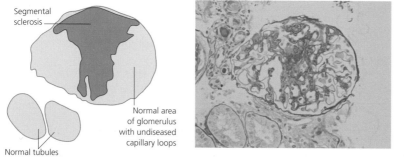

(b) Typical biopsy changes in FSGS

Figure 13.3 Renal biopsy changes in FSGS. (a) Nomenclature used when defining glomerular lesions. (b) Typical biopsy changes in FSGS.

Studies suggest that the incidence of ORG has increased more than 10-fold in recent years, making up 0.2% of all renal biopsies in the 1980s but 2% of biopsies in the late 1990s.

Her biopsy is shown in Figure 13.3(b). Which of the above listed glomerulonephritides is the biopsy compatible with?

Focal segmental glomerular sclerosis, with sclerosis of the central segment of the glomerulus. In patients with obesity-associated FSGS, there is often also glomerulomegaly.

The diagnosis of FSGS requires the presence of areas of glomerular sclerosis and tuft collapse that are both focal (some but not all of glomeruli affected) and segmental (a segment, but not all, of the glomerulus is affected). In idiopathic FSGS, immunostaining is often positive for IgM and C3, and there is epithelial cell (podocyte) foot process effacement on electron microscopy.

How should Miss Price be managed?
General management measures

• Diuretics in order to reduce oedema. Typically high-dose loop diuretics are used, e.g. furosemide 80–150 mg. If the patient has established oedema, this may include gut mucosal oedema, making oral diuretics ineffective and necessitating the use of intravenous diuretics together with fluid restriction, e.g. 1 L/day.
• Antiproteinuric medications including ACEI or ARB.
• Blood pressure control (usually achieved with an agent that has a combined antihypertensive and antiproteinuric effect, i.e. ACEI, ARB).

Specific management of ORG

• Weight loss has been shown to bring about dramatic improvements in proteinuria. Restoration of weight to the normal range can lead to a complete remission. Methods of treating obesity include strict diet, appetite suppressants, behaviour therapy or even more radical measures such as gastric bypass surgery.
• Treatment of elevated cholesterol with statins.

Specific management of idiopathic FSGS

In idiopathic FSGS, a trial of immunosuppression is often undertaken. Immunsuppressants which have been used include steroids, ciclosporin-A, tacrolimus, chlorambucil, cyclophosphamide, azathioprine and mycophenolate mofetil. A recent (2008) Cochrane review of FSGS treatment showed that although corticosteroids remain the mainstay of treatment in idiopathic FSGS, only about 20% of patients experience a partial or complete remission of nephrotic syndrome with treatment. Three studies of ciclosporin-A (CSA) treatment were analysed and showed that there was a significant increase in the number of participants who obtained complete or partial remission with CSA plus low-dose prednisone versus prednisone alone.

Some nephrologists would give a trial of immunosuppressants to patients with ORG if the above basic management techniques of antiproteinurics and weight loss were unsuccessful.

Miss Price asks about the likely outcome of her kidney disease and whether the condition can be cured. What would you say?

Overall, the prognosis for ORG is better than for idiopathic FSGS, with a much slower progression to ESRF. For example, in one of the largest studies of this disorder, 4% of patients with ORG progressed to ESRF in a median of 93 months, in contrast to 42% of patients with idiopathic FSGS who progressed to ESRF in a median of 63 months. The proteinuria in patients with ORG is frequently very responsive to ACEI or ARB. In addition, normalisation of BMI or even a modest reduction in weight can significantly improve disease

What is known about the pathophysiology of obesity-related glomerulopathy?

The pathophysiology of ORG is thought to be related to hyperfiltration injury. Adipose tissue can produce a number of potentially vasoactive components, including angiotensinogen. In addition, adipose tissue also produces adiponectin, a protein which reduces insulin resistance. In obesity, adipose tissue produces less adiponectin and serum levels are low. This is of interest because adiponectin appears to be important for normal podocyte function, with adiponectin-deficient mice showing podocyte foot process effacement and proteinuria. Even modest weight loss can increase adiponectin levels in obese subjects, and this may well contribute to the improvement in proteinuria seen in such subjects.

In association with which other major disease does focal segmental glomerular sclerosis occur, which has markedly increased in prevalence in the last two decades?

Human immunodeficiency virus (HIV) infection. HIV-related renal diseases are the third most common cause of ESRF among African-Americans aged 20–64 years. The most common lesion seen on biopsy is HIV-associated nephropathy (HIVAN), a glomerulopathy demon-

Box 13.1 Secondary causes of FSGS

- Obesity
- HIV
- Reflux nephropathy
- Sickle cell disease

Table 13.1 Genes mutated in familial FSGS

Gene	Chromosome	Protein	Inheritance
NPHS1	19q	Nephrin	AR
NPHS2	1q	Podocin	AR
ACTN4	19q	α-actinin 4	AD
TRPC6	11q	Transient receptor potential cation channel 6	AD

strating FSGS with marked collapsing features (collapse of the glomerular capillary tuft). Other renal lesions observed in HIV include amyloidosis, minimal change disease, cryoglobulinaemia and various forms of immune-complex glomerulonephritis, such as IgA nephropathy, membranous nephropathy and MPGN. HIVAN is more common in Afro-Caribbeans with HIV and tends to improve when HIV is aggressively treated with highly active antiretroviral therapy (HAART).

The secondary causes of FSGS are listed in Box 13.1.

Why is it important to ascertain whether there is a family history of renal disease in patients with focal segmental glomerular sclerosis on biopsy?

A number of inherited/familial forms of FSGS have been identified in the last decade (summarised in Table 13.1). These include both autosomal dominant and recessive forms. The best defined include the following.

• *Nephrin mutations (congenital nephropathy of the Finnish type):* this is an autosomal recessive condition which presents with nephrosis *in utero*. Mutations have been identified in the nephrin gene, NPHS1 on chromosome 19q. The nephrin protein is found within slit diaphragms of podocytes (Figure 13.4). Nephrin knockout mice also develop severe early FSGS.

• *Podocin mutations (steroid-resistant nephrotic syndrome):* this is an autosomal recessive form of nephrotic syndrome. The causative gene is found on chromosome 1q (NPHS2) and encodes a protein podocin. In the

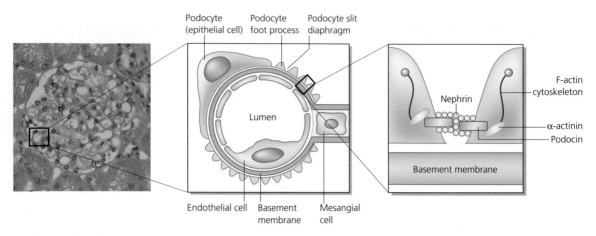

Figure 13.4 The podocyte slit diaphragm.

kidney it is exclusively expressed in podocytes and is localised to the base of foot processes on either side of the slit diaphragm (see Figure 13.4). Podocin-deficient mice also develop early nephrotic syndrome.

Does focal segmental glomerular sclerosis recur in renal transplants?

Inherited forms of FSGS will not recur in transplants because the transplanted kidney will have non-mutated podocin, nephrin, α-actinin-4 or TRPC6 because they are encoded by the donor's genes.

In patients with secondary FSGS, the disease will not recur, providing the primary problem is dealt with, e.g. the BMI of an obese person is restored to somewhere near normal range. Most transplant centres would not list patients for a transplant unless their BMI was

$<35\,kg/m^2$. In some centres criteria are stricter, in an attempt to avoid an excess operative mortality.

In patients with idiopathic FSGS, the recurrence rate post transplant is around 30%. Recurrent disease is characterised by the development of heavy proteinuria in the early post-transplant period. This can occur rapidly, even within hours of transplantation, and untreated has a poor prognosis, with 50–80% graft loss within 1 year. Treatment is with plasma exchange. In patients with a history of aggressive primary FSGS with treatment-resistant nephrosis, some centres advocate pre-emptive plasma exchange prior to transplantation.

If FSGS recurs in the first transplant then recurrence in subsequent transplants is between 80% and 100%, so repeat transplantation is not recommended.

CASE REVIEW

This is a case of a young, obese woman who presented with nephrotic syndrome. Investigations, including a renal biopsy, demonstrated FSGS or ORG. The renal biopsy was complicated by haemorrhage which required radiological intervention with coiling. The patient's nephrosis improved with ACEI and weight loss.

KEY POINTS

- Focal segmental glomerular sclerosis may be primary or familial or may occur secondary to obesity, HIV or reflux nephropathy.
- The first report of an association between obesity and nephrotic range proteinuria (termed obesity-related glomerulopathy (ORG)) was published in the 1970s, with renal biopsy showing glomerulomegaly and FSGS.

- Patients with FSGS (with associated proteinuria) should be treated with ACEI and ARB. Those with ORG should lose weight, as this can lead to dramatic improvements in proteinuria. Primary (idiopathic) FSGS may respond to immunosuppression with prednisolone and ciclosporin.
- Primary FSGS recurs in renal transplants in around 30% of patients.

A 15-year-old girl with facial swelling and frothy urine

Roberta Howley is a 15-year-old girl with a 2-week history of facial swelling. It is worse first thing in the morning and gradually improves throughout the day. She has also noticed some swelling of her ankles in the last 3 days and that her urine has become quite frothy. She has no past medical history and is not taking any medications.

What does a history of frothy urine suggest?

This is in keeping with heavy proteinuria.

On examination she is slim, comfortable and afebrile. BP is 110/65 mmHg, there is mild periorbital swelling and pitting oedema to the mid shins. Examination is otherwise unremarkable.

Investigations show:

Urine dipstick proteinuria 4+. Negative for haematuria, nitrites and leucocytes
Albumin 18 g/dL
Na 136 mmol/L, K 4.0 mmol/L, Urea 4 mmol/L, Creatinine 50 µmol/l
24-hour urine protein – 5 g
US renal tract – two unobstructed, normal-sized (10 cm) kidneys

What is the most likely diagnosis?

The patient has the clinical features of nephrotic syndrome (oedema, hypoalbuminaemia, heavy proteinuria >3.5 g/24 h). In younger children, nephrotic range proteinuria is considered to be present if there is >50 mg/kg/day. In children, the most common cause of nephrotic syndrome is minimal change GN, occurring in 80–90% of cases of childhood nephrosis.

Nephrology: Clinical Cases Uncovered. By M. Clatworthy.
Published 2010 by Blackwell Publishing.

In children, nephrotic syndrome tends to present with facial and particularly periorbital oedema. The latter can be so severe that the child may have difficulty opening their eyes, and can be wrongly diagnosed as a severe allergic reaction. Peripheral oedema and ascites can develop quite rapidly and result in hypovolaemia. Younger children frequently complain of abdominal pain which is presumed to be due to oedema of the gut mucosa.

Some paediatricians assess the selective protein excretion in urine. How is this measured and what is its potential significance?

Selective protein excretion indicates that the glomerular barrier is partially intact; that is, only low molecular weight proteins are being filtered, e.g. transferrin, whereas higher molecular weight proteins such as IgG remain in the circulation. It is calculated as follows

$$\frac{\text{Urine IgG (mol wt 150 kDa)}}{\text{Urine transferrin (mol wt 40 kDa)}}$$

A value of <0.1 is indicative of highly selective proteinuria, which tends to occur only in minimal change. In other primary glomerulonephritides, proteinuria tends to be non-selective.

Should Roberta undergo a renal biopsy to confirm the diagnosis of minimal change glomerulonephritis?

As with all glomerulonephritides, the only way to confirm the diagnosis of minimal change is to undertake a renal biopsy. However, in children with nephrotic syndrome, minimal change is by far the most likely diagnosis, so the risks of biopsy are generally considered to outweigh potential diagnostic benefit, particularly in children aged 1–8 years. There are a number of features which might make a nephrologist consider biopsy in a nephrotic child prior to empirical treatment. These include:

- presence of microscopic or macroscopic haematuria
- presence of significant hypertension
- presence of renal insufficiency
- presence of systemic features suggestive of secondary nephrosis, e.g. rash or joint pain consistent with SLE.

Renal biopsy is also considered in children who fail to respond to treatment or in those who respond to treatment initially but then develop frequent relapses.

Roberta has no features to suggest anything other than a diagnosis of minimal change GN. She is therefore started on treatment empirically, without a biopsy.

What treatment should be started?

Roberta should be started on high-dose oral corticosteroids (e.g. $60\,mg/m^2$/day, maximum $60\,mg$/day). Calcium and vitamin D therapy are often prescribed with steroids, as is some gastric protection (ranitidine or proton pump inhibitor). This treatment should be continued for 1 month. Some physicians would also give antifungal prophylaxis with nystatin or amphotericin. If there is an adequate response, the steroids should be reduced gradually (usually by initially moving to an alternate-day regimen for 1–2 months) and are weaned by around 4 months.

Diuretics such as furosemide may be helpful in managing oedema.

Her parents ask about the potential side-effects. What do you tell them?

High-dose, long-term corticosteroids have a number of unwanted side-effects as shown in Box 14.1. However, provided Roberta responds to the first course of treatment, there are unlikely to be any long-term adverse effects from treatment. Problems tend to arise if children have steroid-resistant disease or frequent relapses.

Box 14.1 Side-effects of corticosteroids in children

- Weight gain
- Growth impairment
- Osteoporosis
- Gastric ulceration
- Skin changes – acne, poor wound healing, easy bruising
- Hypertension
- Impaired glucose tolerance
- Proximal myopathy
- Increased susceptibility to infection

Her parents ask you whether steroid treatment is likely to cure the problem

More than 90% of children will respond to corticosteroids. Indeed, complete remission is considered to be almost diagnostic of minimal change GN in the absence of biopsy. Response tends to occur within 1–2 weeks of starting treatment. However, only 30% of children will continue in remission; the remaining 70% will have a relapse of some sort. In 10% this occurs more than 3 months after withdrawal of treatment. These patients should be re-treated as for primary presentation; 60% will relapse whilst on reducing therapy or less than 3 months following cessation of steroids.

Roberta is started on oral corticosteroids. She is reviewed in clinic 10 days later and her urine dipstick is now negative for protein. She continues on high-dose steroids for 1 month and then moves onto a reducing regimen at this stage. On review at 6 weeks, there is now 4+ protein on dipstick and she has once again developed periorbital oedema.

How should Roberta be managed following her relapse?

Given her age (>10 years) and the presence of a relatively rapid relapse, some nephrologists would perform a biopsy at this stage to confirm the diagnosis. Others would increase her oral corticosteroids once again and biopsy only if there was a second relapse.

Roberta is biopsied. This shows changes typical of minimal change GN (Figure 14.1).

Describe the changes seen

As the name 'minimal change' suggests, the renal biopsy looks completely normal on light microscopic examination (Figure 14.1a). Immunostaining is entirely negative. The only changes visible are on electron microscopy which shows podocyte foot process fusion (Figure 14.1b).

How would you treat Roberta now?

The corticosteroids should be increased again until complete remission is achieved. Steroids can again be reduced at this stage. If there is a further relapse then a steroid-sparing agent such as levamisole or ciclosporin should be considered. Levamisole is an agent recently introduced which was shown to have a steroid-sparing effect in children with minimal change in a British Association for Paediatric Nephrology study in the early 1990s and has a relatively good side-effect profile.

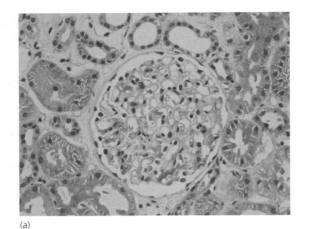

(a)

Normal renal biopsy

Patient's renal biopsy

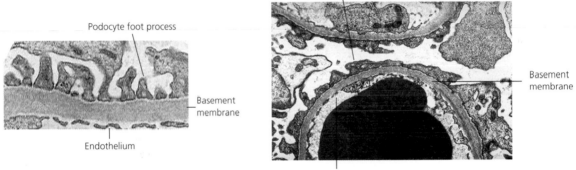

(b)

Figure 14.1 Minimal change GN. (a) H+E staining showing a normal glomerulus. (b) Electron microscopy showing podocyte effacement and fusion of foot processes.

If there is persistant nephrotic range proteinuria and hypoalbuminaemia, then anticoagulation should be considered in order to prevent thromboembolic disease (see case 11). However, this is rarely required in children.

Roberta goes into remission again after just a week of treatment. Steroids are weaned over a more prolonged period (6 months). She remains in remission at 6 months post steroid withdrawal.

Minimal change is associated with a number of diseases. What are they and which is the most commonly observed association in children?

Minimal change GN is associated with:
- Atopy (hayfever/eczema/asthma)
- Hodgkin's disease
- carcinoma (in older adults).

Atopy is the most common association in childhood. In addition, minimal change can be associated with drugs, such as NSAID, and with bee stings.

CASE REVIEW

Roberta is a 15-year-old girl who presents with facial and peripheral oedema and frothy urine. Investigations show nephrotic range proteinuria and a low albumin. In children with nephrotic syndrome, the most likely diagnosis is minimal change. She is therefore treated empirically with oral corticosteroids and responds quickly. She relapses during corticosteroid withdrawal but responds to a second course of high-dose steroids.

KEY POINTS

- Minimal change is the most common cause of nephrotic syndrome in children.
- As in adults, the main complications are infection, thrombosis, hypovolaemia and those related to treatment.
- Children with nephrotic syndrome do not need to undergo renal biopsy unless there are atypical features such as haematuria, significant hypertension and renal impairment.
- More than 90% of children will respond to corticosteroids, although around 70% will have some sort of relapse.

- Relapses should be treated with a further course of high-dose corticosteroids. Steroid-sparing agents such as levamisole or ciclosporin should be considered in these cases, particularly if children have growth impairment or other steroid-associated side-effects.
- Around 5–10% of children will be truly steroid resistant and may go on to to develop lesions consistent with FSGS. Some of these will develop ESRF.

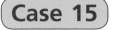 **A 50-year-old woman with hypertension**

Mrs Colleen Charvis is a 50-year-old factory worker who attends her GP practice after an employment medical showed a BP of 165/95 mmHg.

Is this one-off reading sufficient to diagnose Mrs Charvis with hypertension?

No. There should be at least 2–3 readings which are consistently high. Every effort should be made to measure blood pressure accurately. Ideally, the patient should be relaxed (difficult for some patients with so-called white coat hypertension). They should not have any tight clothing and the sphygmomanometer cuff should be an appropriate size (the bladder should encircle at least 80% of the arm).

Mrs Charvis comes to see the practice nurse on two separate occasions, 1 month apart, to have her BP checked. On the first occasion it is 155/90 mmHg, on the second it is 165/95 mmHg.

How would you classify this blood pressure?

Blood pressure is classified according to Table 15.1. If systolic BP and diastolic BP fall into different categories then the higher category should be taken.

Mrs Charvis is reviewed by her GP, who decides that she has Grade 2 (moderate) hypertension and that this is most likely to be essential (primary) hypertension.

What questions should the GP cover in this consultation?

Ninety-five percent of patients who present with elevated blood pressure have essential hypertension (EH). In <5%

there is an underlying cause. Risk factors for EH include:
- increasing age
- BMI >25
- sedentary lifestyle (on average less than 30 minutes of brisk exercise/day)
- high alcohol intake (>3 units/day (men), 2 units/day (women))
- salt intake greater than 6.0 g/day (2.g of sodium)
- environmental stressors.

Mrs Charvis should therefore be asked about these lifestyle factors. In addition, hypertension is a risk factor for atherosclerosis, therefore she should be assessed for other risk factors so that these can be optimally managed. These include:
- smoking
- family history of vascular disease
- cholesterol
- diabetes mellitus
- previous MI/PVD/CVA

Are there any symptoms or signs which might indicate a secondary cause for hypertension?

As stated above, the majority of patients with high blood pressure will have EH. However, in younger patients (<40 years) or in those with severe hypertension, a secondary cause should be sought. Secondary causes of hypertension are listed in Box 15.1 and are mainly due to renal disease (renovascular or chronic kidney disease of any cause), endocrine diseases which affect renal sodium excretion, e.g. Cushing's disease, or pregnancy.

Mrs Charvis works in an electronics factory. Her job largely involves sitting down. She does no regular exercise and smokes 20 cigarettes/day. She tells you that she only drinks on weekends, and then only a gin and tonic or two on a Saturday night. She has no past medical history, and rarely attends the GP surgery. On examination, Mrs Charvis is a

Nephrology: Clinical Cases Uncovered. By M. Clatworthy.
Published 2010 by Blackwell Publishing.

portly lady with a BMI of 32 kg/m². She does not have any tendon xanthomata or xanthelasma visible. Her pulse is 90 bpm and regular, JVP is not elevated. Her apex beat is difficult to palpate but her heart sounds are audible. There is a soft systolic murmur at the lower left sternal edge which does not radiate. Chest is slightly hyperinflated but clear to auscultation. Abdominally, there is a central distribution of adiposity but no organomegaly or masses, and no audible bruits. Her fundi have retinal changes consistent with Grade 3 hypertensive retinopathy (see Box 15.2), including AV nipping and flame haemorrhages.

Table 15.1 BHS classification of hypertension

	Systolic BP (mmHg)	Diastolic BP (mmHg)
Normal	<130	<85
High-normal	130–139	85–89
Grade 1 (mild)	140–159	90–99
Grade 2 (moderate)	160–179	100–109
Grade 3 (severe)	>180	>100

Box 15.1 Secondary causes of hypertension

Renal diseases
- CKD of any cause
- Renal artery stenosis (due to atheromatous disease in 90% of cases and fibromuscular dysplasia in 10% of cases, usually young women)
- Chronic pyelonephritis
- Adult polycystic kidney disease (autosomal dominant, therefore there may be a positive family history, see case 20)
- Acute glomerulonephritis (hypertension is one of the presenting features of nephritic syndrome, seen in IgA nephropathy, postinfectious GN, lupus nephritis)
- Autoimmune diseases – vasculitis (particularly polyarteritis nodosa (PAN)), systemic sclerosis (can present with scleroderma crisis in which there is accelerated hypertension)

Endocrine disease
- Cushing's syndrome
- Conn's syndrome
- Phaeochromocytoma
- Acromegaly
- Diabetes mellitus

Drugs
- Corticosteroids
- Erythropoietin
- Fludrocortisone
- Non-steroidal anti-inflammatory drugs
- Oral contraceptive
- Sympathomimetics (in some cold cures)
- Liquorice

Pregnancy
- Pre-eclampsia
- Eclampsia
- Haemolysis, elevated liver enzymes, low platelets (HELLP)

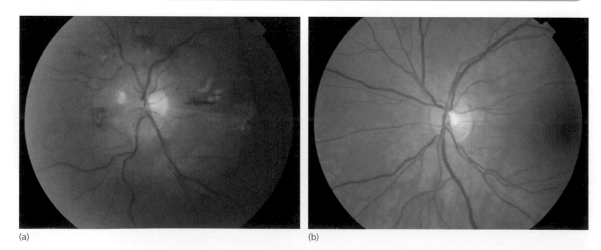

(a)   (b)

Figure 15.1 (a) Retinal changes in malignant hypertension including papilloedema and flame haemorrhage Grade 4 retinopathy. A normal retina is shown in (b) for comparison.

Chronic hypertension can also cause end-organ damage elsewhere including the heart and kidneys.

The heart

Chronic hypertension provides an increased pressure against which the left ventricle (LV) must pump. Like any other muscle consistently exercised, it will hypertrophy. Left ventricular hypertrophy (LVH) can be detectable clinically as a hyperdynamic, heaving apex beat (the term 'heaving' is usually used to describe a pressure-over-loaded LV and the term 'thrusting' to describe a volume-overloaded LV). The ECG may show signs of left axis deviation and LVH (sum of S in V1/2+ R in V5/6 >35 mm) (Box 15.3) and there may be cardiomegaly on CXR. As LVH progresses, the cardiac muscle may outstrip its blood supply, leading to ischaemic cardiomyopathy and LV dilation. The apex beat may then become displaced from its normal position in the fifth intercostal space, midclavicular line. If there is significant LV dilation, then cardiomegaly becomes readily visible on CXR (Figure 15.2).

The kidneys

Hypertension is a major cause of CKD. Typical biopsy changes include thickening of arterioles and interstitial fibrosis in advanced disease (Figure 15.3).

Box 15.2 Retinal changes in hypertensive retinopathy

Grade 1
- Silver wiring and AV nipping (vein is squashed/nipped by thickened artery)
- Narrowing of retinal arterioles (normal ratio of artery:vein is 1/1.1)

Grade 2
- Variable calibre of retinal arterioles (areas of constriction and dilation)

Grade 3
- Haemorrhages – flame haemorrhages and blot haemorrhages
- Cotton wool exudates

Grade 4
- Papilloedema – consistent with malignant hypertension (Figure 15.1a)

Box 15.3 ECG changes associated with chronic hypertension

- Left ventricular hypertrophy – sum of S in V1or V2 + R in V5 or V6 >35 mm
- Left axis deviation (LAD) – a simple way to determine this is to look at whether the complexes are predominantly downwards in II and III. If so, there is likely to be LAD. To precisely determine axis, look at leads I, II, III, aVR, aVL, aVF. The axis of the heart lies at a right angle to the most isoelectric lead
- Left heart 'strain pattern' – ST depression/T wave inversion in V5/V6

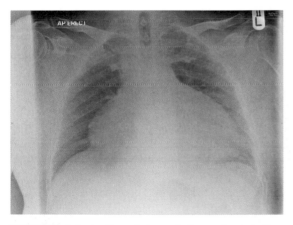

Figure 15.2 A chest radiograph demonstrating cardiomegaly. Even though this is an AP film (and therefore not ideal to assess heart size), the cardiac shadow is abnormal and occupies significantly more than 50% of the total thoracic diameter.

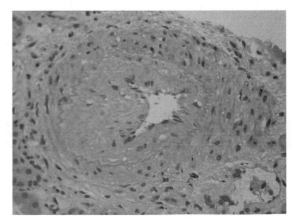

Figure 15.3 Renal biopsy showing an artery with intimal thickening which significantly reduces the luminal diameter. Such changes are typically seen in patients with chronic hypertension.

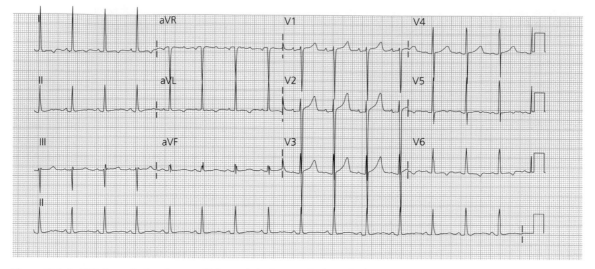

Figure 15.4 An ECG demonstrating changes of left ventricular hypertrophy (sum of S in V2+R in V5 >35 mm).

What investigations would you perform?

Routine investigations in hypertension include:
- Urine dipstick for blood and protein which may indicate CKD
- serum creatinine and electrolytes
- blood glucose (assess for impaired glucose tolerance or diabetes)
- serum total cholesterol/HDL ratio
- ECG.

Investigations show:

Hb 12.1 g/dL, WBC 6.2 × 10⁹/L, Platelets 259 × 10⁹/L

U+E: Na 139 mmol/L, K 4.5,mmol/L, Urea 6.3 mmol/L,
  Creatinine 88 μmol/L (eGFR = 63 mL/min/1.73 m²)

Glucose 5.8 mmol/L

Total cholesterol 5.7 mmol/L

Urine dipstick shows protein trace, negative for blood,
  leucocytes, nitrite, and glucose

Comment on Mrs Charvis' ECG (Figure 15.4)

The ECG is in sinus rhythm but shows LVH (sum of S in V2 + R in V5 >35 mm) and strain (T wave inversion in V5–6, aVL).

Could lifestyle changes be effective in reducing Mrs Charvis' blood pressure?

Modifying lifestyle factors such as diet, alcohol intake and exercise can significantly lower blood pressure. In the

Dietary Approaches to Stop Hypertension (DASH) study, hypertensive patients increased the fruit and vegetables in their diets from two to seven portions per day and reduced the average systolic BP by 7 mmHg and diastolic BP by 3 mmHg. If this is a low-fat diet then the reduction achieved may be as great as 11 mmHg in the systolic BP and 6 mmHg in the diastolic BP.

Alcohol moderation to less than or equal to 21 units in men and 14 units in women per week can reduce the systolic BP by around 3–4 mmHg.

Weight loss is also associated with a reduction in the systolic BP. For each 10 kg loss (above a BMI of 25 kg/m²) the expected fall in the systolic BP is 5–10 mmHg.

The current British Hypertension Society guidelines recommend that younger patients should do three vigorous aerobic training sessions a week and older patients should be encouraged to do 20–30 minutes of brisk walking as long as the blood pressure is mild/moderate and reasonably well controlled. Examples of aerobic activity include walking, cycling and swimming.

Dietary salt should be restricted to 6 g per day. This equates to 2.4 g of sodium per day (1 g sodium = 2.5 g of salt). Although food labels are often unclear, the average salt intake for the general population is nearer 10 g.

Should Mrs Charvis' hypertension be treated?

Yes. Trials indicate that drug therapy should be offered to patients with persistently raised blood pressure of 160/100 mmHg or more, or patients with blood pressure

> **Box 15.4 Recommended targets for blood pressure treatment**
>
> - Non-diabetic without CKD <140/85 mmHg
> - Diabetic without CKD <140/80 mmHg
> - Diabetic with CKD <125/75 mmHg
> - Non-diabetic with persistent proteinuria >1 g/24 h <125/75 mmHg

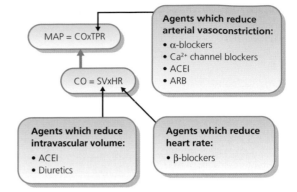

Figure 15.5 The action of anti-hypertensive agents.

of greater than 140/90 mmHg with either a raised cardiovascular disease risk or target organ damage. In Mrs Charvis' case, the aim should be to get her BP to <140/85 mmHg. Current British Hypertension Society recommended targets are shown in Box 15.4.

Which anti-hypertensives might you start Mrs Charvis on?

Mrs Charvis should be started on an ACEI. She has a reduced GFR and protein+ on dipstick (CKD stage 3), therefore an ACEI has additional anti-proteinuric and renal preservation benefits. There are a number of different classes of anti-hypertensive agents.

- Angiotensin-converting enzyme inhibitors (ACEI)
- Angiotensin receptor II blockers (ARB)
- β-Blockers
- Calcium channel blockers
- Diuretics (thiazide, potassium sparing)
- α-Blockers

Each class acts by reducing either CO (by lowering HR or SV) or TPR (Figure 15.5).

The British Hypertension Society has provided guidelines for the use of anti-hypertensives, which are summarised in Figure 15.6. The indications and contra-indications of different anti-hypertensive medications are summarised in Table 15.2.

Given her additional cardiovascular risk factors, Mr Charvis is also commenced on aspirin 75 mg and a statin to reduce cholesterol.

What is malignant hypertension?

Malignant hypertension is said to occur when there is severe diastolic hypertension (>120 mmHg) with Grade

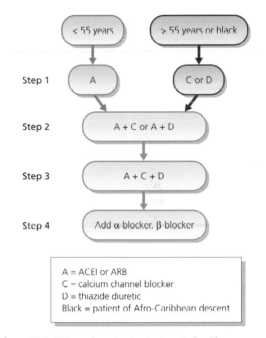

Figure 15.6 BHS new hypertension treatment algorithm.

3 or 4 retinopathy. Patients may have associated renal impairment, proteinuria, encephalopathy or cardiac failure. The characteristic histological feature on renal biopsy is arterial fibrinoid necrosis. It is a medical emergency and requires hospitalisation and specialist management.

Table 15.2 Indications and contraindications for antihypertensive medications

Class of drug	Indications	Caution/contraindications

ACEI	Patients with early CKD and proteinuria
	Patients with LV dysfunction post MI
	Diabetes mellitus
		Pregnancy
		Renovascular disease/renal artery stenosis (RAS)
		  (young, black males tend to have a poor
		  response)

ARB	Patients intolerant of ACEI Diabetes mellitus	Pregnancy Renovascular disease/RAS
α-Blockers	Benign prostatic hypertrophy	Postural hypotension Urinary incontinence
β-Blockers	Post MI Angina	Asthma /COPD Peripheral vascular disease Heart block
Calcium channel blockers	Elderly Angina	Can exacerbate peripheral oedema
Thiazide diuretics	Elderly Isolated systolic hypertension	Gout Can worsen impaired glucose tolerance

CASE REVIEW

A 50-year-old lady presents with persistent moderate hypertension and signs of end-organ damage with early retinopathy and left ventricular hypertrophy. Secondary causes of hypertension are considered unlikely, given that she has a number of risk factors for EH including an increased BMI and sendentary lifestyle. She is managed by giving lifestyle advice (stop smoking, more exercise, lose weight) and is started on an ACEI.

KEY POINTS

- Hypertension should not be diagnosed on a one-off reading. There should be at least two measurements, using an appropriate sized cuff.
- Blood pressure should be monitored every 5 years in all adults until the age of 80 years. Those who are known to have a high/normal BP (see Table 15.1) should be monitored annually.
- Ninety-five percent of hypertension is essential or primary, with no obvious secondary cause. Risk factors for EH include an increased BMI, older age, high alcohol intake, high salt (sodium) intake, sedentary lifestyle and environmental stressors. Modification of these factors can significantly improve BP.
- Hypertension is a major risk factor for other morbidities. Specifically:
  - CVA (7× increase)
  - coronary artery disease (3× increase)
  - cardiac failure (4× increase)
  - peripheral vascular disease (2× increase)
- Treatment is advised if BP is persistently >160/100 mmHg or >140/90 mmHg with evidence of target organ damage. In diabetics, treatment should be given if BP >140/90 mmHg.
- Start with an ACEI/ARB or β-blocker (for <55 years, non-black) or a calcium channel blocker or diuretic if >55 years or Afro-Caribbean.
- Consider giving aspirin and statins if there are other cardiovascular risk factors.

Case 16 A 60-year-old male smoker with hypertension and renal impairment

Mr Bob Shanklin is a 60-year-man who presents to his GP with hypertension. He has been referred to the renal services because the GP started him on an ACEI but this produced a sharp rise in his creatinine from its baseline of 129 μmol/l to 250 μmol/L. The ACEI was therefore stopped and he has been referred to the nephrologists.

Mr Shanklin's past medical history includes an MI at the age of 58 years, hypertension (diagnosed at the time of the MI) which has been poorly responsive to medications, and COPD (for which he takes prn salbutamol inhalers). He also gets symptoms of claudication (cramping pain in the calves) on walking 50 yards, which are worse in the left leg than in the right.

He is a smoker of 40/day (since the age of 16 years), drinks around 30 units of alcohol a week, and works as taxi driver.

His medications include:
- *aspirin 75 mg od*
- *bendroflumethiazide 2.5 mg od*
- *amlodipine 10 mg od*
- *simvastatin 20 mg od*

What examination features are often found in patients with a history of claudication?

• Tar staining of fingers from long-term cigarette smoking.

• Tendon xanthomata, xanthelasma or arcus senilis due to hyperlipidaemia.

• Signs of vascular disease in other parts of the body. For example, the presence of carotid bruits or abdominal aortic/renal artery bruits.

• The abdomen should be examined for the presence of an expansile, pulsatile mass (which may indicate an abdominal aortic aneurysm (AAA)).

Nephrology: Clinical Cases Uncovered. By M. Clatworthy.
Published 2010 by Blackwell Publishing.

• Absent or reduced pulses with audible bruits. Particularly peripheral pulses in the lower limbs (popliteal, dorsalis pedis + posterior tibial pulses; Figure 16.1).

• Ischaemic changes in the skin at the peripheries, e.g. feet may look white or dusky, have hair loss, reduced capillary refill (>4 s) or even ulceration. Ischaemic ulcers tend to occur peripherally over bony prominences, particularly the lateral malleoli. The typical appearance of an ischaemic ulcer is one with a deep base and vertical punched-out edges. In cases of severe ischaemia, the foot may become necrotic and gangrenous.

On examination there is arcus senilis of the cornea. The patient's pulse is 85 bpm and regular, BP is 160/95 mmHg, heart sounds are normal but there is a bruit audible over the right carotid artery. His chest is mildly hyperinflated, with an increase in resonance on percussion throughout his chest. On examination of the abdomen, there is no obvious AAA but there is a definite bruit. The left femoral pulse is present but on auscultation has a loud bruit. Both foot pulses (dorsalis pedis + posterior tibial pulses) are missing on the left, as is the popliteal pulse. On the right, all pulses are palpable, except for the posterior tibial. The left foot looks slightly mottled and has poor capillary refill (6 s). There are no obvious ulcers on the feet.

In a patient with a history of claudication it is useful to assess for critical ischaemia by performing Buerger's test. How is this performed?

The patient is placed supine on an examination couch. Legs are raised at 45° for 2–3 minutes. The patient is then sat up and the legs allowed to hang over the side of the bed. Buerger's test is positive if the feet become white on elevation and hyperaemic when hanging dependent.

Measurement of the Ankle Brachial Pressure Index (ABPI) is also useful (compare the systolic blood pressure in the arm with that in the leg). The ankle pressure will be lower if there is ischaemia in the limb. If the ABPI is

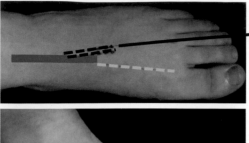

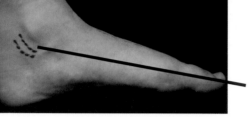

Dorsalis pedis pulse
The artery normally travels between the 1st and 2nd metatarsals (red bar) and branches at this point. It can be identified by tracking up the medial edge of the 1st metatarsal (dashed green line).
In this subject, it is situated quite medially (dashed black lines).

Posterior tibial pulse
Lies posterior to the medial malleolus.

Figure 16.1 Lower limb peripheral pulses. These become impalpable if there is peripheral vascular disease.

<0.5 (i.e. systolic blood pressure in the ankle is less than 50% of that in the arm), then critical ischaemia is said to be present.

Which antihypertensive agents are contraindicated in patients with peripheral vascular disease?

β-Blockers – these can worsen claudication symptoms.

Mr Shanklin has a number of investigations performed in clinic (results shown below).

Hb 16.0 g/dL, WBC 5.4 × 10⁹/L, Platelets 357 × 10⁹/L

Na 139 mmol/L, K 3.8 mmol/L, Urea 10.3 mmol/L, Creatinine 135 μmol/L

Cholesterol 6.5 mmol/L

Normal Ca/PO₄/LFT

Urine dipstick: protein+, negative for blood, leucocytes, nitrites

CXR: hyperinflated lung fields (>6 anterior ribs visible with flattening of the diaphragm)

ECG: LVH

Comment on these results

These show mild polycythaemia (in keeping with chronic hypoxia secondary to COPD). His U+E demonstrate renal impairment with an eGFR of 50 mL/min/1.73 m². His CXR shows hyperinflation, consistent with COPD. His ECG shows that he is in sinus rhythm but has LVH (sum of S in V1 or V2+R in V6 or V5 is >35 mm).

Do you think Mr Shanklin's hypertension is idiopathic/ primary or do his history and examination suggest a secondary cause?

Mr Shanklin is an arteriopath, with multiple vascular risk factors. Examination demonstrates arterial disease throughout his peripheral vascular tree. In addition, he has an abdominal bruit. He also has a history of a significant decline in renal function following introduction of an ACEI. All of these features are suggestive of RAS as the likely cause of his hypertension.

Atherosclerosis is the underlying cause of renovascular disease in >90% of patients with RAS. Ninety percent of lesions are ostial (i.e. occur within 1 cm of the renal artery origin). Many patients will also have atherosclerotic disease in intrarenal vessels in addition to the main renal artery. Risk factors include:

- increasing age
- hypertension
- smoking
- dyslipidaemia
- diabetes mellitus.

Hypertension occurs because the macula densa interprets the reduced intrarenal pressure associated with RAS as systemic hypotension. Renin will therefore be released, which will activate the angiotensin-aldosterone pathway in an attempt to increase blood pressure. The ultimate effect is vasoconstriction and sodium retention (hence water retention, and an expansion in intravascular volume). This will lead to a rise in blood pressure by increasing TPR and SV and hence CO (see Box 16.1).

Box 16.1 Determinants of mean arterial pressure (MAP)

$$MAP = CO \times TPR$$
$$CO = SV \times HR$$

Patients with RAS frequently have CKD or even ESRF. Amongst elderly patients with ESRF, it is a common finding (10–15%), although it may not be the cause of ESRF in some but an incidental finding which occurs as a result of the chronic hypertension and accelerated atherosclerosis observed in CKD of any cause.

Renal artery stenosis can also be caused by fibromuscular dysplasia (FMD), a disease of unknown aetiology characterized by fibrous thickening of the intima, media or adventitia of the renal artery. FMD accounts for just 10% of RAS and usually occurs in young (15–30 years) women. Thus, this is unlikely to be the diagnosis in Mr Shanklin's case. Rarer causes of RAS include vasculitis, aneurysms of the aorta and compression by tumours.

Why is there a marked decline in renal function in patients with renal artery stenosis who are commenced on angiotensin-converting enzyme inhibitors?

The GFR is critically dependent on the tonic constriction of the efferent arteriole to maintain intraglomerular pressure. This constriction is maintained by angiotensin. Introduction of an ACEI reduces angiotensin concentration and thus efferent arteriolar constriction, and GFR.

What further investigations would you perform?

• *US renal tract:* this frequently shows asymmetrical kidneys in patients with renovascular disease (asymmetry is usually considered significant if there is >2 cm difference in bipolar length). Other indicators of RAS on ultrasound include the Arterial Resistance Index, but this can be technically difficult to measure in patients with a high BMI.

• *MR angiography:* both MRI and CT provide a way of non-invasively imaging the renal arteries. MR (requires the use of gadolinium-containing contrast agents) was the preferred method, but is now contraindicated in patients with an eGFR of <60 mL/min/1.73 m^2, due to the occurrence of nephrogenic systemic fibrosis (NSF) in some patients with renal impairment. NSF is a rare but serious fibrosing condition that most often affects the skin overlying the limbs but can also affect other internal organs, including the lungs. The first report on NSF was published in 1997 and there is mounting evidence that this condition is associated with renal failure and the administration of some types of gadolinium. It is thought that gadolinium can accumulate, causing an increase in proliferation of dermal fibroblasts, with deposition of collagen and elastin. Research suggests that the gadolinium-containing contrast agents most likely to release gadolinium, and thus most closely associated with disease, have a linear non-ionic structure. Those least likely (safest) to release free gadolinium ions have a cyclical structure. Many patients with suspected renovascular disease will have a GFR of <60 mL/min/1.73 m^2, so this technique is now of limited use in such patients.

• *CT angiogram:* can allow visualisation of vessels, but a high load of iodine-containing contrast agents may be required.

• *Conventional intra-arterial angiography:* although this is an invasive technique, it is useful in patients with complex anatomy and also allows intervention, such as angioplasty and stenting (where appropriate), which can be performed at the same time.

Mr Shanklin's ultrasound shows that the right kidney is 9 cm and the left 11 cm, with no obvious hydronephrosis. He has an angiogram performed. His U+E are performed the next day and show a marked decline in renal function, with Na 142 mmol/L, K 4.6 mmol/L, Urea 18.3 mmol/L and Creatinine 324 μmol/L.

Why has Mr Shanklin's renal function declined so rapidly?

The most likely reason is contrast-induced nephropathy. This is defined as a >25% increase in serum creatinine following administration of a contrast agent (usually post CT or angiography). It is a relatively common cause of acute renal dysfunction in hospitalised patients. Risk factors include:

• CKD
• diabetes mellitus
• dehydration
• poor LV function
• high dose of contrast
• administration of nephrotoxins.

Alternatively, instrumentation of the aorta and renal artery can lead to the production of cholesterol emboli. This is less likely here, as Mr Shanklin did not have any intervention during the procedure. Cholesterol emboli are thought to break off from arterial plaques (spontaneously or in association with instrumentation or thrombolysis) and can become lodged in the renal tubules, causing interstitial inflammation and a decline in renal function. This may be associated with a peripheral eosinophilia +/− eosinophiluria and obvious emboli elsewhere (often evidenced by purpuric lesions or livedo reticularis in the peripheries).

What measures can be taken to reduce the risk of contrast-induced nephropathy?

High-risk patients should be prehydrated, e.g. 1 litre of normal saline over 4–6 hours before the procedure. Note: care must be taken not to give large volumes of fluid too quickly in these patients who frequently have co-existing LV dysfunction. Other strategies used to prevent contrast-induced nephropathy (CIN) include the administration of N-acetyl cysteine or sodium bicarbonate before the procedure.

Contrast-induced nephropathy usually causes reversible renal failure, and with hydration and removal of other nephrotoxins renal function normally improves. Occasionally the associated decline in GFR is severe enough to require temporary renal support with one or two sessions of haemodialysis.

Mr Shanklin's angiogram shows right renal artery stenosis (Figure 16.2).

How should this patient be managed?

- Lifestyle advice – stop smoking, low cholesterol diet, increase exercise, reduce alcohol intake.
- Increase dose of statin (simvastatin 40 mg).
- Revascularisation procedure. If there is a >75% occlusion of the artery, with declining renal function, then most nephrologists would advocate intervention; 95% of lesions can be dealt with by renal artery angioplasty +/− stenting. Only a minority require surgery and vascular reconstruction. Following revascularisation, there is usually an improvement in blood pressure control but only a tiny minority become normotensive. Improvement in renal function is much more variable. This is because such patients have widespread atherosclerotic disease throughout their vascular tree, including in smaller vessels within the kidneys. In addition, they may also have changes associated with chronic hypertension, such as thickening of intrarenal vessels.

In contrast to atherosclerotic RAS, lesions in FMD tend to be distal to the origin of the renal artery, and appear as a string of beads on angiography. Following angioplasty, patients with FMD tend to have a complete resolution of hypertension and a normal renal function (because the vessels in the kidney distal to the stenosis are usually non-diseased).

Whilst waiting for his angioplasty, Mr Shanklin is admitted as an emergency on the medical take with acute severe shortness of breath and coughing up frothy pink sputum. His CXR is shown in Figure 16.3.

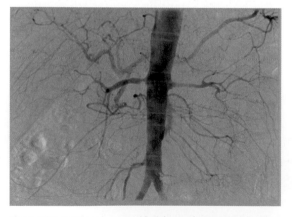

Figure 16.2 Renal angiogram with right renal artery stenosis. The narrowing occurs close to the origin of the artery and is therefore likely to be due to atherosclerosis rather than fibromuscular dysplasia.

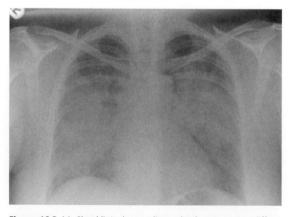

Figure 16.3 Mr Shanklin's chest radiograph, demonstrating diffuse bilateral 'bats wing' shadowing in the lung fields.

What does his chest X-ray show?

Pulmonary oedema – typical X-ray findings include upper lobe venous diversion (vessels supplying upper lobes look thicker and more prominent than those in lower zones of lung), alveolar oedema (so-called 'bat's wings'), the presence of fluid in the horizontal fissure, and interstitial oedema (evidenced by Kerley B lines). There may also be small pleural effusions (evidenced by blunting of the costophrenic angle). Patients with pulmonary oedema may also have cardiomegaly (heart shadow >50% of total thoracic width).

This should be treated by sitting the patient up and giving them oxygen. In this case, Mr Shanklin has a history of COPD and may be a CO_2 retainer, so start with 28% oxygen and then measure blood gases after 30 minutes to rule out significant CO_2 retention. Acute shortness of breath can be relieved with intravenous diuretics (e.g. furosemide 80 mg) and diamorphine (e.g. 2.5 mg). A nitrate infusion may be required in severe cases (acts to vasodilate and thus reduce the afterload).

What are the possible causes of pulmonary oedema in this gentleman?

- Myocardial infarction – Mr Shanklin is an arteriopath at high risk of a further acute coronary event. This can lead to acute LV dysfunction with associated pulmonary oedema. Therefore serial ECG and troponin levels should be performed.
- 'Flash pulmonary oedema' which occurs in around 10% of patients with RAS due to acute left ventricular impairment. It frequently occurs at night (neurohumoral mechanisms, such as altered levels of brain-type natriuretic peptide, are thought to play a role), and can indicate severe bilateral renal artery disease. Flash pulmonary oedema is a definite indication for revascularisation.

CASE REVIEW

This 60-year-old vasculopath presented with hypertension, CKD and a marked decline in renal function following the introduction of an ACEI. Investigations demonstrated a renal artery stenosis. He was advised to stop smoking and his statin was increased. He underwent revascularisation by angioplasty and stenting. This improved his blood pressure control but he continued to have significant CKD.

KEY POINTS

- Atherosclerosis accounts for more than 90% of renovascular disease. Clinical presentation is with hypertension, CKD (with a steep rise in creatinine following introduction of an ACEI) or even ESRF. Around 10% of patients with renal artery stenosis (RAS) develop flash pulmonary oedema.
- Risk factors for RAS include increasing age, hypertension, smoking, dyslipidaemia and diabetes mellitus. Lesions are typically within 1 cm of the origin of the renal artery.
- Renal artery stenosis is a common finding in patients with CKD, but is not always the cause of renal dysfunction and may be an incidental finding, particularly in the elderly.

- Treatment of atherosclerosis-associated RAS is by reducing risk factors (smoking, cholesterol), adding in aspirin and, in some cases, a revascularisation procedure. Angioplasty +/– stenting can be used to treat patients with RAS. A small minority require surgery. Treatment often improves blood pressure control but may not greatly affect renal dysfunction.
- Ten percent of RAS is caused by fibromuscular dysplasia. This tends to give rise to distal renal artery lesions and occurs in young women.

A 25-year-old woman with dysuria and urine dipstick abnormalities

Gabrielle Llewelyn is a 25-year-old woman who presents with a 4-day history of urinary frequency and dysuria. On examination, her temperature is 37.7°C, pulse 90 bpm and BP 125/75 mmHg. She is mildly tender in the right flank and suprapubically but there is no rebound or guarding. Urine dipstick (Figure 17.1) shows protein-, blood+, nitrite+++, lecuocyte+++

What is the most likely diagnosis?

The symptoms are typical of a urinary tract infection (UTI). Characteristic features are urinary urgency, frequency, nocturia and dysuria (usually a burning sensation when passing urine). Some patients develop urinary incontinence or, conversely, urinary retention (more common in men). The presence of flank tenderness and a mild fever raises the possibility that the infection is not confined to the lower urinary tract (i.e. a cystitis) but also involves the upper urinary tract (pyelonephritis). In men, systemic features of infection may accompany prostatitis or pyelonephritis.

The urine dipstick is also typical (usually nitrite and leucocyte positive). The presence of nitrite is relatively specific for a UTI but can occur in the absence of a UTI if the patient has a very high-protein diet.

Some patients present with recurrent urinary symptoms (urgency/frequency/dysuria) but have no evidence of infection (i.e. leucocyte/nitrite/culture negative). This is called the 'urethral syndrome' and indicates urethral inflammation but not cystitis. However, this is a diagnosis of exclusion and care should be taken to rule out infection, particularly with atypical organisms.

What investigations would you perform?

• Pregnancy test: it is wise to rule out pregnancy in any woman of child-bearing age who presents with abdominal or urinary symptoms.

• A midstream urine (MSU) sample for microscopy, culture and sensitivities. (MSU is not taken from the first void of the day. It is obtained by starting the void and catching urine part way through without stopping flow.)

What is the most likely causative organism?

In primary UTI in the community, *Escherichia coli* is the causative organism in >70% of cases. In hospital infections, it makes up only 40%. The pathogens responsible for UTI are summarised in Table 17.1.

The pregnancy test is negative. The urine microscopy shows >100 white cells/mm³.

Is the presence of leucocytes always indicative of urinary tract infection?

No. Leucocytes can be found in the urine in the absence of infection in conditions such as renal or bladder stones, urothelial tumours, chronic interstitial nephritis (secondary to chronic NSAID ingestion or analgesic nephropathy) and chemical cystitis (secondary to cytotoxins, e.g. cyclophosphamide). In such cases, the MSU will be culture negative, ie. there is sterile pyuria.

Sterile pyuria can also occur in some situations when there is actually infection. This occurs if:

• the patient self-medicates prior to culture

• the infection is caused by an organism which does not grow in standard culture media, e.g. chlamydia, candida, mycobacterium.

Nephrology: Clinical Cases Uncovered. By M. Clatworthy.
Published 2010 by Blackwell Publishing.

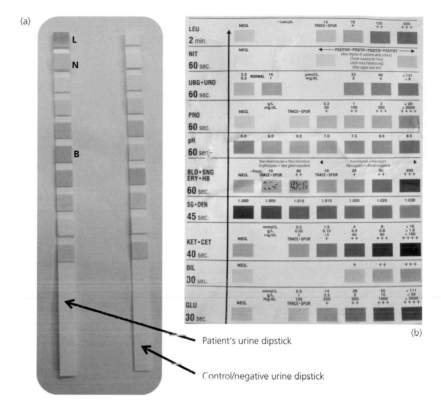

Figure 17.1 The patient's urine dipstick is positive for leucocytes (L), nitrites (N) and blood (B). (b) Reference colours for interpretation of dipstick (found on the side of the dipsticks pot).

Patient's urine dipstick

Control/negative urine dipstick

Table 17.1 Frequency of bacteria causing UTI

Causative organism	% primary infection	% early relapse	% Hospital acquired
E. coli	70–90%	60%	48%
Proteus	2%	15%	10%
Klebsiella, enterobacter	7.5%	20%	15%
Enterococcus	2.5%	–	6%
Staphylococcus	5%	–	6%
Pseudomonas	–	–	15%
Other	2.5%	5%	<1%

The urine culture yields >10^6 E. coli. Gabrielle is started on trimethoprim 200 mg tds. You review Gabrielle's records and find that she has had two similar episodes previously, one 6 months ago and one 9 months ago.

What factors predispose to the development of recurrent urinary tract infections?

Factors which can lead to recurrent UTI are varied and are summarised in Box 17.1.

> **Box 17.1 Factors predisposing to recurrent UTI**
>
> **Local factors**
> - Impaired bladder emptying, e.g. due to prostatic hypertrophy or neuromuscular problems
> - Bladder or renal calculi
> - Renal cysts
> - Anatomical anomaly, e.g. horseshoe kidney
> - Indwelling urinary catheter or recurrent bladder instrumentation
> - Postmenopausal vaginal atrophy
>
> **Systemic factors**
> - Diabetes mellitus
> - Immunosuppression
> - Pregnancy

What general measures would you advise given Gabrielle's history of recurrent urinary tract infections?

- *Drink lots:* many patients with recurrent UTI are chronically dehydrated. They should be advised to drink two cups of fluid an hour whilst they have an infection and aim for 2–3 litres/day on a regular basis.

• *Double voiding:* this involves attempting to urinate a second time, around 5 minutes after initial urination, and ensures there is no residual urine left in the bladder. Stagnant urine and poor bladder emptying are risk factors for recurrent infection.

• *Voiding after intercourse:* intercourse can precipitate UTI by facilitating retrograde movement of bacteria from the urethra. Voiding after intercourse can reduce the risk of coital-associated UTI.

• *Cranberry juice:* a Cochrane meta-analysis published in 2008 showed that cranberry products significantly reduced the incidence of UTI at 12 months (RR 0.65, 95% CI 0.46–0.90) compared with placebo/control. Cranberry products were more effective in reducing the incidence of UTI in women with recurrent UTI than elderly men and women or people requiring catheterisation.

> On going over these points with Gabrielle, she admits that she doesn't normally drink much at all during the day whilst at work. In fact, her fluid intake appears to be limited to five or six cups of tea/day.

What additional investigations would you perform in Gabrielle, given the history of recurrent urinary tract infections?

• *Glucose:* to screen for diabetes.

• *Renal function:* recurrent episodes of pyelonephritis can lead to renal scarring.

• *Plain abdominal film:* to screen for a renal stone. Around 90% are radio-opaque (i.e. they contain calcium).

• *US renal tract:* to screen for stones and structural abnormalities of the urinary tract which may predispose to recurrent UTI.

> The results of her blood tests are shown below.
>
> Hb 12.9 g/dL, WBC 7.9 × 10⁹/L, Platelets 361 × 10⁹/L
> U+E: Na 141 mmol/L, K 4.2 mmol/L, Urea 6.3 mmol/L,
>   Creatinine 85 µmol/L
> Glucose 4.8 mmol/L
>
> The US is performed and demonstrates the presence of a stone in the right kidney. It is radio-opaque.

What is the most likely composition of this stone?

Calcium oxalate stones are the most common and are radio-opaque, so this is the most likely composition of Gabrielle's stone. The other types of renal stone are summarised in Table 17.2 and include triple (calcium, ammonium and magnesium) phosphate stones, uric acid/urate stones and cystine stones. The only way to determine the composition of the stone with complete certainty is to catch it and analyse it. Patients should therefore be encouraged to try and do so by listening for the tinkle of a stone in the pan or, more effectively, by sieving the urine.

What factors predispose to the development of stones?

This obviously depends on the type of stone. For calcium oxalate stones, the main predisposing factors are low urine volume, hypercalciuria and hyperoxaluria. Diseases

Table 17.2 Types of renal stone

	Calcium oxalate stones	Triple phosphate stone	Uric acid/urate stone	Cystine stone
% of stones	60–70%	15–20%	5%	1%
Predisposing factors	Hypercalciuria (e.g. hyper PTH) Hyperoxaluria	Stagnant urine Chronic infection Foreign bodies (sutures, plastic)	Hyperuricaemia (primary/secondary)	Cystinuria (rare inherited disorder)
Radiological appearance	Radio-opaque	Radio-opaque	Radiolucent	Semi-opaque
Macroscopic appearance	Sharp and spiky	Grey-white in colour, can grow quite large	Brown in colour	Small, grey-white

---

Box 17.2 Causes of calcium urolithiasis

Hypercalcaemia leading to hypercalciuria
- Primary hyperparathyroidism
- Sarcoidosis
- Malignancy
- Acromegaly

Isolated hypercalciuria (with normocalcaemia)
- Distal RTA (congenital or acquired)
- Drugs: loop diruetics, lithium, corticosteroids
- Endocrine problems: Cushing's disease, Conn's disease

Hyperoxaluria
- Primary oxaluria (genetic disorder, types I–II are both autosomal recessive)
- Enteric hyperoxaluria (e.g. in Crohn's disease; this occurs if there is ileal inflammation. Malabsorbed fat binds intraluminal calcium which is then not available to complex oxalate)
- Oxalate-rich diet (tea, chocolate, rhubarb, spinach)
- Low dietary calcium intake

Hypocitraturia
- Chronic diarrhoea (laxatives)
- High animal protein intake

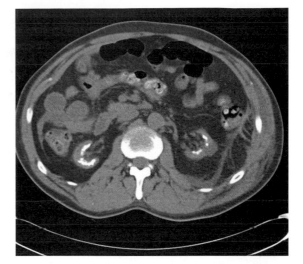

Figure 17.2 An abdominal CT scan showing bilateral medullary calcification (nephrocalcinosis).

Box 17.3 Causes of uric acid urolithiasis

Hyperuricosuria with hyperuricaemia
- Myelo/lymphoproliferative disorder with rapid cell turnover and production of purines
- Inborn error of purine metabolism, e.g. Lesch–Nyhan syndrome
- Idiopathic hyperuricaemia (patients with gout)

Uricosouria with normouricaemia
- Uricosuric drugs
- Proximal RTA

Persistently acidic urine
- Chronic diarrhoeal disease
- Ileostomy

---

associated with these metabolic abnormalities are summarised in Box 17.2. In this particular case low fluid intake, most of which is tea (high in oxalate), is likely to be contributory. Chronic hypercalciuria can lead to nephrocalcinosis, a condition in which there is diffuse medullary +/– cortical calcification (Figure 17.2). The main causes of uric acid stones are summarised in Box 17.3.

What other investigations would you perform?

Give the presence of a stone, Gabrielle should have the following investigations.
- Blood biochemistry
  - Calcium, phosphate, uric acid
  - Chloride, bicarbonate
  - Total protein
- Urine (spot, first-voided morning specimen)
  - Specific gravity
  - pH (pH of 5.3–6.8 makes renal tubular acidosis (RTA) unlikely)
  - Crystalluria (the types and shapes of crystals are shown in Figure 17.3)

- Urine (24-hour collection)
  - Calcium, phosphate, uric acid
  - Creatinine, urea, sodium
  - Oxalate, citrate, magnesium

How should this patient be further managed?

She should be referred to the urologists for management of her current stone. Many pass spontaneously, although this can be extremely painful. Percutaneous nephrolithotomy can be used to retrieve stones in the kidney or upper ureter, assisted by lithotripsy (ultrasonic dissolution) which can be used to break up the stone. Rarely, surgical intervention is required.

Calcium oxalate   Calcium/   Uric acid   Cystine
                   triple phosphate

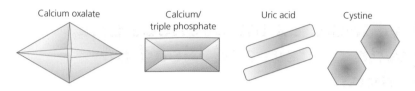

Figure 17.3 Appearance of different types of crystal visible on urine microscopy.

Aim to prevent further stone formation by increasing fluid intake and reducing oxalate and milk intake.

In patients with hypercalciuria, thiazide diuretics such as bendroflumethiazide help to reduce urinary calcium. Oral potassium citrate will reduce the likelihood of stone formation in these patients.

For triple phosphate stones, antibiotic treatment may be required.

Urate and cystine stone formation is inhibited by alkylinising the urine. Aim for a urine pH >6.5 (give oral sodium bicarbonate). Hyperuricaemia should be treated with allopurinol.

Gabrielle is referred to the urologists who perform lithotripsy and percutaneous removal of the stone. There are no obvious abnormalities in Gabrielle's 'stone screen'. She is therefore advised to cut down on tea and greatly increase her fluid intake to prevent any future problems.

CASE REVIEW

A 25-year-old woman presents with dysuria and urinary frequency. On examination, she is febrile and tender in the right flank and suprapubic area. Urine dipstick is positive for leucocytes and nitrites. A MSU sample is taken and has pus cells and grows >10^6 *E. coli*. She is treated with trimethoprim. This is the third UTI in 9 months, so she undergoes further investigations which show the presence of a calculus in the right kidney. She is referred to the urologist for further management of the stone and advised to drink more fluid and reduce her oxalate intake (less tea-drinking).

KEY POINTS

- Urinary tract infections (UTI) are common and make up around 2% of a GP's workload.
- Most UTI are simple or uncomplicated; that is:
  - they occur in an anatomically normal urinary tract
  - they do not involve the kidneys or prostate (i.e. an isolated cystitis as opposed to pyelonephritis or prostatitis)
  - they resolve with a single course of antibiotics and do not frequently recur.
- Seventy to 90% of simple UTI occurring in the community are caused by *E. coli*.
- Management of simple UTI includes a short course of antibiotics (there are usually local guidelines but 5 days of trimethoprim or amoxicillin should suffice), an increased fluid intake and advice on 'toilet hygiene' such as double voiding.

- Patients with pyelonephritis or prostatitis may be febrile and have systemic features of sepsis such as hypotension.
- Patients with recurrent episodes of UTI (3–4 times/year) or those with pyelonephritis should be investigated for an underlying cause, for example renal stones.
- There are four main types of renal stones:
  - calcium oxalate stones (most common, 60–70% of total)
  - phosphate stones, calcium or triple (calcium, magnesium, ammonium)
  - uric acid/ urate stones
  - cystine stones.
- Patients with renal tract stones should be investigated for an underlying cause.

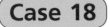

A 40-year-old ex-intravenous drug user with protein and blood on urine dipstick

Mr Mark Phillips is a 40-year-old man who presents with a 6-week history of arthralgia and malaise. He also noticed blotches of light purple discolouration which appeared on his thighs when he went jogging on a cold morning and then disappeared later in the day. He previously used intravenous drugs for around 5 years in his late 20s but has been clean for a number of years. Examination shows no obvious arthropathy. He looks slightly pale and there is a single palpable right cervical lymph node (LN) but no other lymphadenopathy. He is afebrile, pulse 90 bpm, BP 155/90 mmHg, normal HS. Respiratory and abdominal examination are unremarkable except that the liver edge is palpable at 2 cm below the costal margin. He has pitting oedema, limited to his ankles, but there is no obvious rash.

Urine dipstick (of a MSU sample) shows blood +++, protein ++++, leucocytes+, nitrite–

What does the urine dipstick suggest?

The urine has significant blood and protein, indicative of an active urinary sediment. This points towards likely renal (and probably glomerular) pathology.

Investigations show:

Hb 11.1 g/dL, MCV 82, WBC 7.2 × 10⁹/L, Platelets
$Hb\ 11.1\ g/dL,\ MCV\ 82,\ WBC\ 7.2 \times 10^9/L,\ Platelets$
   369 × 10⁹/L
   $369 \times 10^9/L$
PT 14 s, APTT 32 s
U+E: Na 142 mmol/L, K 4.5 mmol/L, Urea 10.3 mmol/L,
   Creatinine 154 μmol/L (eGFR 46 mL/min/1.73 m²)
LFT: normal
Albumin 28 g/dL, Glucose 4.8 mmol/L, CRP 45 mg/L
Urine microscopy: red cell casts
Urine protein/creatinine ratio (PCr): 175
CXR: NAD
Infection screen awaited

Nephrology: Clinical Cases Uncovered. By M. Clatworthy.
Published 2010 by Blackwell Publishing.

How would you interpret these investigations?

Mr Phillips is mildly anaemic (normocytic), in keeping with the pallor found on examination. Clotting is normal. There is renal impairment which may be acute or chronic. Albumin is low; this may be due to chronic disease, liver disease, malabsorption, malnutrition or renal loss of protein. The latter is most likely given 4+ protein on urine dipstick.

Red cells casts on urine microscopy are diagnostic of GN. His urine PCr is elevated, although proteinuria is not within the nephrotic range.

What are the main chronic infections typically associated with intravenous drug use?

- Hepatitis B
- Hepatitis C
- HIV

Can any of these infections cause renal disease?

All three are associated with renal disease, as summarised in Table 18.1. Hepatitis B is typically associated with membranous GN, hepatitis C with mesangiocapillary GN (MCGN) and HIV with a nephropathy with the histological features of FSGS, so-called HIV-associated nephropathy (HIVAN).

The infection screen returns showing negative serology and polymerase chain reaction (PCR) for hepatitis B and HIV. However, the patient is positive for hepatitis C antibodies and RNA. This is found to be genotype 1, with a viral load of 7.6 × 10⁵ copies/mL.

What other investigations would you perform?

- Cryoglobulins
- Rheumatoid factor
- Complement levels (C3/C4)

Table 18.1 Infections and renal disease

Infection	Typical renal pathology	Typical presentation	Other renal manifestations
Hepatitis B	Membranous GN	Nephrotic syndrome +/– microscopic haematuria	MCGN PAN
Hepatitis C	MCGN type I due to cryoglobulinaemia	Dipstick proteinuria/haematuria or nephrotic syndrome	Membranous GN
HIV	HIV-associated nephropathy (HIVAN or collapsing FSGS)	Nephrotic syndrome or proteinuria+/– haematuria	IgA nephropathy MCGN Membranous GN Diffuse proliferative GN

- Renal US
- Renal biopsy

What are cryoglobulins and why are they difficult to detect?

Cryoglobulins are immunoglobulins (antibodies) which agglutinate or precipitate in the cold (at temperatures <37°C). Thus blood must be taken and kept warm (usually taken to the lab in a Thermos flask) or else they will precipitate out and will not be detectable by the time the sample gets to the laboratory. The serum is then stored at 4°C for 1–3 days, after which the cryoprecipitate is visible in the bottom of the tube and is quantified to give the cryocrit. The antibodies may be IgG, IgM or IgA. Cryoglobulins are classified according to whether the antibodies have a single specificity (monoclonal) or multiple specificities (polyclonal) or a mixture of the two (Table 18.2, Figure 18.1).

If the cryocrit is >1 g/L then patients may become symptomatic because significant quantities of cryoglobulin precipitate in peripheral blood vessels. This is frequently manifest as cutaneous vasculitis, as vessels supplying the skin are blocked or complement is activated by the cryoprecipitate. Other manifestations include neuropathy, arthropathy and renal impairment.

The monoclonal IgM in type II (mixed) cryoglobulinaemia is frequently specific for the Fc portion of IgG, i.e. it is a rheumatoid factor antibody. Thus, it is worth doing a test for the presence of rheumatoid factor if cryoglobulinaemia is suspected as this is technically easier and often returns before the cryoglobulin result. The binding of these RF antibodies to the polyclonal IgG making up IgM-IgG complexes is one mechanism by which precipitation is thought to occur.

Table 18.2 Classification of cryoglobulinaemia

Classification	Antibody specificity	Associations
Type I	Monoclonal	Multiple myeloma Waldenstrom's macroglobulinaemia Lymphoproliferative disorders
Type II	Mixed	Hepatitis C infection Autoimmune disease, e.g. SLE
Type III	Polyclonal	Autoimmune disease, particularly primary biliary cirrhosis Infections, e.g. HCV, mycoplasma

Mr Phillips has detectable cryoglobulins in his blood with a cryocrit of 15% (quantified at 1.5 g/L, and found to be mixed). His rheumatoid factor is also positive at 510 IU/L and his C3 is very low and C4 borderline low (0.19 g/L; normal range 0.2–0.5).

What might be the cause of his rash?

The description is typical of livedo reticularis, a lace-like purplish discoloration, usually affecting the lower limbs. It occurs as blood slows down in the cutaneous vascular network because of cryoprecipitation. It is also seen in patients with anticardiolipin antibodies. Other cutaneous manifestations of cryoglobulinaemia include purpura and ulceration.

Mr Phillips' renal US shows two normal-sized kidneys so he undergoes a renal biopsy.

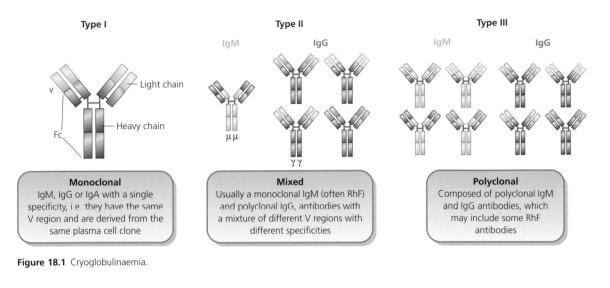

Figure 18.1 Cryoglobulinaemia.

What would you expect the renal biopsy to show?

Mesangiocapillary GN (MCGN) type I (also known as membranoproliferative GN). Typical features include:

- mesangial and endocapillary proliferation
- intraluminal thrombi
- mesangial and luminal deposition of IgM, IgG and C3
- EM demonstrates subendothelial deposits.

How is mesangiocapillary glomerulonephritis classified?

Mesangiocapillary glomerulonephritis is classified according to differences in histological appearance into types I–III, mainly according to differences in EM appearance as summarised in Table 18.3. Type I is most common.

As with all glomerulonephritides, MCGN can occur as a primary/idiopathic disease or secondary to a number of other conditions, mainly infections, as in the case of Mr Phillips. Secondary MCGN tends to show a type I pattern with subendothelial deposits and activation of the classic complement pathway (low C4). This may be because the associated diseases all produce persistent antibody responses which can activate complement via the classic pathway (Figure 18.2). Associations include the following.

- Infection
  - Streptococcal including endocarditis (type I+II)
  - Shunt nephritis (associated with staphylococcal infection of atrioventricular shunts, used for treatment of hydrocephalus)
  - Mycobaterial disease (TB/leprosy)
  - Hepatitis B and C
  - Malaria
- Autoimmunity
  - SLE (type I+II)
  - Systemic sclerosis
  - Sjögren's syndrome
  - Mixed cryoglobulinaemia (may be caused by HCV)
- Dysgammaglobulinaemia
  - Lymphoma
  - Myeloma
  - Leukaemia
- Factor H mutations

In most patients MCGN is primary/idiopathic. In such cases, a general observation is that patients have activation of the classical or alternative complement pathway (evidenced by low C3 and C4). In some cases, specific factors have been identified which mediate alternative complement activation and are termed 'nephritic factors'. Two nephritic factors have been characterised.

- C3NeF$_a$: first factor identified. Found in patients with type II MCGN. C3NeF$_a$ (the 'a' being for the amplification loop) is an IgG autoantibody which binds to an epitope of the activated form of factor B, to form a complex C3bBbNeF$_a$. This complex is more stable than the native C3bBb and is also resistant to inactivation by factor H. In some patients it is associated with partial (upper body) lipodystrophy (atrophy of fat). This is because adipocytes play a role in controlling complement by producing factor D (a protease which breaks down factor B). C3NeF$_a$ inhibits this process, causing local lysis of adipocytes.

Table 18.3 Classification of MCGN

Classification	Biospy (light microscopy)	Biopsy (immunostaining)	Biopsy (EM)
Type I	Mesangial proliferation Double contour BM	Peripheral C3, IgG +/–C4, C1q	Subendothelial deposits
Type II ('dense-deposit disease')	Mesangial proliferation Thickened BM	Mesangial C3	Deposits within the basement membrane
Type III	Mesangial proliferation	Peripheral C3, IgG	Subendothelial deposits Subepithelial deposits

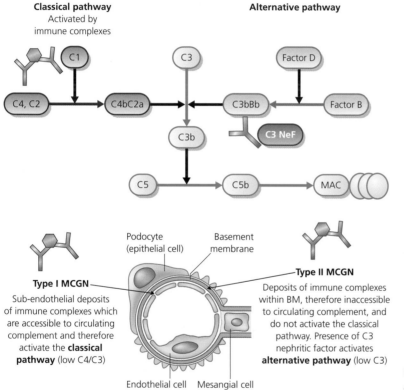

Figure 18.2 Complement pathway activation in MCGN.

Table 18.4 Clinical features of different types of MCGN

Classification	Complement pathway	Complement levels	Other features
Type I	Classical pathway	Low C3, C4	Associated with cryoglobulinaemia Rarely associated with Factor H associations
Type II ('dense-deposit disease')	Alternative pathway	Very low C3	C3NeF$_a$ identified in some patients Partial lipodystrophy
Type III	Terminal pathway	Boderline low C3, C4, C5	Older patients Prognosis better C3NeF$_t$ identified in some patients

• C3NeF$_t$: the nephritic factor of the terminal (t) pathway is found in patients with type III MCGN. It principally activates the terminal complement components, and patients with C3NeF$_t$ have depressed levels of both C3 and C5.

How should Mr Phillips be treated?

General managment includes BP control and control of proteinuria. This is probably best achieved by using ACEI or ARB.

His hepatitis C infection needs to be worked up further. He should therefore be referred to a hepatologist. Treatment of his hepatits C infection should lead to an improvement in cryoglobulinaemia and renal disease.

Mr Phillips is referred to the hepatologists. He undergoes a liver biopsy which shows mild chronic hepatitis. His HCV infection is treated with interferon-α and ribavirin. The viral load responds well to this treatment.

What is the prognosis of Mr Phillips' problem?

The prognosis of HCV-associated cryoglobulinaemic MCGN is not well defined because prior to the identification of HCV, many patients were treated with immunosuppressive therapy (steroids+/−cytotoxins such as cyclophosphamide) and did quite poorly. A study in the pre-HCV treatment era showed that 45% gained some improvement in renal function, in 20% it stayed the same and 35% progressed to ESRF. Outcomes are very much better with the use of antiviral treatment. Some nephrologists advocate the use of immunosuppressant and antiviral treatment in patients who have significant or progressive renal impairment.

Six months following treatment, Mr Phillips' creatinine was 118 μmol/L and his cryocrit was <5%. Urine dipstick showed protein+ and no blood.

CASE REVIEW

This is a case of an ex-intravenous drug user who presented with hypertension and blood and protein on urine dipstick and a history of livedo retiularis on his thighs. Investigations showed renal impairment, hepatitis C infection and the presence of cryoglobulins in the blood. Renal biopsy confirmed the diagnosis of cryoglobulin-associated MCGN. His HCV infection was treated with interferon and ribavirin, which improved both renal function and dipstick abnormalities.

KEY POINTS

• Patients with chronic infections such as hepatitis B, C and HIV can develop GN. In patients with hepatitis C, this is typically type I MCGN and is frequently associated with the presence of cryoglobulins.
• Cryoglobulins are antibodies which precipitate at <37°C. They are classified according to their specificity (monoclonal or polyclonal).
• In HCV infection, cryoglobulins are usually a mixture of a monoclonal IgM and polyclonal IgG and are present in up to 50% of patients. Only a minority are symptomatic (1%).
• Patients with HCV-associated cryoglobulinaemia often have +ve RF and low circulating C3 and C4 levels.
• MCGN is classified into three types according to histological appearances, and each type can be primary/idiopathic or can occur secondary to other problems such as cryoglobulinaemia or infection. Type I is the most common followed by Type II.
• Type I MPGN is characterised by subendothelial immune deposits on EM and activation of the classical complement pathway (low C3 and C4).
• Type II MPGN is characterised by immune deposits within the basement membrane on EM and activation of the alternative complement pathway (low C3). In some patients with type II MPGN, a nephritic factor is identified (C3NeF$_a$). This is an IgG autoantibody which stabilises C3bBb, thus causing excessive activation of the alternative complement pathway. It can also be associated with partial lipodystrophy.
• In the case of HCV-associated cryoglobulinaemia with type I MCGN, both problems can respond well to treatment of the underlying hepatitis C infection.

Case 19 A 35-year-old man with macroscopic haematuria

Mr Nigel Jenkins is a 35-year-old man who is admitted to A+E with macroscopic haematuria. He had been playing rugby and was struck by an opposition player's knee in the right flank. This was followed by severe flank pain and heavy macroscopic haematuria. On examination, his pulse is 100 bpm and his BP is 175/105 mmHg. O_2 sats are 100% on air and his chest is clear. He is tender in the right flank but has no rebound or guarding. Initial investigations performed in the emergency department show a creatinine of 120 μmol/L (eGFR 66 mL/min/1.73 m³). A US scan of his renal tract reveals multiple cysts (>5) in both kidneys.

What is the most likely cause of his pain and macroscopic haematuria?

The most likely underlying diagnosis is adult polycystic kidney disease (APKD), also known as autosomal dominant polycystic kidney disease (ADPKD). APKD is relatively common, affecting around one in 800 individuals in caucasian populations. Although cyst formation begins in childhood, it doesn't usually become clinically evident until adulthood. Patients with APKD have multiple fluid-filled cysts in both kidneys (Figure 19.1). These may fill with blood following trauma, resulting in severe abdominal pain and macroscopic haematuria, as in this case. The cysts may also become infected, causing pain, fevers, rigors and systemic sepsis. Infections in cysts may be difficult to clear.

Renal stones (uric acid > calcium oxalate) are twice as common in patients with APKD as in the general population and may also cause flank pain in this patient group.

What further aspects of the history would you explore?

Adult polycystic kidney disease can cause hypertension and CKD, so any history of headaches/visual disturbance

(hypertension), tiredness or breathlessness (anaemia), itchiness (hyperphosphataemia) or nausea (uraemia) should be obtained.

Patients with APKD may have cysts in other organs including the liver (80%), pancreas, ovaries, lungs and thyroid. They may therefore have symptoms (most likely pain) related to these. In some patients, liver cysts predominate, leading to liver failure which can be so severe as to require liver transplantation.

Adult polycystic kidney disease can also be associated with valvular heart disease, diverticular disease and berry aneurysms. Any history consistent with these associated features of APKD, including history of stroke/cerebral haemorrhage, should be sought. Some patients also develop coronary artery aneurysms.

Why is it important to take a careful family history?

Adult polycystic kidney disease is an autosomal dominant condition. New mutations occur in only 5% of cases, although many patients will not be aware of a positive family history of disease. Closer questioning or discussion with older relatives may prompt recall of a family member who died of 'kidney trouble' or 'brain haemorrhage'. Associated berry aneurysms do not occur in all affected families.

Autosomal dominant polycystic kidney disease is caused by mutations in one of two genes, PKD1 (chromosome 16p) and PKD2 (chromosome 4q), encoding polycystin 1 and polycystin 2 respectively. Mutations in PKD1 are more common than PKD2, accounting for 85% of cases of APKD. Mutations in either gene lead to cyst formation but PKD1 mutations tend to be associated with an increased number of renal cysts and the development of renal failure at a younger age. On average, this occurs 20 years earlier in patients with PKD1 mutation (median age of ESRF 50 years versus 70 years in patients with PKD2 mutations).

Nephrology: Clinical Cases Uncovered. By M. Clatworthy. Published 2010 by Blackwell Publishing.

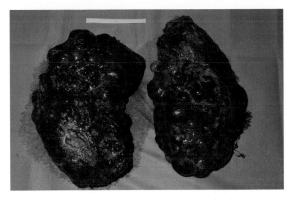

Figure 19.1 Polycystic kidneys post-nephrectomy (undertaken because of recurrent cyst haemorrhage and discomfort).

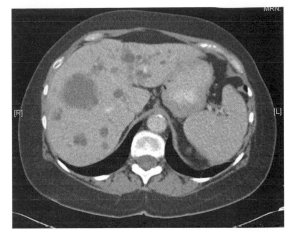

Figure 19.3 An abdominal CT scan showing liver cysts in a patient with APKD.

Mr Jenkins' pulse is now 90 bpm (post co-codamol for pain). He is euvolaemic and repeat BP is 160/95 mmHg. He has no obvious murmurs. He is still tender in his right flank and deeper palpation reveals a fullness there. His left kidney is not obviously palpable but the liver is slightly enlarged, with the edge lying 2 cm below the costal margin. Fundoscopy shows early hypertensive changes of silver wiring and AV nipping.

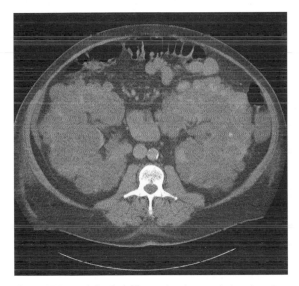

Figure 19.2 An abdominal CT scan showing massively enlarged, cystic kidneys in a patient with APKD.

What additional examination findings would you seek?

• Signs associated with chronic hypertension, e.g. retinopathy, left ventricular hypertrophy (hyperdynamic, heaving apex beat +/− systolic flow murmur).

• Signs consistent with valvular pathology: careful auscultation of the praecordium to rule out murmurs, particularly mitral valve prolapse, although patients may have MR or AR.

• Signs consistent with cysts in other organs: in patients with a large number of renal or liver cysts, organomegaly will be detectable on abdominal examination (Figures 19.2 and 19.3 show a CT from a patient with massively enlarged kidneys and liver cysts).

What investigations would you perform?

• Blood tests
  ○ Full blood count: he has macroscopic haematuria and so could have had a significant fall in his haemoglobin. Platelet count should also be checked as thrombocytopaenia may predispose to easy bleeding.
  ○ PT and APTT: clotting abnormalities may lead to haemorrhage with minimal trauma.
  ○ U+E: to confirm elevated creatinine documented on admission bloods, and to assess for abnormalities of potassium and urea.
  ○ LFT, albumin.
  ○ Calcium and phosphate: if he has significant CKD as a result of his APKD then there may be a reduced production of $1,25(OH)_2$Vit D and hence hypocalcaemia. This stimulates the release of PTH from the parathyroids (secondary hyperparathyroidism).

• ECG: to assess for signs of LVH which might be associated with chronic hypertension (i.e. left axis deviation, and sum of S in V1 or V2 plus the R in V5 or V6 >35 mm).

• CXR: to assess heart size (looking for cardiomegaly secondary to LVH in chronic hypertension).

Investigations show:

Hb 15.1 g/dL, WBC 7.4, Platelets 410 × 10⁹/L

Clotting normal

U+E: Na 139 mmol/L, K 5.4 mmol/L, Urea 8.3 mmol/L,
     Creatinine 122 µmol/L (eGFR 62 mL/min/1.73 m²)

LFT: normal

Albumin 36 g/L

cCa 2.25 mmol/L, PO₄ 0.9 mmol/L

Urine dipstick shows protein++, blood++++, negative for
     leucocytes, nitrites and glucose

CXR: NAD

ECG: LVH

What immediate management steps would you undertake?

Mr Jenkins is haemodynamically stable with no respiratory compromise. The main issue is therefore pain control. Haemorrhage into cysts and cyst rupture can be very painful, in part due to the presence of clots in the renal collecting system causing renal colic. Management includes bed rest and analgesia (often opiates). Intravenous fluids should be given to increase urine output to 2–3 litres/day, in an attempt to wash the clot out of the kidney.

Mr Jenkins should be informed of the possibility of recurrent episodes of macroscopic haematuria and given advice on how to manage these episodes at home with simple analgesia and oral hydration. He may not require admission for all episodes, if managed in this way. He should also be advised to avoid contact sports in which abdominal trauma may occur (e.g. rugby or boxing).

What other issues need to be addressed during follow-up?

Mr Jenkins is hypertensive (even when pain free). He also has ECG changes consistent with LVH, i.e. end-organ damage resulting from hypertension, which should be treated. In APKD, treatment of blood pressure is recommended for adults with a BP >130/80 mmHg. ACEI inhibitors or ARB are preferred because there is some evidence that treatment with these agents is associated with a preservation of renal function in patients with APKD (see later).

Patients with APKD can develop hypertension in childhood (said to occur in 35% of patients) which, if untreated, can contribute to declining renal function

as well as the development of LVH (which is associated with cardiovascular morbidity and mortality later in life).

Mr Jenkins asks whether his 3-year-old daughter can be screened for the disease. What advice would you give?

Although the two genes causing APKD have been identified, genetic screening for PKD1 mutations is not a particularly useful tool unless a large number of family members with disease are available for linkage analysis. Even then, this is difficult because the gene is very big, with areas of duplication, and a large number of mutations have been described. Some centres screen for PKD2 mutations (if there is a sufficient family pedigree) but this gene is abnormal in only 10% of cases.

In adults with a positive family history of APKD, radiological screening with ultrasound (which can detect cysts of >1 cm) is useful. The proposed criteria for diagnosis include:
- age <30 years: two or more unilateral or single bilateral cysts in patients
- age 30–59 years: 2+ cysts in each kidney
- age >60 years: at least four cysts in each kidney.

However, the absence of cysts in patients <30 years does not rule out the diagnosis.

In patients with a positive family history of cerebral haemorrhage or aneurysm, MR angiography is recommended. In the absence of a positive family history of aneurysm, screening is not routinely recommended for asymptomatic patients.

In the case of Mr Jenkins' daughter, a reasonable strategy would be to screen on an annual basis for elevated BP or urine dipstick abnormalities. Any hypertension should be treated. Once she is in her late teens, a US scan could be performed. The absence of cysts at this stage would make disease unlikely. The scan should then be repeated when she is >30 years and if there are still no cysts at this time, APKD is virtually excluded. Pursuing a diagnosis more aggressively in younger individuals currently has little benefit because of the lack of proven disease-modifying agents, although careful BP control in individuals with disease is important as early as possible.

Prior to screening at any age, patients should undergo appropriate counselling about the nature of the disease and the implications of a positive diagnosis on their life, for example, getting life insurance.

Mr Jenkins' macroscopic haematuria resolves within 3 days but he continues to have microscopic haematuria and proteinuria. He is started on ramipril 2.5 mg, which is gradually increased by his GP following discharge. During a subsequent renal outpatient appointment, his BP is much better controlled on ramipril 10 mg od (BP 125/80 mmHg). However, he does get the occasional twinge in both flanks and feels that his abdominal girth is expanding. He wants to know if there are any medications which can prevent the further progression of cyst formation.

What would you say?

There are currently (2009) no proven treatments which have been shown to reduce cyst formation or progression in a randomised controlled trial. The Halt Progression of Polycystic Disease study, currently recruiting, should determine whether a combination of ACEI and ARB can reduce the rate of increase of kidney volume as well as decline in renal function.

There are some data to suggest that sirolimus (rapamycin) may reduce cyst formation. This was first noted in patients who had undergone kidney or liver transplantation and were placed on sirolimus as their anti-rejection medication. Serial abdominal scans showed a reduction in renal cyst volume. Currently, there is insufficient evidence to routinely start patients with APKD on this immunosuppressant, which has a number of significant side-effects.

Other agents being evaluated include tolvaptan (ADH analogue) and octreotide.

What is the likelihood that Mr Jenkins will need renal replacement therapy?

Renal failure requiring RRT occurs in at least 50% of patients, and typically develops in the fourth to sixth decades of life. In patients with APKD, compensatory hyperfiltration in surviving nephrons may maintain a normal GFR for a number of decades, in spite of significant cyst formation. APKD accounts for 10% of patients requiring RRT in the UK.

Imaging studies (with US, MR or CT) allow an estimation of kidney volume, which can be useful in predicting the risk of development of renal failure. The combined volumes of both polycystic kidneys frequently exceeds 1000 mL, compared with 300 mL for normal female kidneys and 400 mL for male kidneys. Combined kidney volumes of >1500 mL are associated with a decrease in GFR.

Mr Jenkins already has a significant number of cysts and a reduced GFR. Serial monitoring of his renal func-

tion should be performed to allow optimal preparation for RRT when required, as well as for the treatment of complications associated with CKD, e.g. anaemia and hyperphosphataemia.

Ideally, he should be placed on the renal transplant waiting list 6 months prior to the anticipated dialysis start-date. In some patients, native polycystic kidneys can be so big that there is no space within the abdomen for the transplant. In such cases a native nephrectomy may be required to make room for the renal allograft prior to the patient being listed for transplantation.

Why do polycystic kidney disease mutations lead to cyst formation?

The precise mechanisms of cyst formation are unclear but we do know something about the normal functions of the polycystin proteins. Polycystin-1 is a large (>4000 aa) membrane protein with 11 transmembrane domains, a short cytoplasmic domain and a long extracellular domain. It is located at desmosomal and adherens junctions in renal epithelial cells and is thought to play some role in cell–cell adhesion. Polycystin-1 and polycystin-2 also form part of the primary cilium, an organelle thought to be important as a flow sensor in renal tubular epithelial cells. Cell cilia are also essential for cell division, acting as organizers of the mitotic spindle poles during mitosis. The cytoplasmic domain of polycystin-1 appears to interact with polycystin-2, as well as with a number of other molecules including TSC2 (tuberin). TSC2 forms part of the tuberous sclerosis complex, which lies in the mTOR pathway and may explain the observed beneficial therapeutic effect of sirolimus (which inhibits the mTOR complex 1, mTORc1) in APKD.

The processes which initiate cyst formation are unclear, but intrafamilial heterogeneity and the focal nature of cyst formation have led to the 'two-hit hypothesis' for cyst formation, which suggests that cysts form in cells with an inherited mutation in one allele and a somatic mutation occurring in the other allele. Once cyst formation is under way, dysfunction of polycystin-1 or -2 allows dysregulated proliferation of the tubular epithelial cells lining cysts, promoting cyst growth.

What other renal cystic diseases do you know?

Autosomal dominant polycystic kidney disease is the most common renal cystic disease. Others include von Hippel–Lindau syndrome and tuberous sclerosis. Their features are summarised in Table 19.1.

Table 19.1 Renal cystic diseases

	Frequency	Aetiology	Clinical features
APKD	1/500–1/1000	Autosomal dominant. Mutations in PKD1, ch16 (encoding polycystin-1) & PKD2, ch 4 (polycystin-2)	Hypertension/haemturia/loin pain in early adulthood. ESRF in mid-late adulthood
Infant PKD	1/10,000	Autosomal recessive. Gene on ch 6	ESRF in childhood. Associated with severe hepatic fibrosis. Poor prognosis
Von Hippel–Lindau syndrome	1/30,000–1/50,000	Autosomal dominant. VHL gene located on ch 3 and is a tumour suppressor gene	Renal cysts are premalignant, therefore nephrectomy may be required. Also develop phaeochromocytoma and spinocerebellar haemangiomas
Tuberous sclerosis	1/10,000	Autosomal dominant. Mutations in TSC1, ch 9 (hamartin) and TSC2, ch16 (tuberin). Both are tumour suppressor genes and function as a complex in the mTOR pathway	Characterised by CNS tubers (epilepsy), skin lesions (shagreen patches, angiofibromas) Renal involvement includes cysts, angiomyolipoma and renal cell carcinoma
Medullary sponge kidney	1/5000–1/10,000	Sporadic, unknown aetiology. Cysts develop from ecstatic collecting ducts	Cysts may calcify, leading to nephrocalcinosis. Associated with renal calculi and recurrent UTI
Simple cysts	Increases with age	Sporadic, unknown aetiology	Single or multiple fluid-filled cysts. Usually asymptomatic incidental finding on US

CASE REVIEW

A 35-year-old man presents with loin pain and haematuria after trauma to his flank during a rugby game. He has a fullness in his right flank and a palpable liver edge. Investigations show mild renal impairment and more than five cysts in both kidneys on ultrasound, consistent with a diagnosis of APKD. He is treated with analgesia and intravenous fluids. Further management included blood pressure control, monitoring of renal function and counselling of family members.

KEY POINTS

- Autosomal dominant polycystic kidney disease is characterised by the development of cysts in all parts of the nephron. It is relatively common, occurring in one in 800 in caucasian populations. Around 10% of patients requiring RRT in the UK have ESRF secondary to APKD.
- Clinical presentation includes flank pain, macroscopic haematuria, hypertension and renal impairment. Many patients are diagnosed as a result of family screening.
- Cysts form not only in the kidneys but also in other organs including the liver, pancreas and ovaries. Other manifestations include mitral valve prolapse, berry aneurysms and intestinal diverticulae.

- Mutations in two genes have been identified: PKD1 (chromosome 16p), accounting for 85% of cases, and PKD2 (chromosome 4q) in 10% of cases.
- No treatments have been proven to reduce cyst formation.
- Patients should be monitored for hypertension, and this should be treated with ACEI where possible.
- Other cystic renal diseases include autosomal recessive (infantile) PKD, von Hippel–Lindau syndrome and tuberous sclerosis.

Case 20   An 82-year-old woman with dark urine

Mrs Marjorie Ring is a 82-year-old woman who is found by a neighbour having had a fall. She lives in her own home and is normally independent. She tripped over her bedroom rug on the previous evening and couldn't get up because of pain in her right hip. She dragged some blankets onto the floor to keep herself warm but remained there until the next afternoon when her friend called around and let herself in. Mrs Ring has very little past medical history for a lady of her age; she has some mild arthritis in her finger joints and had a TIA 10 years ago after which she was found to be hyperlipidaemic. Medications include aspirin 75 mg and a statin.

On examination, Mrs Ring is a slim woman whose temperature is 36°C. She has dry mucous membranes and reduced skin turgor. Her pulse is 98 bpm, regular and of normal character. BP 105/65 mmHg. JVP is not visible. HS normal but an ejection systolic murmur is evident in the aortic area. It does not radiate to the carotids. O_2 saturations are 98% on air. Chest is clear to auscultation and abdominal examination is unremarkable. She has a large bruise on her right buttock and inferior to her right iliac crest and significantly reduced range of movement of her right hip.

Mrs Ring passes some urine in A+E whilst waiting to see a doctor. The nursing staff note that the urine is dark brown in colour (Figure 20.1) and shows 4+blood on dipstick and protein 1+ but no other abnormalities.

What is your first management priority?

Mrs Ring's airway and breathing are satisfactory but she is intravascularly volume depleted as evidenced by tachycardia, a relatively low BP for an elderly lady, JVP not visible, reduced skin turgor and dry mucus membranes. She should therefore be rehydrated with intravenous fluids. In elderly patients, these should not be given too quickly in case of left ventricular dysfunction and the

Nephrology: Clinical Cases Uncovered. By M. Clatworthy. Published 2010 by Blackwell Publishing.

likelihood of precipitating pulmonary oedema e.g. give 1 litre of normal saline over 4 hours.

A cannula is placed and Mrs Ring is started on some normal saline. Some routine blood tests are sent (results shown below) and a urine sample for microscopy.

Investigations show:

Hb 11.8 g/dL, MCV 85, WBC 6.5 × 10⁹/L, Platelets 259 × 10⁹/L

Hb 11.8 g/dL, MCV 85, WBC 6.5×10^9/L, Platelets 259×10^9/L

U+E: Na 150 mmol/L, K 7.1 mmol/L, Urea 16.3 mmol/L, Creatinine 185 μmol/L (eGFR 24 mL/min/1.73 m²)

LFT: normal Ca 2.02 mmol/L (normal range 2.12–2.60), PO_4 2.7 mmol/L (normal range 0.8–1.4)

Albumin 35 g/dL, Glucose 5.0 mmol/L, CRP 7 mg/L

Urine microscopy: no red cells, no casts

CXR: NAD

Right hip X-ray: no fracture.

ECG: 90 bpm, sinus rhythm, peaked T waves

What treatment should Mrs Ring receive as a matter of urgency?

She is hyperkalaemic with ECG changes (peaked T waves). This needs to be treated to prevent potentially fatal cardiac arrhythmias.

Mrs Ring is given 10 mL 10% calcium gluconate and 10 units of Actrapid together with 50 mL of 50% dextrose. The peaked T waves resolve and a repeat K+ taken on a venous gas in A+E is 5.8 mmol/L.

Why is Mrs Ring hypernatraemic?

The most likely cause of hypernatraemia in this case is dehydration or water depletion. Other causes are shown in Box 20.1.

Given her hypernatraemia, the normal saline is stopped and replaced with a 1 L bag of 5% dextrose, prescribed over 4 hours.

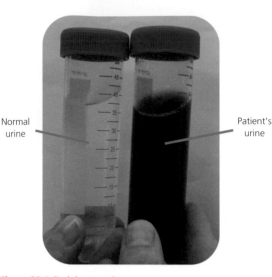

Normal urine

Patient's urine

Figure 20.1 Dark brown urine.

Box 20.1 Causes of hypernatraemia

- Fluid loss without water replacement, typically fever, vomiting, diarrhoea, burns.
- Incorrect IV fluid replacement (if patient is NBM and maintained on IV fluids then N saline should be alternated with 5% dextrose).
- Diabetes insipidis: inability to concentrate urine, therefore dilute urine produced and plasma becomes increasingly hyperosmostic.
- Hyperaldosteronism: can be primary, as in Conn's syndrome. This is associated with hypokalaemia.

What is the most likely cause of her dark urine, given that she is dipstick blood 4+ but has no red cells on microscopy?

This is most likely to be due to the presence of myoglobin in the urine. Myoglobin is a muscle protein which is freely filtered at the glomerulus. It leads to dark urine and gives a false positive for blood on urine dipstick (as does haemaglobinuria).

True haematuria can also give dark urine, particularly if it is glomerular in origin, giving so-called 'coke-coloured' urine. However, in cases of glomerular haematuria, dipstick will be positive for blood, but there will also be red cell casts or misshapen/fragmented red cells visible on urine microscopy. Macroscopic haematuria from the lower urinary tract can lead to red-brown discolouration of the urine, becoming darker if the urine

remains in the bladder for a longer period. In such cases, the dipstick is positive for blood and morphologically normal red cells can be visualised on microscopy. Red-brown discoloured urine can also be seen with rifampicin treatment, beetroot ingestion and in some cases of porphyria. In these conditions the dipstick will be negative for blood.

Mrs Ring's GP calls to ask how she is getting on. You take the opportunity to ask about her past medical history, in particular whether she has ever had any U+E performed previously. He tells you that she is usually very sprightly but did have some U+E performed at the octogenarian well-woman clinic 2 years ago. At this time her creatinine was 65 μmol/L (eGFR 81 mL/min/1.73 m².).

Why has she developed acute renal impairment?

The most likely differentials are as follows.

- Pre-renal failure/ATN secondary to volume depletion.
- Rhabdomyolysis: a number of features make this a possibility.
  - The probable presence of myoglobin in the urine.
  - Hypocalcaemia: in part due to binding of calcium to damaged muscle cells. In rhabdomyolysis, hypocalcaemia does not usually become so severe as to require corrective treatment.
  - Elevated K+, disproportionate to the degree of renal impairment. Potassium is released from damaged muscle cells as they die.
  - A compatible history with a prolonged period of immobility and exposure to statins.

What additional investigations would you perform?

- *Creatine kinase (CK):* CK is a muscle enzyme which is released following damage by any cause. In rhabdomyolysis levels are usually raised at least five times the normal range and can be 100 times normal. CK levels rise 12 hours after the initial damage and the higher the peak level, the more likely that renal impairment will occur.
- *US renal tract:* to exclude any other cause of acute renal failure such as obstruction or in this case haematoma (less likely).

Mrs Ring's CK is 68,000 iu/L (normal range 25–195 iu/L). US shows 2 × 9.8 cm kidneys with no hydronephrosis. This is consistent with a diagnosis of rhabdomyolysis secondary to

> **Box 20.2 Causes of rhabdomyolysis**
>
> **Physical trauma**
> - Compression of muscles: crush syndrome (e.g. in earthquakes), car accident, confinement in a fixed position (e.g. after a stroke, due to drunkenness or in prolonged surgery).
> - Muscle ischaemia: arterial thrombosis or embolism, arterial clamping during surgery, generally reduced blood supply if patient is profoundly hypotensive, e.g. severe sepsis.
> - Excessive muscle activity: extreme physical exercise (particularly when poorly hydrated), muscle tetany, prolonged seizures or status epilepticus.
> - Electrocution: for example, lightning strike, high-voltage electric shock.
>
> **Non-physical causes**
> - Disorders of muscle energy supply (usually hereditary enzyme problems), for example, carnitine deficiency, McArdle's disease, phosphofructokinase deficiency
> - Toxins
>   - Heavy metals
>   - Snake/insect venom
>   - Foodborne toxins, e.g. coniine from quail that have consumed hemlock (coturnism), some wild mushrooms contain rhabdo-causing toxins
> - Recreational drugs
>   - Alcohol
>   - Metamphetamines
>   - Cocaine
> - Heroin
> - 3,4-Methylenedioxymethamphetamine (MDMA or Ecstasy)
> - Medications
>   - Statins, especially when prescribed in combinations with fibrates. The risk is said to be 0.44 cases per 10,000 patients annually, which increases to 5.98 if a fibrate is added.
>   - Antipsychotic medications: neuroleptic malignant syndrome, can cause severe muscle spasms and rhabdomyolysis.
>   - Neuromuscular blocking agents, used in anasthesia, may cause malignant hyperthermia, also associated with rhabdomyolysis.
> - Infections
>   - Coxsackie
>   - *Plasmodium falciparum*
>   - Herpes viruses
>   - Legionella
>   - Salmonella
> - Electrolyte and metabolic disturbances
>   - Hyper- and hyponatraemia
>   - Hypokalaemia
>   - Hypocalcaemia
>   - Diabetic ketoacidosis
>   - Hypothyroidism
> - Autoimmune muscle damage: polymyositis, dermatomyositis

her fall and prolonged period of immobility on the hard floor with a possible contribution from the statins she takes.

What are the causes of rhabdomyolysis?

Rhabdomyolysis can occur secondary to physical trauma to muscle or due to non-physical causes, such as drugs (summarised in Box 20.2). The most common pharmacological culprit is statins. In many cases of rhabdomyolysis it is likely that there are contributions from both physical and non-physical causes (as seen in this case), for example, if a patient has a history of heavy exercise followed by heavy alcohol intake. In all cases, swelling of damaged muscle can lead to compartment syndrome; that is, the swelling of muscle within a fascial compartment can compromise its blood supply by compressing incoming vessels. This leads to further muscle damage and a vicious cycle which can only be interrupted by surgical decompression.

Mrs Ring is rehydrated with a further bag of 5% dextrose. Twelve hours after admission, her JVP is visible and she feels much less thirsty. Unfortunately, she has not passed a great deal of urine since admission (see chart, Figure 20.2). Repeat bloods show Na 138 mmol/L, K 5.0 mmol/L, Urea 22.3 mmol/L, Creatinine 357 µmol/L.

Why does rhabdomyolysis lead to renal failure?

Myoglobin is thought to be directly toxic to renal tubules. It is small enough to be freely filtered at the glomerulus. Under acidic conditions myglobin precipitates with Tamm Horsfall protein and forms casts within tubules which obstruct the normal flow of filtrate through the nephron. Cast formation is facilitated by high levels of uric acid and acidification of the urine. In addition, iron released from the myoglobin is thought to generate reactive oxygen species, which can further damage the tubular

Date:

Ward:

Adult daily fluid balance chart (simple)

Pump asset numbers:

Pump 1

Pump 2

Previous days	Weight:	Fluid restriction:
Balance:		

For staff use only:
Surname: RING
First names: MARJORIE
Date of birth: 4/12/26
Hospital no: 123456
~~Male~~/Female: F
(Use hospital identification label)

Time	Oral fluid volume	Enteral feed volume	Input 1		Running input total	Urine	NG drainage/ aspiration	NG pH	Diarrhoea		Running output total	Balance	Initial
	Input in mL					Output in mL							
01:00													
02:00													
03:00													
04:00													
05:00													
06:00													
07:00													
08:00													
09:00													
10:00													
11:00	Admission												
12:00			250	60	310	40					40	+270	
13:00			250										
14:00			→ 250		810								
15:00			250			50					90	+720	
16:00			250		1310								
17:00			250		1560						90	+1470	
18:00			167		1727						90	+1637	
19:00	150		167		2044	70					160	+1884	
20:00			167										
21:00	150		167		2528	30					190	+2338	
22:00			167										
23:00			167		2862	40					230	+2632	
24:00			125		2987	10					240	+2747	
Total	300		2625	60	2987	240					240	2747	⊕

Figure 20.2 Mrs Ring's daily fluid balance chart.

cells. Renal biopsy usually shows acute tubular necrosis in addition to casts.

How should Mrs Ring be treated?
• Stop statin.
• Continue rehydration: the aim is to promote a diuresis so that lots of dilute urine is produced, making cast formation less likely. Thus once the patient is adequately hydrated, diuretics such as furosemide can be used.
• Alkalinisation of urine: some nephrologists advocate the use of intravenous bicarbonate in an attempt to alkalinise urine. This should reduce the likelihood of cast formation.
• Supportive therapy including haemodialysis if necessary. Many patient end up requiring a period of renal support, particularly if the peak CK levels are very high.

Mrs Ring becomes increasingly oliguric. A temporary dialysis line is inserted and she is commenced on haemodialysis.

What is Mrs Ring's overall prognosis?
Mrs Ring's renal failure should be reversible, although she may need a period of renal support whilst her ATN recovers. However, any patient admitted with single-organ renal failure has around a 10% 1-year mortality.

Depending on the development of other complications, such as compartment syndrome requiring surgical intervention, mortality in cases of rhabdomyolysis may be as high as 20%.

Mrs Ring remains dialysis dependent for a week, after which her urine output begins to improve. She is discharged 2 weeks later with a creatinine of 120 μmol/L but requires a temporary care package to assist at home, including a carer calling morning and night.

Final note: historical description of rhabdomyolysis
It is thought that the Bible may contain the earliest account of rhabdomyolysis. In the Old Testament Book of Numbers, the Jews demanded meat whilst travelling in the desert. God sent quail in response to the complaints, and people ate large quantities of quail meat. This was followed by a plague which killed numerous people. Rhabdomyolysis after consuming quail was formally described more recently and termed 'coturnism', after Coturnix, the main quail genus. It is known that migrating quail consume large amounts of hemlock, which contains the poisonous alkaloid coniine, which has been shown to cause rhabdomyolysis.

CASE REVIEW

An 82-year-old woman is admitted after a fall and a period of immobility in a fixed position on the floor. Medications include aspirin and a statin. Urine is dark brown in colour and dipstick positive for blood, but there are no casts or red cells visible on urine microscopy. Investigations reveal acute renal impairment and an elevated CK, in keeping with a diagnosis of rhabdomyolysis with associated myoglobinuria. She is treated with intravenous fluid, but requires a period of haemodialysis. She recovers her renal function and is discharged with an appropriate care package.

KEY POINTS

• Dark urine which is dipstick positive for blood but contains no red cells or casts on microscopy is likely to be due to myoglobinuria.
• Myoglobin is a muscle protein released following damage to muscle fibres (rhabdomyolysis).
• Rhabdomyolysis can be caused by physical damage to muscle, for example, compression, excessive exercise, prolonged seizure activity or electrocution.
• Rhabdomyolysis can also be caused by other factors including infections (e.g. coxsackie, legionella),

recreational drugs (e.g. alcohol) and prescription drugs (statins).
• The classic clinical picture is of elevated CK, high K+ (released from damaged muscle cells), low calcium (bound to damaged muscle) and acute renal impairment.
• Treatment is rehydration with the aim of encouraging diuresis and preventing myoglobin cast formation within tubules. This may be facilitated by alkalinising the urine.
• Patients often require a period of renal support but can fully recover renal function. Mortality is around 10–20%.

Case 21 A 28-year-old type I diabetic man with abdominal pain and vomiting

Mr Ian Harris is a 28-year-old man with type I diabetes mellitus (DM) who presents to his GP with abdominal pain and vomiting. He is referred to the Medical Assessment Unit.

What questions would you ask?

• Abdominal pain: duration, onset, site, nature, severity, exacerbating and relieving factors?
• Vomiting: duration, what is he bringing up, does it sound like haematemesis?
• Other abdominal symptoms: Bowel open? Passing flatus (if not, may point to intestinal obstruction)? Abdominal distension (also associated with obstruction)?
• Systemic symptoms or symptoms suggestive of infection? Fever, sweats, cough, sputum, dysuria, frequency, foot/leg ulcers? Diabetics are at increased risk of developing sepsis which can become severe very rapidly.
• Past medical history: how long has he had DM? Are his blood sugars well controlled?
• Drug history: current insulin regimen and other drugs.
• Smoking history: smoker? Exacerbates diabetic micro- and macrovascular disease

Mr Harris has been vomiting for 5 days. This is mainly brown/green-coloured liquid which does not contain blood. For the past 2 days he has had almost constant gnawing, epigastric pain which does not radiate. He is passing flatus and his abdomen is not particularly distended. Over the last day he has also become more lethargic and sleepy.

Mr Harris has been diabetic since the age of 4 years. This has been fairly poorly controlled since his teens. He tells you that his last HbA1c performed in clinic a month ago was 9.9%. His current insulin regimen is Human Mixtard (insulin) bd. He is a smoker who works as a supermarket shelf stacker.

What is HbA1c and what does it reflect? Comment on Mr Harris' HbA1c

HbA1c is a glycosylated form of Hb which normally makes up around 5% of all Hb. If there are persistently elevated levels of blood glucose, this proportion increases. Glycosylation of Hb is irreversible so, once glycosylated, HbA1c will remain in the circulation for the remaining lifespan of the red blood cell (approximately 120 days). Thus it reflects glycaemic state over a period of months. Mr Harris' HbA1c is significantly elevated – it should be <6.5%. Therefore, it is likely that his diabetes is poorly controlled with frequent hyperglycaemia.

What are the important points to address on examination?

• Is the patient well and haemodynamically stable (i.e. not tachycardic, hypotensive, peripherally shut down)?
• Is his temperature elevated, which might point towards an infection as the possible cause of presentation.
• Is there any source of sepsis? Infected ulcers on feet? Signs consistent with a chest infection? Suprapubic tenderness or loin pain suggestive of UTI?
• Abdomen: site of maximal tenderness? Peritonitic? Bowel sounds?

On examination, Mr Harris is unwell, drowsy and peripherally cool and mottled. Pulse is 125 bpm, blood pressure 85/50 mmHg, fingerprick glucose 26.1 mmol/L, Temperature 37.2 °C, RR 32/min, oxygen saturations 95% on air. JVP not seen, heart sounds normal. Chest clear. Abdomen – generalised tenderness, no rebound, no guarding.

List some appropriate investigations

• U+E: patients with a long history of type I DM, with poor control, may have microvascular complications, including diabetic nephropathy with renal impairment.
• Arterial blood gas: to assess whether the patient is acidotic.

Nephrology: Clinical Cases Uncovered. By M. Clatworthy. Published 2010 by Blackwell Publishing.

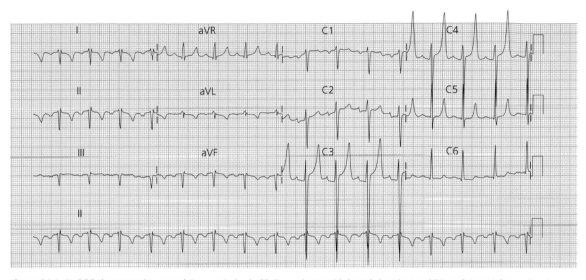

Figure 21.1 An ECG demonstrating tented T waves in leads C3–5, consistent with hyperkalaemia. In addition, there is left axis deviation, and borderline LVH with T wave inversion in the limb leads.

- Full blood count: white cell count may be elevated if there is infection.
- Blood cultures.
- Urinalysis: in particular looking for the presence of ketones (associated with ketoacidosis), or of leucocytes and nitrites (consistent with a UTI).
- Chest radiograph.
- HbA1c.
- ECG.

The investigation results were as follows:

Na^+ 130 mmol/L, K 7.1 mmol/L, Urea 30.3 mmol/L, Creatinine 368 μmol/L, Cl 102 mmol/L

Hb 16.8 g/dL, WBC 24.7 × 10⁹/L, Neutrophils 23.3 × 10⁹/L

Urinalysis: ketones 4+, glucose 4+, protein++, negative for blood, nitrites, leucocytes

ABG: pH 7.12 (7.35–7.45), pO_2 19.6 kPa (8–12), pCO_2 2.6 kPa (4–6), HCO_3 10 mmol/L (22–28)

ECG: shown in Figure 21.1

What sort of acid–base disturbance is present?

Blood pH is normally very tightly regulated and is kept between 7.35 and 7.45. The two organs responsible for regulating H^+ ion concentration are the lungs and the kidneys. Acidosis is defined as a pH < 7.35 and alkalosis as a pH of >7.45.

When interpreting arterial blood gases, start with pH, then look at pCO_2, then look at bicarbonate.

- Look at the pH. Is the patient acidotic (pH < 7.35) or alkalotic (>7.45)?
- Look at the pCO_2. Is CO_2 consistent with the pH? Remember, CO_2 is an acidic gas ($CO_2 + H_2O \leftrightarrow H_2O_2 \leftrightarrow H^+ + HCO_3^-$). In the case of acidosis, if the primary problem is respiratory then the CO_2 will be elevated.
- Look at the bicarbonate. This gives information about the metabolic component of the acid–base disturbance.

In this case, pH < 7.35 so this is acidosis. pCO_2 is low, so the primary problem is metabolic, with respiratory compensation. The HCO_3^- is low, confirming that this is a metabolic acidosis.

Compensation is the process by which the body attempts to correct an acid–base imbalance (Table 21.1). If the primary problem is respiratory, then the kidneys will try to correct the pH. This is achieved by retaining HCO_3^- if there is a respiratory acidosis and secreting HCO_3^- if there is a respiratory alkalosis. If the primary problem is metabolic, then the lungs will try to correct the pH. This is achieved by blowing off CO_2 if there is a metabolic acidosis and retaining CO_2 if there is a metabolic alkalosis.

How does the body sense acid–base disturbances?

- Peripheral chemoreceptors are located in the carotid and aortic bodies (which detect changes in H^+, O_2, CO_2). Signals are then carried via glossopharyngeal nerve to the

Table 21.1 HCO_3^- and pCO_2 levels in partially compensated acid–base disturbances

	pH	HCO_3^-	pCO_2
Respiratory acidosis	<7.35	↑	↑
Respiratory alkalosis	>7.45	↓	↓
Metabolic acidosis	<7.35	↓	↓
Metabolic alkalosis	>7.45	↑	↑

respiratory centre in the medulla and the respiratory rate is then altered.

• Central chemoreceptors are situated in the ventrolateral medulla (which detect changes in CO_2). Again, these lead to changes in respiratory rate according to whether there is acidosis (increased respiratory rate to blow off CO_2) or alkalosis (reduced respiratory rate to maintain CO_2).

What is the anion gap in Mr Harris' blood?

$$\text{Anion gap} = (Na^+ + K^+) - (HCO_3^- + Cl^-)$$
$$= (130 + 7.0) - (10 + 102)$$
$$= 137 - 112$$
$$= 25\, mmol/L$$

Normal anion gap is 10–18 mmol/L and represents the unestimated anions in the blood which consist of albumin, phosphate and other organic acids. It can help in distinguishing the cause of a metabolic acidosis. In this particular case, there is a metabolic acidosis with a high anion gap.

What are the causes of metabolic acidosis with high anion gap?

Metabolic acidosis with a high anion gap occurs due to increased production/reduced clearance of acids.

• Lactic acidosis (shock, hypoxia, sepsis)
• Ketoacidosis (diabetes, alcohol)
• Renal failure
• Liver failure
• Drugs/toxins (salicylates, ethylene glycol, methanol)

What is the most likely diagnosis in this case?

Diabetic ketoacidosis (DKA). DKA only occurs in type I DM, not in insulin-treated type II DM. Clinical features

of DKA include a reduced levels of consciousness, abdominal pain (which may mimic an acute abdomen), fever, polyuria, polydipsia. Haematological and biochemical features include high glucose, urinary ketones, acidosis, hyperkalaemia, high white cell count (even in the absence of infection) and an elevated amylase (up to 10× upper limit of normal). The triad of hyperglycaemia, ketonuria and acidosis are the diagnostic features of DKA.

What are the most appropriate immediate management steps?

The life-threatening problems are dehydration and lack of insulin. Therefore give:

• *intravenous fluids:* normal saline (1 litre stat, 1 litre over 1 hour, 2 hours, 4 hours, 6 hours). Add 20 mmol KCl to all bags (except first, if K^+ >6 mM). The rate of administration of intravenous fluid needs to be adjusted if the patient is known to have left ventricular dysfunction

• *intravenous insulin:* 10 units insulin stat IV. Run at 6 units/h until ketosis resolved (if blood glucose <15, use dextrose saline). Then use a standard sliding scale.

Total body potassium is low and potassium ions are simply in the 'wrong space' due to insulin insufficiency. Potassium levels will drop with the administration of intravenous fluids and insulin and will therefore need to be replaced. In fact, although most patients with DKA will have hyperkalaemia on presentation, hypokalaemia can become a problem once insulin is started. Therefore potassium should be added to replacement fluid and regular monitoring of serum potassium is mandatory.

You see Mr Harris on the ward later in the day. K^+ is now 3.6 mmol/L. He is receiving N saline with 40 mM KCl. His BM is now 15 mM and falling. He is catheterised and has a good urine output but he remains drowsy.

What two other management options will you undertake to prevent complications?

Severe acidosis leads to gastric atony which makes Mr Harris likely to develop vomiting. He has a reduced Glasgow Coma Score (GCS) and is therefore less able to protect his airway. This means that he is at risk of aspiration if he does develop vomiting. Hence, a wide-bore nasogastric tube for gastric decompression is indicated in patients with DKA with a GCS of <15.

Mr Harris is also at risk of venous thromboembolism. Severe dehydration and immobility both predispose to DVT. Therefore all patients should receive prophylactic anticoagulation with low molecular weight heparin unless there is a specific contraindication.

Other general measures which should be considered in patients with DKA include:
- ICU/HDU referral
- exclude and treat sepsis
- monitor U&E regularly
- catheterise if not passing urine regularly
- consider CVP line if fluid balance hard to assess or CCF
- oxygen if hypoxaemic (SpO$_2$ <94%)
- consider i.v. bicarbonate if pH < 7.

A nasogastric tube is inserted and Mr Harris is started on enoxaparin 40mg subcutaneously. Fluid replacement and sliding scale are continued and he slowly improves. Five days later, he is feeling much better and is ready to go back on his regular insulin. His repeat U+E are now as follows.

Na$^+$ 141 mmol/L, K 5.0 mmol/L, Urea 10.3 mmol/L, Creatinine 158 µmol/L (eGFR 48 mL/min/1.73 m^2, CKD stage 3). On reviewing his notes, you see that his creatinine has been abnormal for at least a year.

What aspects of the history would be useful in determining the cause of renal impairment?

In a patient like Mr Harris with a long history of poorly controlled diabetes, the most likely cause of renal impairment is diabetic nephropathy. This is one of the three microvascular complications of diabetes, the others being neuropathy and retinopathy. Microvascular complications usually develop in tandem and their severity is related to overall glucose control. Patients who have renal impairment secondary to diabetic nephropathy will usually have a history of retinopathy, and will often have had some form of retinal photocoagulation. In patients with renal impairment, fundoscopy should be performed to look for signs of diabetic retinopathy (Box 21.1).

Patients with diabetic nephropathy may also have a history of neuropathy (lack of sensation in fingers or feet) or of autonomic neuropathy, particularly a history of postural hypotension (they get dizzy when they stand), impotence or gastroparesis (history of vomiting after meals). The different types of neuropathy observed in diabetes are summarised in Box 21.2. Autonomic neu-

> **Box 21.1 Diabetic retinopathy**
>
> 1 Background – microaneurysms (dots) and microhaemorrhages (blots), hard exudates
> 2 Preproliferative – cotton wool spots (soft exudates indicative of retinal infarcts), more extensive microhaemorrhage
> 3 Proliferative – new vessel formation (requires urgent ophthalmological opinion)
> 4 Maculopathy – changes described in 1 or 2 affecting the macula

> **Box 21.2 Different forms of neuropathy observed in diabetes mellitus**
>
> 1 Peripheral sensory neuropathy ('glove and stocking' neuropathy, vibration sensation lost early)
> 2 Painful neuropathy
> 3 Autonomic neuropathy
> 4 Mononeuritis multiplex
> 5 Diabetic amyotrophy (painful wasting and weakness of quadriceps muscles of the thigh)

ropathy can also lead to chronic urinary retention. This can result in recurrent UTI and intermittent obstruction, both of which may exacerbate renal impairment. It is therefore useful to perform a bladder scan post micturition to ensure the patient is fully emptying their bladder if there is any history suggestive of retention.

What are the clinical features of diabetic nephropathy?

Early diabetic nephropathy is characterised by microalbuminuria. In type I diabetics, this usually occurs 7–10 years after diagnosis. As lesions progress, proteinuria increases and can even become so heavy as to be in the nephrotic range. Microalbuminuira is defined as 30–300 mg/24 h and is not detectable by standard urine dipstick. It may be detected using a specialised (and more expensive) urine dipstick kit or can be quantified by estimating the albumin/creatinine ratio (ACR) in a single urine sample. This has proved useful in monitoring patients with diabetes who are at risk of developing diabetic nephropathy. An ACR of >2.5 mg/mmol in men or >3.5 mg/mmol in women is indicative of microalbuminuria. An ACR of >30 mg/mmol indicates there is proteinuria which will be identifiable on regular dipstick. An ACR of 30 mg/mmol is approximately equivalent to a protein/creatinine ratio (PCr) of 50 mg/mmol.

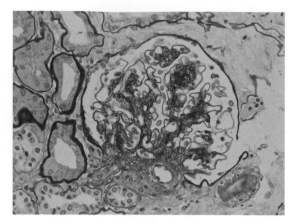

Figure 21.2 A renal biopsy showing a glomerulus with typical diabetic changes including mesangial expansion and nodular sclerosis. Other changes observed include arteriolar hyalinosis and interstitial expansion and fibrosis.

In the early stages of diabetic nephropathy, there is hyperfiltration and elevated GFR and an overall increase in the volume of kidneys. As nephropathy progresses, there is a decline in GFR, measurable as a gradually increasing creatinine.

What are the histopathological manifestations of diabetic nephropathy?

Diabetes mainly affects the glomeruli, leading to thickening of the basement membrane and glomerulosclerosis, which may be diffuse or nodular (Kimmelstiel–Wilson lesions). There is mesangial expansion and mesangiolysis can occur. Figure 21.2 shows a typical renal biopsy taken from a patient with advanced diabetic nephropathy.

The development of nephropathy is clearly related to chronic hyperglycaemia. One of the pathological mechanisms involved is the non-enzymatic glycation of proteins to produce advanced glycosylation end products (AGE). AGE can stimulate the production of type IV collagen and reactive oxygen species by mesangial cells, endothelial cells and macrophages, contributing to the glomerulosclerosis observed.

How should Mr Harris' nephropathy be treated?

• Tight glucose control is useful in slowing the progression of microalbuminuria and early renal dysfunction. However, once there is heavy proteinuria, there is irreversible damage in the kidney which is self-perpetuating.

• Antiproteinurics: ACEI and ARB have been demonstrated to reduce microalbuminuria and slow the progression of renal impairment. Screening for microalbuminuria should allow early detection and treatment.

• Tight blood pressure control: hypertension worsens diabetic glomerulopathy and should therefore be aggressively treated. ACEI and ARB are the first-line treatment, as described above, but some patients may require additional agents. Aim for a BP of <125/75 mmHg in a diabetic with CKD.

• Treatment of dyslipidaemia with diet, statins, +/– fibrates.

• Advise to stop smoking.

To summarise, the risk factors for progression of diabetic nephropathy are poor glucose control, hypertension, dyslipidaemia and smoking. Each of these should be maximally corrected.

What is the prognosis of Mr Harris' renal disease?

At least 25% of diabetics diagnosed before the age of 25 years will go on to develop ESRF. In the UK, diabetes is the most common cause of ESRF requiring RRT, making up around 25% of patients on dialysis. In the US, they make up nearer 45% of patients reaching ESRF.

What is the best form of renal replacement therapy for Mr Harris, should he progress to ESRF?

Transplantation is the best form of RRT for diabetics. However, some will not be fit enough for transplantation by the time they reach ESRF if they have already accrued significant macrovascular disease in the form of coronary artery disease, cerebrovascular disease and peripheral vascular disease.

For those starting dialysis, the survival is much poorer than for age- and sex-matched non-diabetics starting dialysis. For example, UK renal registry data in 2007 showed a 92% 1-year survival for non-diabetics <65 years of age starting dialysis compared with an 83% 1-year survival in diabetics of the same age. This is because most diabetic patients starting dialysis already have significant vascular disease, which dialysis seems to accelerate. Cardiovascular events including MI, cardiac arrest and CVA are the most common causes of death in this population, followed by infection. There is some suggestion that peritoneal dialysis (PD) may be a better option than haemodialysis (HD), at least for younger, fitter diabetics. An analysis of US Medicare data between 1995 and 2000 demonstrated that, among diabetic patients with no co-morbidities, patients on PD had a lower relative death rate at ages below 45 years. In diabetic patients more than 45 years old, with or without co-morbidities, PD patients had a higher relative death rate as compared with the rate in HD patients. The overall survival of diabetic patients with different forms of RRT is shown in Table 21.2.

Table 21.2 Survival of diabetics with renal replacement therapy

Renal replacement therapy	5-year survival	10-year survival
Cadaveric renal transplant	75%	50%
Living renal transplant	85%	60–65%
Kidney-pancreas transplant	80%	60–65%
Dialysis (PD or HD)	30%	<1%

Data courtesy of UK Blood and Transplant

CASE REVIEW

A 28-year-old man with poorly controlled type I diabetes presents with abdominal pain and vomiting. On examination, he is unwell, hypotensive and tachycardic. Investigations show a metabolic acidosis with a high anion gap. He also has ketonuria and a high blood glucose in keeping with a diagnosis of diabetic ketoacidosis. He is treated with intravenous fluids and a sliding scale. On recovery, he is noted to have renal impairment, with a reduced GFR and CKD stage 3. He also has a history of diabetic retinopathy and proteinuria on urine dipstick. Thus his renal impairment is most probably due to diabetic nephropathy. He should be commenced on an ACEI or ARB and encouraged to improve his glucose control. It is likely that in the long term the patient will progress to ESRF and will require RRT.

KEY POINTS

- Acidosis is defined as a blood pH < 7.35 and alkalosis as a pH of >7.45.
- If a patient presents with metabolic acidosis then the anion gap should be calculated as follows: $(Na + K) - (HCO_3^- + Cl)$.
- Metabolic acidosis with a high anion gap can be caused by lactic acidosis, renal failure, liver failure, drugs/toxins (salicylates, ethylene glycol, methanol) and ketoacidosis.
- Diabetic ketoacidosis (DKA) is characterised by the triad of acidosis, ketonuria and hyperglycaemia.
- Only type I diabetics develop DKA. It is a serious illness which can be life-threatening and may require nursing in a high-dependency or critical care unit. Patients should be treated with aggressive intravenous rehydration and intravenous insulin. Complications include

thromboembolism (due to immobility and dehydration) and aspiration pneumonia (due to gastroparesis and impaired consciousness).
- Patients with type I diabetes frequently develop renal involvement, with diabetic nephropathy of some degree occurring almost universally after >15 years of disease. At least 25% of diabetics diagnosed before the age of 25 years will go on to develop ESRF. In the UK, diabetes is the most common cause of ESRF requiring RRT.
- Diabetic patients on dialysis have a worse prognosis than non-diabetics. The preferred form of renal replacement therapy for diabetics is transplantation. For long-term survival, a kidney-pancreas or living donor kidney transplant is the best option.

Case 22 A 22-year-old man with weakness and lethargy

Mr Iestyn Gough is a 22-year-old man who is currently an inpatient on the oncology ward. He had an osteosarcoma excised 2 years ago. He has been relatively well but now has recurrent disease in his pelvis. He received chemotherapy 1 week ago and has been admitted with weakness and lethargy.

What aspects of the history would you explore?

- Duration of symptoms?
- What is meant by weakness? Focal neurological symptoms (which might occur if there were brain or spinal cord metastases) or generalised muscle weakness? Are there systemic symptoms suggestive of infection? Cough, sputum, shortness of breath, diarrhoea, dysuria, frequency which might account for lethargy?
- Past medical history: details of osteosarcoma, particularly of recurrence. Does he have any other past medical history, e.g. similar symptoms or of neurological disease?
- Drug history: what chemotherapy did he get? What are his current meds? Recreational drugs?
- Smoking history: smoker? Alcohol?
- Family history: any medical problems, including neurological problems.

Mr Gough was previously completely fit and well until he developed the osteosarcoma in his right femur. This was treated surgically and with standard combination chemotherapy. Since then, he has not had any further medical problems, until the development of recurrent disease in his pelvic bone. There is no evidence of disease elsewhere.

He had combination chemotherapy 1 week ago, which included ifosfamide. After the first few days of treatment he felt slightly nauseated and weak, but in the last week or so

he has felt increasingly unwell. He described himself as 'tired and washed-out' and feels like his muscles are generally weak. He has had difficulty walking any distance and getting from sitting to standing. He has not had any focal neurological symptoms nor any systemic or localising symptoms suggestive of infection. His current medications include amphotericin lozenges and omeprazole.

Examination shows that he is afebrile. Pulse 80 bpm, BP 120/70 mmHg, RR 15 rpm, O₂ saturations 98% s/v air. Chest clear, abdomen soft, non-tender. No organomegaly.

What investigations would you perform on initial assessment?

- FBC, U+E, CRP, Ca/PO$_4$, LFT
- Urine dipstick
- CXR
- ECG

Investigations show:

Hb 10.5 g/dL, WBC 3.3 × 10^9/L, Platelets 164 × 10^9/L

Na 137 mmol/L, K 2.5 mmol/L, Urea 5.3 mmol/L, Creatinine 90 μmol/L

Normal Ca/PO$_4$/LFTs

Urine dipstick: no glycosuria, no proteinuria

CXR normal

What changes might be present on the electrocardiogram?

Mr Gough has significant hypokalaemia which is associated with U waves on ECG (Figure 22.1).

What are the causes of hypokalaemia?

- Renal losses: diuretics (loop and thiazide), renal tubular acidosis (RTA), excess aldosterone
- GI losses: diarrhoea, laxative abuse, villous adenoma
- Alkalosis: hydrogen ions transported out of cells at the expense of K$^+$ flowing in

Nephrology: Clinical Cases Uncovered. By M. Clatworthy. Published 2010 by Blackwell Publishing.

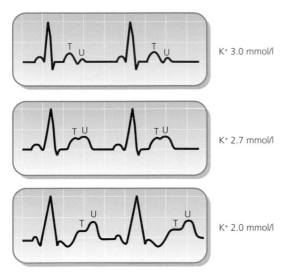

K⁺ 3.0 mmol/l

K⁺ 2.7 mmol/l

K⁺ 2.0 mmol/l

Figure 22.1 ECG changes in hypokalaemia. The QRS complexes begin to widen when the serum potassium drops to 2.5–3 mmol/l, the ST segments may become depressed and the T waves may begin to flatten. The U waves also begin to increase in size, becoming as tall as the T waves. The U waves reach 'giant' size and fuse with the T waves when the level drops to 1.5–2 mmol/l. Symptoms of hypokalaemia range from polyuria in mild cases to muscle weakness.

What additional investigations may be useful?

- Magnesium and chloride levels
- ABG

These tests are performed and the results are shown below.

- Cl 116 mmol/L (normal range 96–104)
- ABGs : pH 7.24, HCO_3 9 kPa, CO_2 3.3 kPa

What acid–base disturbance is shown?

Metabolic acidosis. When interpreting arterial blood gases:

- look at the pH – is the patient acidotic (pH < 7.35) or alkalotic (pH > 7.45)?
- look at the PCO_2 – is the primary problem respiratory or metabolic? Remember, CO_2 is an acidic gas. $CO_2 + H_2O \leftrightarrow H_2O_2 \leftrightarrow H^+ + HCO_3^-$
- look at the bicarbonate – this gives information about the metabolic component of the acid–base disturbance. In this case pH < 7.35 so this is acidosis. pCO_2 is low/normal, so the primary problem is metabolic. The HCO_3^- is low and this confirms that this is a metabolic acidosis.

What is the anion gap in this case?

14.5 (normal)

$$\begin{aligned} \text{Anion gap} &= (Na + K) - (HCO_3^- + Cl) \\ &= (137 + 2.5) - (9 + 116) \\ &= 139.5 - 125 \\ &= 14.5 \, nmol/L \end{aligned}$$

A normal anion gap is 10–18 mmol/L. This represents the unmeasured anions which consist of albumin, phosphate and other organic acids. It can help in distinguishing the cause for a metabolic acidosis.

So, this is a case of metabolic acidosis with a normal anion gap.

What are the causes of a metabolic acidosis with a normal anion gap?

- Type 1 renal tubular acidosis ('classic distal')
- Type 2 renal tubular acidosis ('proximal')
- Chronic diarrhoea

The patient does not have a history of GI disturbance/diarrhoea, so this picture is likely to be due to renal loss of K⁺ and inappropriate acid handling. RTA usually presents as a hyperchloraemic, metabolic acidosis, with a normal anion gap. The aetiology is a failure of urinary acidification (defective reabsorption of bicarbonate in the proximal tubule or a failure of H⁺ secretion in the distal tubule). This may occur as a primary disease due to mutations in genes encoding the pumps controlling bicarbonate and acid transport, or may be due to acquired dysfunction of damaged tubular function (mainly due to drugs and toxins such as heavy metals).

What further investigation may be useful in confirming the possibility of a renal tubular acidosis?

Urine pH. Normal urine pH is variable and generally runs between 4.5 and 7.5. Patients with distal RTA are unable to acidify urine to a pH of <5.3.

Mr Gough's urine pH is 7.6, which is inappropriately high, given the presence of systemic acidosis. This makes RTA the likely diagnosis.

Renal tubular acidosis is divided into two main subsets: type I (distal) RTA, in which there is a failure of H⁺ or ammonium secretion in the distal tubule, and type II (proximal) in which there is defective reabsorption of bicarbonate in the proximal tubule. Distal RTA is more

Table 22.1 Features of distal and proximal RTA

	Type I (distal)	Type II (proximal)
Urine pH	>5.3 (never acidifies)	Variable
Plasma HCO₃	<10 mmol/L	>14 mmol/L
Plasma K	Low	Normal-low
Complications	Nephrocalcinosis, calculi	Osteomalacia
Other features	UTI	Glycosuria, aminoaciduria

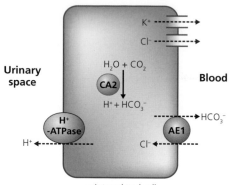

Figure 22.2 Mechanisms involved in acidifying urine in the collecting duct. See text for details.

common than proximal RTA. In addition, proximal RTA usually occurs in children with Fanconi's syndrome with associated aminoaciduria and glycosuria.

Which features suggest that the diagnosis in this case is of distal rather than proximal renal tubular acidosis?

A number of features of this case make distal (type I) RTA the most likely diagnosis, particularly the very low K⁺ and very low bicarbonate. In proximal RTA, the urine acidification is variable, as there is opportunity for attempted acidification in the distal nephron. The features which distinguish distal from proximal RTA are shown in Table 22.1.

The collecting duct is the principal site of urine acidification and is composed of two cell types:
- principal cells – transport Na, K and water
- α-intercalated cells – secrete H⁺ and HCO3⁻.

Acid secretion is performed by the α-intercalated cells, and involves two pumps (H⁺ATPase and the basolateral Cl⁻:HCO₃⁻ anion exchanger 1 (AE-1)) and an enzyme (carbonic anhydrase 2 (CA2)) (summarised in Figure 22.2). Damage to the α-intercalated cells or a specific dysfunction of either of the pumps or the enzyme leads to distal RTA.

What is the likely cause of distal renal tubular acidosis in this patient?

Distal RTA can be caused by mutations in the gene encoding AE-1 (autosomal dominant dRTA) or in the gene encoding one of the subunits of the H⁺ATPase (autosomal recessive RTA, associated with sensorineural deafness). Some patients also have defective CA2, which is also an autosomal recessive condition. In this particular case, the cause is unlikely to be an inherited mutation,

Box 22.1 Causes of distal (type I) RTA

Primary (genetic cause)
- AE-1 (AD)
- H⁺ATPase mutation (AR, associated with sensorineural deafness)
- CA2 mutation (AR, associated with osteopetrosis and cerebral calcification)

Secondary
- Autoimmune disease – Sjögren's disease, SLE, rheumatoid arthritis
- Medullary sponge kidney
- Drugs – amphotericin, lithium, anticancer (ifosfamide), amiloride, triamterene, trimethoprim, pentamidine
- Toxins – vanadate, toluene

Rare – pregnancy, sickle cell anaemia

because these patients will usually present in infancy. Mr Gough is much more likely to have acquired distal RTA. There are a number of secondary causes of distal RTA, shown in Box 22.1. In this particular case, the timing of onset suggests that the tubular dysfunction is related to the ifosfamide he received 2 weeks previously.

How would you treat this patient?

Oral potassium and bicarbonate supplementation.

What is the likely prognosis for this problem?

It is likely that the tubular dysfunction will spontaneously recover over the next week or so.

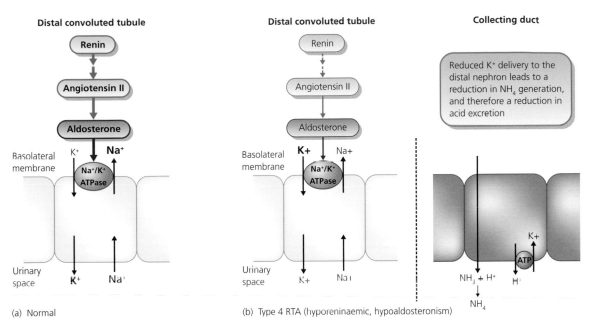

(a) Normal   (b) Type 4 RTA (hyporeninaemic, hypoaldosteronism)

Figure 22.3 Type IV (hyperkalaemic) RTA. (a) Normal. (b) Type 4 RTA (hyporeninaemic, hypoaldosteronism).

What are the other types of renal tubular acidosis and in what context do they occur?

• Type III: rarely used as a classification because it is now thought to be a combination of type I and type II.

• Type IV: type IV RTA ('hyperkalaemic distal') involves the distal tubule and in contrast to the other types of RTA, there is hyperkalaemia. It is associated with a mild (normal anion gap) metabolic acidosis and occurs due to hypoaldosteronism (Figure 22.3).

Causes include the following.

• Primary aldosterone deficiency (rare)
  ○ Primary adrenal insufficiency
  ○ Congenital adrenal hyperplasia
  ○ Aldosterone synthase deficiency
• Hyporeninaemic hypoaldosteronism (due to decreased angiotensin II)
  ○ Renal dysfunction, most commonly diabetic nephropathy
  ○ HIV infection
  ○ Drugs – ACEI, NSAID, ciclosporin
• Aldosterone resistance
  ○ Drugs (amiloride, spironolactone, trimethoprim, pentamidine)
• Pseudohypoaldosteronism

The treatment of type IV RTA is with a mineralocorticoid (such as fludrocortisone), as well as possibly a glucocorticoid for cortisol deficiency, if present. Hypertension and oedema can be a problem in patients with hyporeninaemic hypoaldosteronism so often a diuretic, such as the thiazide diuretic bendromethazide, or a loop diuretic, such as furosemide, is used to control the hyperkalaemia.

CASE REVIEW

A 22-year-old man with a history of recurrent osteosarcoma presents with weakness and lethargy following a recent course of chemotherapy. Investigations demonstrate significant hypokalaemia and a hyperchloraemic, metabolic acidosis with a normal anion gap. The most likely cause of this presentation is an acquired distal renal tubular acidosis secondary to cytotoxic agents which can affect acid secretion by the collecting duct of the kidney. He is treated with potassium and bicarbonate supplements orally. A spontaneous recovery would be expected.

KEY POINTS

- Hypokalaemia usually presents with muscle weakness. The typical ECG change associated with a low potassium is the development of U waves.
- Hypokalaemia can be caused by the loss of K^+ into the gut (e.g. diarrhoea), the renal tubules (diuretics and RTA) or intracellular space (redistribution due to acidosis).
- The classic feature of RTA is hyperchloraemic metabolic acidosis. This occurs because of a failure of either the proximal or distal tubular mechanisms involved in urine acidification. Distal (type I) RTA is more common and biochemical features are more severe, including an inability to lower urinary pH to less than 5.3, severe hypokalaemia and a bicarbonate of <10 mmol/L.
- Distal RTA occurs because of defects in the α-intercalated cells of the collecting duct epithelium, specifically dysfunction of AE-1 and H^+ATPase, pumps involved in acid secretion. These can be congenital or acquired (secondary to autoimmune diseases, drugs and nephrocalcinosis).
- Treatment of dRTA is with oral bicarbonate and potassium supplementation.

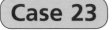 **Case 23** # A 58-year-old type II diabetic with confusion and hyponatraemia

Mr Sanjay Singh is a 58-year-old type II diabetic. He is admitted following a road traffic accident with a head injury and fractured tibia and fibula. Glasgow Coma Score (GCS) on admission was 15 and a CT head did not show any obvious fracture, haematoma or contusion. His lower limb fractures are fixed in plaster of Paris (POP) and he is admitted for observation and analgesia.

Bloods on admission are shown below.

Na 135 mmol/L, K 4.0 mmol/L, Urea 7.3 mmol/L, Creatinine 112 µmol/L, Glc 6.8 mmol/l
Hb 15.8 g/dL, WBC 5.7 × 10⁹/L, Platelets 230 × 10⁹/l

He is seen on ward round the next day and a plan is made to discharge him later in the day. Unfortunately, he becomes increasingly confused during the afternoon. His temperature is 38°C, pulse 90 bpm, BP 145/85 mmHg and JVP is visible. He has no peripheral oedema. O₂ saturations are 93% on air and there are some crackles at the right base. There are no focal neurological signs. Repeat bloods are shown below and Mr Singh's drug chart is shown in Figure 23.1.

Na 125 mmol/L, K 3.8 mmol/L, Urea 5.7 mmol/L, Creatinine 108 µmol/L, Glc 10.6 mmol/L
Hb 15.5 g/dL, WBC 6.2 × 10⁹/L, Platelets 353 × 10⁹/L

What is the most likely cause of Mr Singh's hyponatraemia?

The causes of hyponatraemia are summarised in Box 23.1. Mr Singh's hyponatraemia is acute and he is not obviously oedematous, fluid overloaded or dehydrated (thus CCF, nephrosis, cirrhosis and diarrhoea are unlikely to be the cause of his hyponatraemia). He is not on any medications, particularly diuretics, which might directly affect renal salt handling. We are not told anything about Mr Singh's fluid replacement regimen, therefore if he has

Nephrology: Clinical Cases Uncovered. By M. Clatworthy. Published 2010 by Blackwell Publishing.

been given an excess of 5% dextrose in the past 36 hours, this may have caused hyponatraemia. However, given all of the above exclusions, the most likely diagnosis is the syndrome of inappropriate antidiuretic hormone (SIADH).

Review of Mr Singh's fluid charts shows that he has had free oral intake but no intravenous fluids.

What investigations would you undertake to confirm the diagnosis of syndrome of inappropriate antidiuretic hormone?

Serum and urine osmolalities should be measured. Plasma osmolality is usually kept within a tight range. In SIADH there is dilute plasma with osmolalities of <260 mmol/kg and inappropriately concentrated urine with urine osmolalities of >500 mmol/kg. Urinary sodium levels are usually >20 mmol/L.

Mr Singh's urine osmolality is 549 mosmol/kg and his serum osmolality is 258 mosmol/kg, confirming the diagnosis of SIADH.

What is the likely cause of syndrome of inappropriate antidiuretic hormone in Mr Singh's case?

Syndrome of inappropriate antidiuretic hormone can be caused by many pathologies, as summarised in Box 23.2. In this particular case, it is most likely to be due to head injury. However, there may be other contributory features. His examination findings suggest the possibility of a right basal pneumonia (febrile, crackles at right base). In addition, he has been given opiates for his pain and is receiving chlorpropamide (see drug chart in Figure 23.1).

Where is antidiuretic hormone produced and what are its actions?

Antidiuretic hormone (ADH, also known as vasopressin) is produced in the hypothalamus, stored in vesicles in the

Prescription chart

Surname SINGH First names SANJAY Consultant MRC	Hospital No. A30694 Date of birth Sex 20/6/50 M Ward BEECH	Weight Height	Drug sensitivities Doctor must enter this information on FRONT of case folder		
			Date	Drug/substance	Signature
			22/10	ul	

Regular prescriptions

Month and date ⟶

Tick times or enter other times ⟶

1. Drug (approved name) ASPIRIN				6													
Dose 75mg	Route PO	Start date 22/10	Stop date	⑧													
				12													
Signature: ⌒ Bleep no.: 123			Pharm	14													
Additional instructions				18													
				22													

2. Drug (approved name) ATORVASTATIN				6													
Dose 10mg	Route PO	Start date 22/10	Stop date	8													
				12													
Signature: ⌒ Bleep no.: 123			Pharm	14													
Additional instructions				⑱													
				22													

3. Drug (approved name) CHLORPROPAMIDE				6													
Dose 250mg	Route PO	Start date 22/10	Stop date	⑧													
				12													
Signature: ⌒ Bleep no.: 123			Pharm	14													
Additional instructions				18													
				22													

4. Drug (approved name) COPROXAMOL				6													
Dose Ti	Route PO	Start date 22/10	Stop date	⑧													
				⑫													
Signature: ⌒ Bleep no.: 123			Pharm	14													
Additional instructions				⑱													
				㉒													

5. Drug (approved name)				6													
Dose	Route	Start date	Stop date	8													
				12													
Signature: Bleep no.:			Pharm	14													
Additional instructions				18													
				22													

6. Drug (approved name)				6													
Dose	Route	Start date	Stop date	8													
				12													
Signature: Bleep no.:			Pharm	14													
Additional instructions				18													
				22													

Figure 23.1 Mr Singh's prescription chart.

Box 23.1 Causes of hyponatraemia

- Inappropriate water retention – SIADH. Urine osmolality is usually >500 mosmol/kg (inappropriately concentrated when compared with serum osmolality which tends to be <260 mosmol/kg)
- Excess water intake
  - Psychogenic polydipsia
  - Inappropriate IV fluids
- Combined Na + water retention with an excess of water
  - Congestive cardiac failure (CCF)
  - Nephrotic syndrome
  - Cirrhosis
- Salt loss
  - Renal: diuretics, Addison's disease, salt-losing nephropathy
  - GI: diarrhoea, villous adenoma
- Pseudohyponatraemia
  - Hypercholesterolaemia
  - Hyperproteinaemia

Box 23.2 Causes of SIADH

- Malignancy
  - Pancreatic cancer
  - Lymphoma
  - Small cell carcinoma of the lung
  - Prostate cancer
- CNS/neurological disorders
  - Abscess
  - Meningoencephalitis
  - Subarachnoid/subdural haemorrhage
  - Head injury
  - Guillain–Barré syndrome
- Pulmonary disorders
  - TB
  - Pneumonia
  - Pulmonary abscess/empyema
  - Aspergillosis
- Metabolic causes
  - Porphyria
- Drugs
  - Chlorpropamide
  - Opiates
  - Cytotoxins
  - Chlorpromazine

posterior pituitary and released in response to rising plasma osmolality or a reduction in plasma volume/pressure. Its main action is on the kidneys, causing water retention and thus a more concentrated urine to be produced (as its name suggests).

Antidiuretic hormone causes a more concentrated urine to be produced by increasing the permeability to water of the distal convoluted tubule and collecting ducts, thus allowing an increase in water reabsorption down the osmotic gradients set up by the loop of Henle. This results in the excretion of a smaller volume of more concentrated urine – antidiuresis.

Antidiuretic hormone increases permeability via the insertion of additional water channels (aquaporin-2) into the apical membrane of the tubules/collecting duct epithelial cells. This is achieved through the action of ADH on V2 receptors, G protein-coupled receptors on the basolateral membrane of cells lining the distal convoluted tubules and conducting ducts. Following binding, the G protein triggers the cAMP cascade which triggers the insertion of aquaporin-2 water pores by exocytosis of storage vesicles. The aquaporins then allow water to pass out of the distal convoluted tubules and the conducting tubules into the interstitium and back into the blood, increasing the concentration of urine and expanding blood volume.

Antidiuretic hormone also increases peripheral vascular resistance and thus mean arterial blood pressure. This effect appears small in healthy individuals but may be an important compensatory mechanism for restoring blood pressure in hypovolaemic shock.

Antidiuretic hormone also has a number of actions locally in the brain including:
- memory formation
- maintenance of circadian rhythm
- control of aggressive behaviour.

How would you manage this patient?

The main management of SIADH is to restrict fluid intake to 0.5–1 L per day. This is usually in the form of normal saline, if IV fluids are used (NB: normal (0.9%) saline contains approximately 150 mmol/L of Na). Occasionally hypertonic saline is given but this requires careful management to avoid a rapid increase in sodium levels. The aim is to bring the sodium up by no more than 5 mmol/day. Severe cases may require the use of demeclocycline, an agent which causes nephrogenic diabetes insipidus, i.e. it makes the collecting tubules insensitive to the actions of ADH.

More recently, a new class of drugs has become available in the form of specific V2 antagonists, for example tolvaptan and satavaptan, which may be useful in SIADH.

Why is important not to correct hyponatraemia too quickly?

If plasma Na+ is corrected too quickly then central pontine myelinolysis (CPM) can occur, where neurones in the pontine region become demyelinated. This is thought to be due to rapid fluid shifts out of the brain in response to large increases in plasma sodium. Patients rapidly develop para- or quadraparesis, dysphagia, dysarthria, diplopia and loss of consciousness. Diagnosis is by clinical features and MRI (showing a high signal in the pons).

Aim to correct plasma sodium by 5 mmol/L/24 h. Maximum correction 8 mmol/L/24 h. Reports of CPM have occurred where Na has risen by >10 mmol/L/24 h.

Mr Singh is placed on a 1000 mL fluid restriction over the next 4 days. A chest X-ray confirms a likely right basal

Table 23.1 Causes of hypontraemia according to volume status and urine Na excretion

	Hypovolaemia	Euvolaemia/hypervolaemia
Urine Na+>20 mM	Diuretics Hypoadrenalism / Addison's	SIADH Hypothyroidism Chronic renal failure
Urine Na+<20 mM	Vomiting Diarrhoea	LVF Cirrhosis Nephrotic syndrome

pneumonia and he is therefore commenced on appropriate antibiotic therapy. His sodium rises from 125 to 129 mmol/L on day 1, to 132 mmol/L on day 2 and to 136 mmol/L by day 3. He is finally discharged on oral antibiotics on day 6.

CASE REVIEW

A 58-year-old type II diabetic is admitted following an accident. Over the next 36 hours he becomes confused. Investigations show significant hyponatraemia (Na 125 mmol/L), reduced serum osmolality and increased urine osmolality in keeping with a diagnosis of SIADH.

This has probably been caused by the head injury sustained during the accident. He is fluid restricted to 1 L in 24 hours and his sodium begins to rise. He improves rapidly and is discharged 5 days later with a sodium of 136 mmol/L.

KEY POINTS

- Mild hyponatraemia is common and usually asymptomatic. If the sodium falls to around 120 mmol/L then there is often restlessness, irritability and confusion. Sodium levels of <110 mmol/L lead to progressive coma and seizures.
- Hyponatraemia occurs if there is too little sodium, too much water or both.
- When assessing the cause of hyponatraemia, it is important to establish the volume status of the patient.
- If the patient is hypovolaemic then hyponatraemia may be caused by diuretics, hypoadrenalism, salt-wasting nephropathy (see Table 23.1).
- If the patient is euvolaemic or fluid overloaded then hyponatraemia may be due to SIADH, chronic renal failure, LVF, cirrhosis or nephrotic syndrome (see Table 23.1).

- In SIADH, typical findings are:
  - ○ Na <125 mmol/L
  - ○ patient is normovolaemic
  - ○ urinary Na >20 mmol/L
  - ○ plasma osmo <260 mosmol/kg
  - ○ urinary osmo >500 mosmol/kg.
- Syndrome of inappropriate antidiuretic hormone may be caused by intracranial pathology such as head injury or infection, pulmonary pathologies including pneumonia, malignancies and drugs (particularly chlorpropamide and chlorpromazine).
- Treatment of SIADH is with fluid restriction. The aim should be to bring the sodium up slowly in order to avoid central pontine myelinolysis.

A 49-year-old man with headache and malaise

Mr Evan Davies, a 49-year-old man, is urgently referred by his GP to the nephrology clinic. He presented 2 days ago with a 9-month history of headache and malaise. Examination was unremarkable except that he looked a little pale and his blood pressure was elevated (190/100 mmHg). The GP sent off some routine blood tests which showed Na 138 mmol/L, K 4.8 mmol/L, Urea 18 mmol/L, creatinine 350 μmol/L and Hb 8.5 g/dL (MCV 82), prompting the referral. Prior to the consultation an ultrasound scan of his renal tract is performed. This shows two 8 cm kidneys with thin cortices. There is no evidence of hydronephrosis.

Do you think this patient's renal failure is acute or chronic? Which features of the case support your view?

Anaemia is associated with both acute and chronic renal failure, and therefore is not necessarily a useful guide in this case. Previous documentation of creatinine is extremely helpful. Clearly, if his creatinine was 100 μmol/L 1 month earlier then this is acute renal failure/acute kidney injury. Unfortunately, in many cases, the patient has had no previous contact with the healthcare system and therefore no prior documentation of renal function. In this particular case, the US shows two small kidneys (you would expect them to be around 10–12 cm in an adult male), with thin cortices. This suggests chronic renal failure. In such cases, a renal biopsy is unlikely to be helpful in elucidating the underlying cause of his renal failure and will merely show a fibrotic, scarred kidney.

What are the causes of chronic kidney disease?

The causes of acute renal failure are usually classified as pre-renal, renal and post-renal, and chronic kidney disease can be approached in the same way. It is useful to remember that the most common causes of ARF are

pre-renal +/− acute tubular necrosis and postrenal (obstruction). In contrast, the most common causes of CKD tend to be pathologies which would be classified as renal, rather than pre- or post-renal (Box 24.1). In many cases, it is impossible to determine the precise cause, because the end results of some pathologies are very similar, e.g. chronic GN, pyelonephritis and reflux nephropathy all cause interstitial fibrosis and tubular atrophy on renal biopsy.

What are the complications of chronic kidney disease?

1. Anaemia: due to erythropoietin deficiency.
2. Chronic kidney disease-bone and mineral disorder (CKD-BMD): the kidneys play an important role in maintaining bone and mineral homeostasis. CKD leads to bone and mineral abnormalities at three levels, together termed CKD-BMD.

• Renal bone disease: native vitamin D (cholecalciferol) is hydroxylated first by the liver to 25-hydroxy vitamin D, and secondly by the kidneys to the active hormone 1,25 dihydroxyvitamin D3 (calcitriol). Renal failure leads to reduced 1α-hydroxylase activity and hence low circulating calcitriol levels. Calcitriol is central to calcium homeostasis: its deficiency in CKD leads to decreased intestinal calcium absorption, hypocalcaemia and impaired mineralisation of bone, manifesting as 'renal rickets' in children and osteomalacia in adults.

• Hyperphosphataemia, abnormalities of calcium metabolism and secondary hyperparathyroidism. Healthy kidneys excrete the same amount of phosphate as is consumed, preventing phosphate accumulation. In CKD renal phosphate excretion is impaired and phosphate begins to accumulate. To compensate for this, two hormones are released which increase phosphate excretion by the kidneys: PTH (released by the parathyroid glands) and fibroblast growth factor 23 (FGF23) (released by bone cells). However, FGF23

Nephrology: Clinical Cases Uncovered. By M. Clatworthy. Published 2010 by Blackwell Publishing.

> **Box 24.1 Causes of CKD**
>
> - Diabetic nephropathy
> - Hypertensive nephropathy
> - APKD
> - Chronic GN
> - Chronic pyelonephritis/reflux nephropathy
> - Obstructive uropathy
> - Renovascular disease

stops 1α-hydroxylase in the kidneys from activating vitamin D, and worsens vitamin D deficiency. Low vitamin D levels lead to further increase in PTH release because parathyroid cells sense both calcium and vitamin D. When these are low, more PTH is released to increase calcium and to try and stimulate vitamin D production. The end result is a spiralling increase in PTH, which releases calcium from bone. This process also weakens bone and increases phosphate, perpetuating the vicious cycle and contributing to renal bone disease. If left untreated, parathyroid glands become enlarged and stop responding to the normal inhibitory signals. This leads to hypercalcaemia and is termed tertiary hyperparathyroidism (see Part 1, Figure F).

- Extraskeletal calcification. The abnormalities above lead to the deposition of calcium in soft tissues and arteries. The arterial wall can become heavily calcified and stiff, leading to decreased compliance, increased systolic blood pressure and left ventricular hypertrophy. Calcium deposition is enhanced by hyperphosphataemia and hypercalcaemia, and the metabolic acidosis which often accompanies CKD.

3. Hypertension secondary to chronic intravascular volume overload. Volume overload increases stroke volume (SV). An increase in SV will lead to a rise in cardiac output (CO = SV $\times$ HR). A rise in CO will lead to an increase in mean arterial pressure (MAP = CO $\times$ TPR).

4. Accelerated atherosclerosis/vascular disease. Hypertension and chronic hypercalcaemia lead to accelerated atherosclerosis and vascular calcification, and an increased risk of CAD, PVD and cerebrovascular accidents.

5. Metabolic acidosis. The kidneys excrete the daily acid load generated by amino acid metabolism. As the kidneys fail, patients develop a progressive metabolic acidosis. Chronic acidosis can promote renal bone disease and leads to muscle wasting and malnutrition.

What questions would you ask Mr Davies when taking a history?

The history should include questions which might assist in determining the underlying cause of his CKD.

- Duration: when was he last well? What are his main symptoms?
- Urinary symptoms? In this case those associated with chronic prostatic disease, e.g. hestitancy, poor stream. He is relatively young to develop prostatic disease.
- Past medical history: DM? Hypertension? (The most common causes of ESRF in the UK are diabetic nephropathy and hypertensive nephropathy). MI/CVA/PVD – if the patient has a history of other atherosclerotic diseases then renovascular disease may be the underlying diagnosis. Prostatic hypertrophy? In older males obstructive uropathy can cause CKD.
- Family history: there are a number of inherited causes of CKD, the most common being autosomal dominant polycystic kidney disease. However, the absence of cysts in his kidneys on US rules out this diagnosis. There are also a number of inherited diseases which can cause glomerulonephritis and may present like this with small shrunken kidneys, for example, Alport's syndrome or familial FSGS.
- Drug history: some medications can be associated with chronic kidney damage including NSAID, ciclosporin and lithium.
- Smoking history: smoker (associated with atherosclerosis and therefore renovascular disease)? Alcohol (chronic liver disease and liver failure can be associated with renal impairment)?

It is also helpful to determine whether he has any symptoms associated with the complications of CKD.

- Anaemia: shortness of breath, angina, tiredness
- Hyperphosphataemia: itchiness
- Uraemia: nausea, loss of appetite, symptoms associated with uraemic pericarditis (chest pain, breathlessness), in advanced uraemia patients can become confused and encephalopathic
- Volume overload: ankle swelling, shortness of breath (pulmonary oedema)

Mr Davies tells you that he has felt lethargic and lacking in energy for around 2 months. This has been much worse recently and has been associated with mild nausea and itchiness. The headache has been occurring for much longer, probably around 10 months. He gets it every day, describes it as thumping, of gradual onset and responsive to paracetamol. He has no associated neurological symptoms such as numbness or weakness in the arms and legs, and no visual disturbance. He has not been short of breath on exertion, nor does he give any history of orthopnoeal paroxysmal nocturnal dyspnoea. His ankles have been mildly swollen for a few weeks.

Mr Davies was previously very fit and healthy and has never had any heart, liver or kidney problems. He has not had any urinary or prostatic symptoms. He does not take any regular medications and is a non-smoker who drinks no alcohol. He works as a salesman, but is finding the daily travelling required more and more difficult.

What features are important to seek during clinical examination?

Examination should attempt to confirm or exclude the presence of the complications of CKD.

- Anaemia (pale conjunctivae/palmar creases)
- Hyperphosphataemia (excoriation marks)
- Fluid overload (signs of congestive cardiac failure, e.g. raised JVP, displaced apex beat, left parasternal heave (RVH), murmurs, bibasal crepitations (pulmonary oedema) or peripheral oedema

Clues as to the underlying cause of his CKD.

- Peripheral signs of vasculitis (rashes, nasal crusting, sinusitis), SLE (butterfly rash, arthroapthy)
- Blood pressure: hypertension is both a cause of CKD and can occur as a result of CKD
- PVD, carotid bruits, femoral bruits, poor peripheral circulation with reduced or absent peripheral pulses (may point towards renovascular disease)
- Signs of chronic liver disease: leuconychia, jaundice, hepatomegaly, ascites
- Signs associated with inherited GN, e.g. deafness/hearing aids in Alport's syndrome

Mr Davies is afebrile, with no peripheral signs of an autoimmune or inflammatory process. He is clinically anaemic with pale palmar creases and conjunctivae. His pulse is 72bpm and regular. Blood pressure is elevated at 180/98mmHg, cardiovascular examination is otherwise normal. All pulses are easily palpable and there are no obvious bruits. His chest is clear with no signs of pulmonary oedema. There is no liver or spleen palpable and no signs of chronic liver disease in the peripheries. He has minimal pitting oedema affecting only his feet bilaterally.

What investigations would you request?

- Blood tests
  - Full blood count (to confirm anaemia observed by GP)

- Iron studies (given the GP's initial blood tests showed significant anaemia, it is worth checking that Mr Davies is iron replete at this stage. Chronic uraemia reduces the absorption of iron from the GI tract, so many patients with CKD are iron deficient and are often given intravenous iron to avoid difficulties with absorption and the impalatibility of oral iron supplements)
  - Renal function: to confirm the degree of renal impairment
  - LFT, albumin
  - Glucose (diabetes can cause CKD, although it would probably have been diagnosed prior to presentation with diabetic nephropathy)
  - Calcium and phosphate
  - PTH
  - Autoimmune screen: even in the absence of obvious signs of autoimmune disease, an autoimmune screen can sometimes turn up a surprise positive finding. A renal autoimmune screen includes ANA, ANCA, complement (C3/C4), immunoglobulins, rheumatoid factor, cryoglobulins and anti-GBM antibodies
- Urine dipstick
- 24-hour urine collection for protein or spot ACR if dipstick is positive for protein
- ECG: to assess for signs of hyperkalaemia, a complication of CKD. In addition, the patient is hypertensive; if this is chronic, there may be signs of left ventricular hypertrophy on ECG (i.e. left axis deviation and sum of S in V1/V2 plus R in V5/V6 >35mm)
- CXR: to assess heart size (looking for cardiomegaly secondary to LVH in chronic hypertension), lung fields may show signs of pulmonary oedema (upper lobe diversion, fluid in horizontal fissure, Kerley B lines)

Investigations show:

Hb 8.1g/dL, MCV 82, WBC 8.2 × 10⁹/L, Platelets 369 × 10⁹/L

Clotting normal

U+E: Na 138mmol/L, K 4.4mmol/L, Urea 28.3mmol/L, Creatinine 364μmol/L (eGFR 17mL/min/1.73m²)

LFT: normal

Albumin 29g/dL

Glucose 4.8mmol/L

cCa 2.10mmol/L, PO₄ 2.9kPa, HCO₃ 27mmol/L

PTH 190pg/mL

Urine dipstick shows protein++, blood+, negative for leucocytes, nitrites and glucose

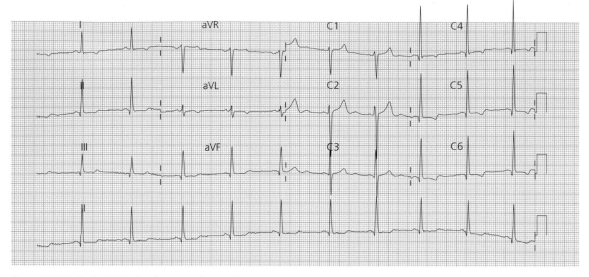

Figure 24.1 Mr Davies' ECG, showing LVH and LV strain (T wave inversion in lateral leads).

24-hour protein collection 2.1 g in 1.5 L
CXR demonstrates mild cardiomegaly, with clear
lung fields
ECG:sinus rhythm, left ventricular hypertrophy (LVH)
(Figure 24.1)

How would you interpret these results?

The investigations are consistent with a diagnosis of CKD stage 4 (see Table 24.1). The cause is unclear given that Mr Davies has presented with near ESRF and two small kidneys. He has a number of complications associated with CKD including anaemia (Hb 8.1 g/dL), hypocalcaemia, hyperphosphataemia and hyperparathyroidism. He is hypertensive and this can cause ESRF or may occur as a result of CKD. The LVH present on ECG suggests long-standing hypertension and therefore this may be hypertensive nephropathy.

What general treatment measures could you begin?

• *Treat hypertension.* An ACEI or ARB will increase both his potassium and creatinine and therefore should be used with caution. A β-blocker or calcium channel blocker would be a reasonable suggestion at this stage. In patients with CKD, a BP <130/80 mmHg is desirable or even lower (125/75 mmHg recommended) if there is proteinuria (as in this case).
• *Treat anaemia.* If he is iron deficient, then intravenous iron is usually administered. Once the patient is iron

Table 24.1 Chronic kidney disease stages

CKD stage	eGFR (mL/min/ 1.73 m²)	Other features
1	90+	Normal renal function but urine dipstick abnormalities or known structural abnormality of renal tract or diagnosis of genetic kidney disease
2	60–89	Mildly reduced renal function plus urine/structural abnormalities or diagnosis of genetic kidney disease
3	30–59	Moderately reduced renal function
4	15–29	Severely reduced renal function
5	<15	End-stage renal failure

replete, he should be commenced on recombinant erythropoietin.
• *Treat hyperphosphateamia.* This is achieved by a combination of dietary advice and phosphate binders. Unfortunately, some of the most tasty foods are high in phosphate, including cheese, milk, yoghurts and chocolate. Patients should also be commenced on a phosphate binder (e.g. calcium acetate or aluminium hydroxide)

which should be taken with food and binds to the phosphate, preventing its absorption from the gut. Calcium-containing agents should not be used in patients who have hypercalcaemia (due to tertiary hyperparathyroidism) or vascular calcification. The long-term use of aluminium-containing binders is now infrequent due to the problems encountered with chronic aluminium toxicity, including so-called 'dialysis dementia' and microcytic anaemia. Sevelamer, a new phosphate-binding agent, is a synthetic polymer which does not contain calcium or aluminium. It binds intestinal phosphate and can be used in patients with hypercalcaemia. All phosphate binders are relatively impalatable (causing diarrhoea, bloating and discomfort) and are therefore poorly tolerated by patients.

• *Treat hypocalcaemia/hyperparathyroidism.* Active vitamin D is the cornerstone of treatment for secondary hyperparathyroidism. Native vitamin D (cholecalciferol) requires 1α-hydroxylation and is therefore less effective in this setting. Widely used treatments are alfa-calcidol (1α-hydroxycholecalciferol), which requires hepatic hydroxylation, or calcitriol (1,25-dihydroxyvitamin D3). Such treatments reduce PTH secretion and parathyroid hyperplasia, correct hypocalcaemia and improve renal bone disease. Unsurprisingly, the main side-effect of active vitamin D preparations is hypercalcaemia. Recently, active vitamin D analogues (e.g. paricalcitol) have become available which are less likely to lead to hypercalcaemia, but their use is limited by cost. In patients with resistant disease, the calcimimetic cinacalcet can also be helpful in managing patients with CKD-associated hyperparathyroidism. It is also costly. Inadequately treated parathyroid hyperplasia progresses to tertiary hyperparathyroidism, which may require surgical intervention. Chronic hypercalcaemia and hyperphosphataemia associated with tertiary hyperparathyroidism make a significant contribution to the increased risk of vascular disease in patients with CKD, and therefore have a significant effect on overall morbidity and mortality.

• Management of traditional vascular risk factors such as cholesterol and smoking.

How often should Mr Davies be seen in renal clinic?

Patients with CKD stage 4 should be seen 3–6 monthly for bloods and assessment. In the UK it is recommended that patients with CKD have their renal function regularly assessed so that any decline in function can be managed in a timely and appropriate manner. Suggested frequency of review is as follows.

• Stage 1 – annual
• Stage 2 – annual
• Stage 3 (known to be stable) – annual
• Stage 3 (newly diagnosed or progressive) – 6 monthly
• Stage 4 (known to be stable) – 6 monthly
• Stage 4 (newly diagnosed or progressive) – 3 monthly
• Stage 5 – 3 monthly

Stable renal function is defined as change in GFR of $<2\,mL/min/1.73\,m^2$ over 6 months or more. Progressive kidney damage is defined as change in GFR of $>2\,mL/min/1.73\,m^2$ over 6 months or more.

In patients with CKD stage 4, it is recommended that the following blood tests are performed on a 3–6 monthly basis: creatinine, Hb, Ca, PO_4, K, HCO_3, PTH. There should also be a dietary assessment (low phosphate +/− low potassium), correction of acidosis (with oral bicarbonate supplements), optimal BP control and treatment of anaemia with iron+/− EPO.

What other issues need to be addressed?

Mr Davies' renal function is poor and it is likely that he will need RRT in the future. He needs to be informed of this and of the various RRT options, which should be discussed in detail. Some patients with ESRF can be managed conservatively (with the measures described above), and this may be appropriate in very elderly individuals with multiple co-morbidities. For most patients RRT is advised – haemodialysis, peritoneal dialysis or renal transplantation. Timely planning for dialysis is important so that access (arteriovenous fistula (AVF) or PD catheter) is in place when the patient needs RRT. Early transplant work-up is also preferable, and many patients are now placed on the deceased-donor transplant waiting list around 6 months before it is anticipated that they will need dialysis. In addition, if they have a friend or relative who may act as a live donor, then pre-emptive transplantation may be possible before they need dialysis.

CASE REVIEW

A 49-year-old man presents with heachache and lethargy. Investigations show an eGFR of 17 mL/min/1.73 m^2 (CKD stage 4) and two small kidneys on ultrasound. The patient's iron stores, PTH, calcium and phosphate are assessed, and appropriately managed with intravenous iron, 1α-calcidol and Calcichew. In addition, the patient is provided with information about end-stage kidney disease and the options available to him, including haemodialysis, peritoneal dialysis and transplantation.

KEY POINTS

- Chronic kidney disease is usually asymptomatic in its early stages, so patients often present late with advanced disease.
- The causes of CKD are generally renal, the most common being diabetic nephropathy, hypertensive nephropathy, APKD, chronic GN, chronic pyelonephritis/reflux, chronic obstruction and renovascular disease.
- The frequency of CKD increases with age. It is thought that around 5% of the population have a GFR of <60 mL/min/1.73 m^2. Screening for CKD in primary care allows timely referral to specialist services and can slow the progression and reduce the complications of CKD.
- UK guidelines suggest that patients at risk of developing CKD should be screened (by measuring serum creatinine) on an annual basis. This includes those with:
  ○ previously diagnosed CKD, ADPKD, reflux nephropathy, biopsy-proven GN, persistent proteinuria, urologically unexplained persistent haematuria
  ○ hypertension, diabetes mellitus, heart failure, atherosclerotic coronary, cerebral or peripheral vascular disease
  ○ bladder outflow obstruction, neurogenic bladder, urinary diversion, recurrent stone disease
  ○ long-term treatment with ACEI, ARB, NSAID, lithium, 5-aminosalicylates, calcineurin inhibitors
  ○ multisystem diseases that involve the kidney
  ○ a first-degree relative with CKD.
- The complications of CKD are anaemia, 1,25(OH)$_2$ vitamin D deficiency (leading to hypocalcaemia and hyperparathyroidism), accelerated vascular disease and renal bone osteodystrophy.
- These complications can be treated with iron and recombinant erythropoietin, 1α-calcidol and phosphate binders.
- Patients should also be informed of, and prepared for, renal replacement therapy. This includes transplant work-up (where appropriate) or the formation of an AVF (in preparation for haemodialysis).

Case 25 A 23-year-old man with shortness of breath

Mr Wayne Halfpenny is a 23-year-old man who presents acutely to A+E with shortness of breath. Examination shows pulse 100 pbm, BP 180/95 mmHg, JVP 6 cm, no murmurs or pericardial rub. Oxygen saturations 90% s/v air, RR 20 rpm. On auscultation, there are coarse inspiratory crepitations to the mid zones.

Initial investigations are shown below:

Hb 6.8 g/dL, WBC 5.0 × 10⁹/L, Platelets 269 × 10⁹/L

Na 146 mmol/L, K 5.9 mmol/L, Urea 56 mmol/L, Creatinine 1250 µmol/L

cCa 2.05 mmol/L, PO₄ 2.5 mmol/l

CRP 12 mg/L

CXR: pulmonary oedema

An ultrasound of his renal tract is shown in Figure 25.1.

How would you interpret these investigations?

The bloods show that he has significant anaemia and severe renal failure. His calcium is low and his phosphate is high, in keeping with secondary hyperparathyroidism (elevated PTH due to hypocalcaemia). In this case, his calcium is likely to be low because of renal failure, which leads to a reduction in the activity of renal 1α-hydroxylase required for the production of active vitamin D.

The ultrasound scan shows two small kidneys (≈8 cm) with cortical thinning and no hydronephrosis. Normal size for kidneys in a young man is around 11–12 cm. The renal failure is therefore likely to be chronic.

He has significant pulmonary oedema on his chest radiograph, which is probably secondary to fluid overload. Patients with renal failure become oliguric and therefore cannot adequately control their volume status.

Fluid taken orally which cannot be removed by the failing kidney will accumulate in both the peripheral tissues (peripheral oedema) and the lungs (pulmonary oedema).

How should Mr Halfpenny be managed?

The cause of renal failure should be sought with an acute renal screen (see Box 25.1) and can be pre-renal, renal or post-renal. Obstruction has been excluded by the US scan (no hydronephrosis) and there is nothing to suggest a pre-renal cause (chronic hypotension, e.g. in patients with severe congestive cardiac failure, can lead to chronic renal impairment or renovascular disease). Therefore, there is likely to be a renal cause, for example a GN or chronic pyelonephritis.

Given the kidney size, his renal failure is unlikely to be reversible. He is significantly fluid overloaded. A bolus of high-dose furosemide may be helpful in promoting a small diuresis in the short term, but it is likely he will need emergency dialysis for removal of fluid. This requires the insertion of a temporary dialysis catheter. He is also significantly anaemic and will require a blood transfusion. However, this is likely to push up his potassium further and give extra volume, so should therefore be given during dialysis.

What risks need to be discussed with the patient prior to insertion?

Temporary dialysis lines are usually placed into the internal jugular vein or the femoral vein. The main complications are:

- pneumothorax (internal jugular line)
- haemorrhage/haematoma formation
- arterial puncture
- mediastinal damage (rare, internal jugular line)
- infection.

Nephrology: Clinical Cases Uncovered. By M. Clatworthy. Published 2010 by Blackwell Publishing.

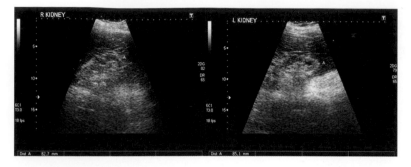

Figure 25.1 Ultrasound scans showing bilateral small kidneys (right 8.27 cm, left 8.51 cm).

> **Box 25.1 Acute immunological renal screen**
>
> - ANA, ANCA, anti-GBM, anti-dsDNA
> - C3/C4
> - C3 nephritic factor
> - IgG, paraprotein, Bence Jones protein
> - Cryoglobulins

Are there any particular problems which can arise when inserting lines in patients with ARF?

In order to insert a central line, the patient needs to be lying relatively flat. Someone like Mr Halfpenny who has significant pulmonary oedema may struggle to lie flat because this will make his breathlessness worse (orthopnoea). Patients with uraemic pericarditis are also often reluctant to lie down, because the chest pain associated with pericarditis is relieved by sitting forward. In addition, severe uraemia can impair platelet function, so the exit site can be quite oozy post-insertion. Finally, during internal jugular line insertion, the end of the wire may tickle the right ventricle and precipitate an arrhythmia (hyperkalaemia makes this more common and more serious).

> *A temporary line is inserted into the left internal jugular vein under ultrasound guidance. The post-insertion chest-X ray is shown in Figure 25 2. You are asked to check the position of the line and to exclude any complications.*

What will you write in the notes?

There is upper lobe diversion (volume overload). There is a left internal jugular temporary dialysis line, the tip of which is lying in the right atrium. There is no obvious pneumothorax (look for this by tracing out the vascular markings in the lung right out to the peripheries).

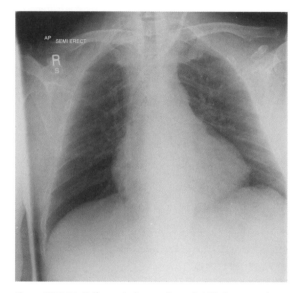

Figure 25.2 Mr Halfpenny's chest radiograph (AP) demonstrating upper lobe diversion and a left internal jugular central line.

| *Mr Halfpenny is started on haemodialysis.*

The first session should be short (usually 2 hours) in order to prevent a rapid drop in urea and the 'dialysis disequilibrium' which can result. When haemodialysis is started in severely uraemic patients, neurological disturbances may occur. Symptoms develop during or immediately after haemodialysis and include nausea, headache, blurred vision, disorientation and increased blood pressure. More severely affected patients can progress to confusion, seizures, coma and even death. The risk of disequilibrium syndrome can be minimized if dialysis is initiated as frequent (daily) short (2-hour) sessions. Symptoms of dialysis disequilibrium syndrome are usually self-limiting and dissipate within several hours.

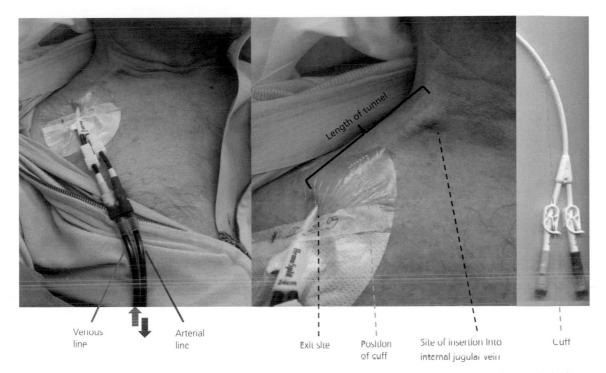

Venous line   Arterial line   Exit site   Position of cuff   Site of insertion into internal jugular vein   Cuff

Figure 25.3 Patient receiving haemodialysis via a tunnelled dialysis line. The line is tunnelled under the skin to reduce the risk of infection. There is a cuff partway up the line which sits in the tunnel. Scar tissue forms around the cuff and assists in stabilizing the line and preventing the proximal migration of skin flora.

How long should the temporary line be left *in situ*?

Seven to 10 days. More permanent access will need to be established for long-term dialysis. Initially this will be in the form of a tunnelled central line. If it is likely that the patient will need chronic haemodialysis, an AVF should also be formed as soon as possible, because this will take around 2 months to mature. This should be borne in mind during the day-to-day management of the patient and if possible, their non-dominant upper limb should be rested from venesection and cannulation in an attempt to preserve the veins for surgery.

His first few dialysis sessions go without difficulty. Given the extent of his anaemia, he is given two units of blood with his second dialysis session. Mr Halfpenny's acute renal screen does not reveal any abnormalities, so it is impossible to identify the precise cause of ESRF. Renal biopsy is not usually helpful as it shows only fibrosis and tubular atrophy.

What are the most likely underlying diagnoses?

In patients presenting with ESRF and small kidneys, with a normal acute renal screen, it is likely that one of the following diagnoses is the underlying cause of chronic kidney damage:
- renal dysplasia
- reflux nephropathy
- IgA nephropathy
- hypertensive nephropathy.

Given that there is no acute cause of renal impairment, it is unlikely that renal dysfunction will be reversible. Therefore, a tunnelled central line is inserted for medium-term haemodialysis (Figure 25.3).

What are the problems associated with long-term use of a tunnelled line for haemodialysis?

The main complications associated with the long-term use of intravascular dialysis catheters include infection,

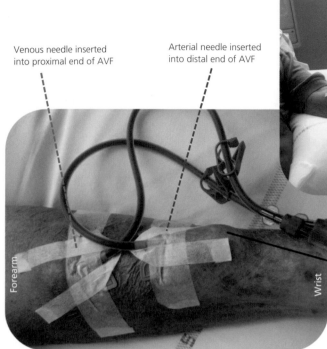

Venous needle inserted into proximal end of AVF

Arterial needle inserted into distal end of AVF

Forearm

Wrist

Blood is removed via the arterial needle/line, dialysed and then returned to the patient via the venous needle/line

This patient has a well-developed radiocephalic AVF

Figure 25.4 Patient receiving haemodialysis via an AVF.

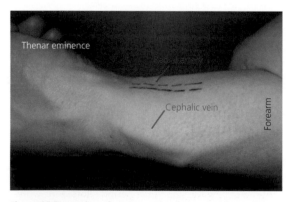

Thenar eminence

Cephalic vein

Forearm

Figure 25.5 Vessels at the wrist used to form an AVF. The radial artery (dotted lines, red arrow) runs close to the cephalic vein (blue arrow) at the wrist. The two can be joined to make an AVF.

particularly with gram-positive organisms. *Staphylococcus epidermidis* and *Staph. aureus* are the most common causative bacteria and are associated with both exit site and tunnel infections. Occasionally such line infections can be complicated by infective endocarditis if there is recurrent bacteraemia during dialysis episodes.

Recurrent or prolonged venous catheterization can lead to stenosis or occlusion of the vein. This precludes further use of the vein for central access and if the subclavian or innominate vein is involved, such stenoses may cause venous hypertension of the limb and make the arterio-venous fistula (AVF) function poorly.

Mr Halfpenny attends a dialysis education session in order to learn about the different options for RRT and decides to opt for long-term haemodialysis. He is therefore referred to the surgeons for AVF formation, which is done prior to discharge from hospital. He is established on dialysis (on a Monday, Wednesday and Friday, for 4 hours at each session) via a tunnelled central line and then an AVF (Figure 25.4).

For patients on maintenance haemodialysis, the vascular access of choice is an AVF. The forearm is usually the site of choice and the standard location for anastomosis is 3–5 cm proximal to the wrist since the radial artery and cephalic vein come close together at this site (Figure 25.5). The first attempt is usually performed in the patient's non-dominant hand. Another suitable site is the anatomical snuff box where the dorsal branch of the radial artery and cephalic vein are closely apposed. The operation is usually carried out under local anaesthetic.

Are there any other issues in this case which need to be addressed, preferably prior to discharge?

• *Anaemia:* provided iron stores are adequate (this should have been checked prior to transfusion), the patient should be commenced on recombinant erythropoietin (EPO) to replace native EPO which would normally be made by the kidneys. The introduction of recombinant human EPO is probably the single most important advance in the management of chronic renal failure in the last 20 years. Prior to this, the only treatment for anaemia was blood transfusion which was associated with a number of complications including sensitisation against HLA antigens (thus limiting the number of suitable organ donors), transmission of infectious agents (mainly hepatitis B and C and HIV), and haemochromatosis due to iron overload. In addition, chronic anaemia led to cardiovascular complications, particularly left ventricular dysfunction and congestive cardiac failure. The correction of anaemia with EPO has a number of beneficial effects including improvement of overall well-being, exercise performance and cognitive function. Several studies have also shown a reduction in the prevalence of LVH and the risk of congestive heart failure.

The shared US and European consensus is that a reasonable target range for correction of anaemia in dialysis patients should be Hct 33–39% (i.e. Hb 11–13 g/dL). EPO can be administered either subcutaneously or intravenously.

• *Secondary hyperparathyroidism:* hypocalcaemia results from a deficiency of renal 1α-hydroxylase activity, which reduces the levels of active vitamin D (see Part 1, Figure F). The patient should be commenced on vitamin D supplementation, for example 1α-calcidol, to correct hypocalcaemia and reduce the drive for the production of PTH in an attempt to prevent the development of tertiary hyperparathyroidism.

• *Work-up for transplantation:* this should be started as quickly as possible, particularly in younger patients as transplantation offers significant survival benefits compared with dialysis. Work-up includes assessment of blood group, HLA type (A, B, DR) and sensitisation

(presence of anti-HLA antibodies) (see case 30). It is likely that Mr Halfpenny will need a period on dialysis to optimise his volume status and cardiovascular function.
• *Lifestyle changes:* low-potassium and low-phosphate diet, fluid restriction, smoking cessation.

Mr Halfpenny is seen at his 6-monthly haemodialysis clinic review.

What issues should be addressed during the review?

• Is dialysis being adequately tolerated by the patient, both physically and mentally? For example, does he become hypotensive during or after sessions, is his vascular access working satisfactorily, how is he coping with the inevitable effect that regular dialysis sessions have on his lifestyle?
• Is the patient complying with fluid restriction and diet restrictions?

Mr Halfpenny seems to be coping relatively well. He comes in for evening dialysis slots and continues to work full time. He is currently dialysing via a left radiocephalic AVF which is working well. However, he does tend to get symptomatic hypotension during dialysis sessions. He has no significant urine output (urine output tends to become negligible when patients have had ESRF for a significant period) and is on 750 mL fluid restriction which he finds difficult.

Why do patients become hypotensive during dialysis?

Hypotension is a common dialysis-associated complication. There may be associated nausea, vomiting and muscle cramps. The main cause is excess volume removal by ultrafiltration which is replaced by refilling from the interstitial fluid compartment. If the ultrafiltration (UF) rate exceeds the refilling rate, intravascular volume contraction will result. If a patient does not adhere to his fluid restriction then he may need a higher volume removed during the same time period allotted for dialysis. Therefore the UF rate is even more likely to exceed the rate of replacement from the interstitium. Another cause of plasma volume contraction is an underestimation of the so-called dry weight to be achieved at the end of the dialysis session. The effect of both is to reduce SV and hence CO, which in turn leads to a reduction in MAP.

In normal circumstances, the autonomic response to the reduction in SV is to increase HR and TPR. However, studies suggest that in dialysis patients there is often an impaired sympathetic response to volume removal, possibly due to the effects of chronic uraemia on the autonomic nervous system. In addition, in older patients with impaired LV function this inability to compensate for dialysis hypotension can lead to a temporary reduction in cardiac output.

The acute management of dialysis hypotension involves stopping or reducing the rate of ultrafiltration. The patient should be placed in the supine position and if he remains hypotensive it may be necessary to give volume replacement, e.g. 250–500 mL bolus of saline or Gelofusine.

A number of factors can exacerbate dialysis hypotension including occult sepsis, myocardial infarction, pericardial disease/effusion and haemorrhage.

General measures to prevent repeated episodes of hypotension include increasing the patient's dry weight (if appropriate) or prolonging dialysis time to reduce the rate of ultrafiltration per hour.

What are the important features to note on reviewing Mr Halfpenny in the haemodialysis clinic?

• General appearance, particularly signs of cachexia: some patients develop so-called dialysis cachexia and can lose muscle mass on starting dialysis. They may also have poor nutrition if they stick rigorously to the low-phosphate and low-potassium diets imposed.
• Intravascular volume status: patients with little urine output often struggle with strict fluid restrictions and become chronically volume overloaded. This may be manifest as a raised JVP, elevated blood pressure, peripheral or pulmonary oedema.
• Dialysis access: lines or AVF should be checked. The line exit site/tunnel should be checked for signs of infection (erythema, tenderness, discharge). A number of problems can arise following fistula formation, including steal syndrome with signs of ischaemia in the limb distal to the fistula. With time, AVF can become quite large and unsightly and may also develop aneurysmal segments.
• Cardiovascular complications of chronic dialysis: these include:
  ○ endocarditis related to recurrent bacteraemia (therefore look for splinter haemorrhages, Osler's nodes, Janeway lesions, new murmur)
  ○ changes associated with chronic volume overload, hypertension and anaemia, particularly LVH and dysfunction

  ○ aortic calcification/sclerosis: patients with chronic hypercalcaemia (due to tertiary hyperparathyroidism) develop medial calcification of blood vessels and calcification of the aortic valve.

There are no peripheral stigmata of endocarditis and Mr Halfpenny is slim but not cachectic. The AVF has a good thrill and is not aneurysmal. His left hand looks healthy and non-ischaemic. His pulse is 80 bpm and BP 165/95 mmHg. JVP is visible at 5 cm above the manubriosternal joint. He has a soft systolic flow murmur which does not radiate. Chest is clear. There is no peripheral oedema.

  His monthly haemodialysis bloods are shown below

Hb 10.8 g/dL, WBC 6.2 × 10⁹/L, Platelets 369 × 10⁹/L

Hb 10.8 g/dL, WBC 6.2×10^9/L, Platelets 369×10^9/L

Na 136 mmol/L, K 5.2 mmol/L, Urea 26 mmol/L, creatinine 550 μmol/L

cCa 2.06 mmol/L, PO$_4$ 1.8 mmol/L, PTH 540 pg/mL

CRP 16 mg/L

His medication list is as follows:

Amlodipine 5 mg od
Lisinopril 10 mg od
Aspirin 75 mg od
Darbepoetin 80 mg SC once a week
Calcichew (calcium carbonate, a phosphate binder) 1 g tds with food

What adjustments would you make to his medications?

There are a number of issues.
• Hypertension: his predialysis BP is elevated (should be <140/90 mmHg). This may be in part due to intravascular volume overload. He should be encouraged to stick to his fluid restriction and it may be necessary to further reduce his dry weight. If this does not improve matters then his antihypertensive meds could be increased (e.g. increase lisinopril to 20 mg).
• His phosphate levels are too high in spite of Calcichew. Therefore it may be useful to switch to an alternative phosphate binder such as sevelamer.
• In addition, he should be commenced on 1α-calcidol as he is now hypocalcaemic and his PTH is elevated (>1.5× normal range).

What do you understand by the term 'dialysis adequacy'?

Dialysis adequacy is a measure of whether the dose of dialysis the patient receives is sufficient to adequately remove waste products. Failure to provide adequate dialysis can have a negative impact on long-term survival of patients on dialysis. Dialysis adequacy is usually assessed by two measures.

- Kt/V (where K is the dialyser clearance of urea, t is the dialysis time, and V is the patient's total volume of body water). Kt/V = 1.0 indicates that a volume of blood equal to the distribution volume of urea has been completely cleared of urea.

- Urea reduction ratio (URR). This is calculated by the formula: $URR = \dfrac{U_{pre} - U_{post}}{U_{pre}} \times 100$

Both measures of dialysis adequacy involve taking blood samples from the patient before and after dialysis and measuring the urea. Current UK Renal Association guidelines suggest that physicians should aim for a target Kt/V of >1.4 or a URR of >70%.

CASE REVIEW

A 23-year-old man presents with severe dyspnoea secondary to pulmonary oedema. Investigations show that he has ESRF with small kidneys and a creatinine of >1000 μmol/L. A temporary dialysis line is placed and he is started on haemodialysis in order to remove fluid. The patient receives appropriate dialysis education and opts for haemodialysis rather than peritoneal dialysis. He is subsequently dialysed via a tunnelled central line and then an arteriovenous fistula. He is also commenced on recombinant erythropoietin. Intradialytic hypotension and secondary hyperparathyroidism are the main ongoing management issues.

KEY POINTS

- For acute haemodialysis, venous access may be temporarily achieved using a temporary central dialysis catheter (which lasts for a week or so). In the medium term, access is provided via a tunnelled central line, which can last for a number of months.
- The main complication of tunnelled lines is infection (exit site, tunnel or even infective endocarditis), which is often caused by staphylococci. Prolonged use of lines (for months or even years) is possible, but may be associated with the development of stenoses in central veins.
- For patients on maintenance haemodialysis, the vascular access of choice is an AVF. The non-dominant forearm is the standard location for the anastomosis.
- A number of complications can limit the long-term survival of AVF. Occlusion/thrombosis of the fistula can occur if the patient becomes hypotensive on dialysis due to excessive removal of fluid, if he/she is hypercoagulable or if there is a pre-existing stenosis of the draining vein.
- Another problem encountered is 'steal syndrome', so named because the AVF 'steals' blood which would

normally flow to the palmar arch. The symptoms of steal syndrome are a cold sensation and pallor of the fingers frequently accompanied by ischaemic pain and, in severe cases, necrosis. Treatment of steal syndrome is to decrease the blood flow through the fistula, thereby ensuring enough blood supply to the peripheral tissues. This may involve closing off the fistula.
- Patients with ESRF on dialysis also have problems with:
  - hypertension (mainly due to fluid overload in anuric patients). This can be addressed by encouraging patients to adhere to fluid restriction (750 mL in 24 hours) and attempting to remove excess fluid during dialysis sessions
  - hyperphosphataemia (treated with a low-phosphate diet and oral phosphate binders)
  - vitamin D deficiency/secondary hyperparathyroidism (usually treated with oral supplementation)
  - anaemia (treated with iron supplementation and recombinant erythropoietin).

Case 26 A 34-year-old man on haemodialysis

Mr Barry Henson is a 58 year old with ESRF of unknown cause who has been on haemodialysis for 18 months. Unfortunately, he frequently misses his regular dialysis slots and struggles to keep to his 750 mL fluid restriction. He also continues to smoke, in spite of advice to the contrary. Mr Henson is unhappy because he feels constantly tired and washed out. Monthly predialysis blood tests are shown below:

Hb 8.1 g/dL, WBC 8.6 × 10⁹/L, Platelets 364 × 10⁹/L
U+E: Na 137 mmol/L, K 5.9 mmol/L, Urea 29.3 mmol/L,
 Creatinine 793 μmol/L, cCa 2.31 mmol/L PO₄ 2.2 mmol/L
CRP 12 mg/L
Glucose 4.2 mmol/L

His medications are:
Doxasosin 8 mg bd
Lisinopril 20 mg od
Aspirin 75 mg od
Simvastatin 20 mg od
Darbepoetin 100 μg SC weekly (self-administered)
Sevelamer tds with food

You note that he has been persistently anaemic over the last 3 months despite having started recombinant erythropoietin (EPO, darbepoetin in this case) and having the dose increased 1 month ago.

What are the causes of persistent anaemia in dialysis patients receiving erythropoietin replacement?

Erythropoietin resistance can result from a number of factors.

• Iron deficiency: this is the most common cause for a suboptimal response to EPO therapy. Assessment of iron stores can be difficult because ferritin levels are often

elevated in dialysis patient, along with CRP. If serum iron is low and total iron-binding capacity is high then iron should be replaced. Oral supplementation is poorly tolerated and poorly absorbed. Therefore iron is frequently administered intravenously, as this can easily be performed during dialysis sessions.

• Uncontrolled hyperparathyroidism: if long standing, this can lead to marrow fibrosis.

• Inadequate quality or quantity of dialysis: optimising the quality of the water used for the preparation of the dialysis fluid may reduce the degree of anaemia and the patient's EPO requirements. Various chemical contaminants (aluminium, copper, lead, chlorine) and bacterial contamination of the dialysis fluid (which trigger the generation of cytokines and enhance an inflammatory state) act as inhibitors of erythropoiesis. The use of pyrogen-free, 'ultrapure' dialysate can result in a significant reduction of EPO dosage.

• Drugs, e.g. ACEI.

• Aluminium overload: this is now uncommon in dialysis patients but can lead to EPO insensitivity. It is usually associated with a normo- or microcytic anaemia.

• Compliance issues: if EPO is self-administered subcutaneously then there may be compliance issues, sometimes because patients genuinely forget to give it because it is only required once every 1–2 weeks. Others do not like self-medicating subcutaneously, although 'pens' are available for ease of administration.

What is the major side-effect encountered following commencement of erythropoietin?

Many patients experience a worsening of pre-existing hypertension or develop new hypertension. Around 20% of patients with ESRF started on EPO will require the institution or increase of antihypertensive medications. The elevation of BP usually develops soon after starting EPO, and is more common in patients with pre-existing hypertension. It is frequently correlated with the rapidity

Nephrology: Clinical Cases Uncovered. By M. Clatworthy.
Published 2010 by Blackwell Publishing.

of the increase of haematocrit. The control of EPO-induced hypertension is facilitated by reducing excessive extracellular volume through more intensive fluid removal during dialysis.

> *On closer questioning, it seems as though Mr Henson is not keen on giving himself EPO injections, and thus his persistent anaemia is probably due to lack of compliance. The EPO is therefore given intravenously, during dialysis sessions. His anaemia improves but he continues to have problems with his fluid restriction and is persistently fluid overloaded. His predialysis blood pressure is generally around 200/100mmHg and he often needs at least 4 litres of fluid to be removed during each dialysis sessions. His named dialysis nurse spends some time trying to emphasise the importance of keeping to his fluid restriction and taking his antihypertensive medications.*
>
> *Two weeks later Mr Henson attends his routine dialysis session but is complaining of headache and lethargy. You are asked to attend the dialysis unit and assess him whilst he is on the machine.*

What questions would you ask on initial assessment?

• Duration: when did the headache start?
• Onset: sudden or gradual? Sudden-onset headache suggests vascular causes, e.g. SAH.
• When is it worse? Headache which is worse at night or first thing in the morning and wakes patient from sleep is suggestive of raised intracranial pressure.
• In terms of headache – site, exacerbating and relieving factors? Worrying features: vomiting, blurred vision, photophobia?
• Any other neurological symptoms? Weakness, numbness, word-finding difficulty, speech difficulty.
• Previous similar episodes?
• Any systemic symptoms, such as fevers or night sweats, which may indicate an infection?
• Any cardiovascular symptoms such as chest pain or shortness of breath?
• What medications is he currently taking?

> *Mr Henson has had an occipital headache for 24 hours. It came on gradually over a period of hours and is not exacerbated by light. Over the last few months he has had a thumping headache intermittently, particularly prior to dialysis sessions, but this current headache is more severe. He has no other neurological symptoms and has not been febrile. His other medications are as noted previously.*

What are the important signs to seek when examining Mr Henson?

Given his history (dialysis-dependent ESRF, poorly controlled hypertension), the most likely diagnoses are:
• dialysis-associated hypotension
• hypertension-associated headache
• CVA – ESRF is a major risk factor for atherosclerosis and vascular disease, therefore CVA and MI can occur in relatively young patients
• intracerebral haemorrhage (hypertension associated).

End-stage renal failure is also an immunosuppressed state (dialysis patients have been shown to have abnormal numbers and function of lymphocytes, possibly due to chronic uraemia), so infections (meningitis/encephalitis) should also be considered.

Appropriate signs to seek on examination include the following.
• GCS
• Purpuric rash (associated with meningococcal septicaemia)
• Temperature
• CVS – BP? Intravascular volume status? Signs consistent with LVH, hyperdynamic apex, which may be displaced, systolic flow murmur
• RS – respiratory rate, pulmonary oedema
• NS – neurological signs, particularly signs of raised intracranial pressure (papilloedema, false localising signs, e.g. VI cranial nerve palsy, and the presence of any focal neurological signs
• Signs of hypertensive retinopathy (silver wiring, AV nipping, flame haemorrhages, papilloedema).

> *Mr Henson is afebrile. His BP is 210/110mmHg and his pulse 100bpm.*
>
> *Neurological examination reveals a GCS of 14, and he seems slightly confused. Peripherally he has a left pronator drift and an upgoing plantar on the left. His fundi are difficult to visualise but his disc margins seem indistinct.*

What are your differential diagnoses?

He has definite localising neurological signs suggestive of right-sided cerebral pathology. In addition, the relatively acute onset is suggestive of a vascular event. Possible causes include a thromboembolic cerebrovascular accident or an intracerebral haemorrhage. Accelerated/malignant hypertension is less likely given the marked focal neurological signs.

Mr Henson has been on the dialysis machine for 30 minutes when you review him, and as you sit to write your notes he deteriorates further and develops worsening headache and more severe weakness.

What are your immediate management steps?

• Ensure airway, breathing and circulation are adequate. If there is concern about any of these features then an urgent intensive care referral is advisable.
• Stop the dialysis session.
• Provided his consciousness level is sufficient to ensure a safe airway and he is cardiovascularly stable, urgent investigations should be organised, including:
  ○ FBC, U+E, CRP, clotting
  ○ ECG
  ○ CT head.

You ask the nurse to stop the dialysis session immediately and reassess Mr Henson's condition. He is adequately maintaining his airway, although his GCS has reduced to 13/15. His respiratory rate is 16 rpm, pulse 110 bpm, BP 205/115.

Investigations are as follows:

Hb 10.1 g/dL, WBC 9.2 × 10⁹/L, Platelets 434 × 10⁹/L
U+E: Na 135 mmol/L, K 5.4 mmol/L, Urea 29.3 mmol/L,
   Creatinine 546 μmol/L
CRP 16 mg/L, glucose 5.0 mmol/L
Clotting: PT 14 s, APTT 42 s
ECG: LVH
CT head is shown in Figure 26.1

What do the investigations show?

• The Hb and U+E are in keeping with a patient on long-term haemodialysis.
• The APPT is prolonged, probably due to the heparin he received during the dialysis session.
• The ECG shows LVH, in keeping with the history of chronic hypertension.
• The CT shows a right-sided intra-cerebral haemorrhage.

Given the prolonged APTT, he is given protamine to normalise his clotting. Mr Henson's case is discussed with the neurosurgeons, who advise admission to the neurointensive care unit where he is intubated and ventilated. An intracranial bolt is inserted to monitor intracranial pressure (ICP). His blood pressure is

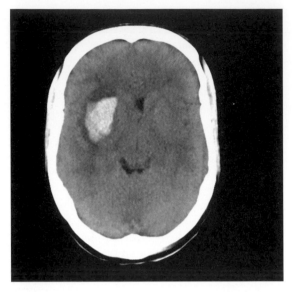

Figure 26.1 Mr Henson's CT head demonstrating right-sided intracerebral haemorrhage with some surrounding oedema and mid-line shift.

controlled with intravenous nimodipine. Mr Henson's ICP remains within the normal range and he is extubated 24 hours later. He makes good progress on the stroke unit, and after a 1 week has some residual left-sided weakness and slurred speech but is able to function independently.

Three years later Mr Henson is still on dialysis, although he is currently active on the transplant waiting list. He still struggles with fluid restriction and continues to smoke. You are asked to review Mr Henson because he has developed symptomatic hypotension during his dialysis session. Predialysis BP was 155/100 mmHg but halfway through the session (after 1 litre of ultrafiltration) he developed headache and dizziness and his BP was 90/50 mmHg. The dialysis nurse stopped ultrafiltration and gave two 500 mL boluses of Gelofusine. In spite of this, his BP remains low at 100/60 mmHg.

Mr Henson denies any chest pain, but does feel slightly short of breath.

The dialysis nurse has sent off some urgent bloods, including a troponin-I.

An ECG is performed (Figure 26.2).

What does the ECG show?

The ECG shows ST elevation inferiorly, consistent with MI.

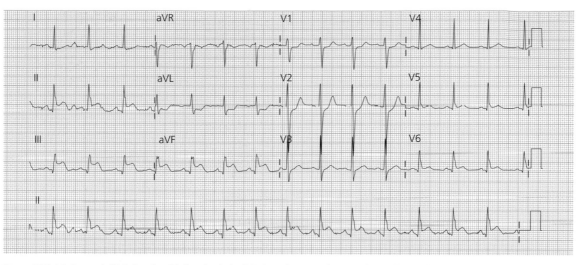

Figure 26.2 Mr Henson's ECG showing ST elevation in leads II, III, and aVF consistent with an inferior infarct. This territory is usually supplied by the right coronary artery, which also supplies the SA node. Therefore, inferior MIs can be associated with conduction abnormalities.

Mr Henson's troponin-I is elevated at 1.4 and rises to 5.1 at 12 hours (normal range = 0–0.4 ng/mL). Dialysis is stopped, and he is transferred to the coronary care unit for further observation and management. He is reviewed by the cardiologists and undergoes primary angioplasty.

Does an elevated troponin reliably indicate myocardial damage in a patient with end-stage renal failure?

Troponin-T and troponin-I are both integral parts of the cardiac muscle infrastructure. Troponin is release into the bloodstream when there is damage to cardiac myocyte cell wall integrity, hence its widespread for the diagnosis of MI. Although patients with ESRF may have supranormal levels of troponin on a regular basis, a rise in troponin-I (from baseline to 12 hours post event) has been shown to be specific for myocardial damage. Furthermore, careful analysis of large studies of patients with acute coronary syndrome e.g. GUSTO IV (Global Use of Streptokinase and Tissue-plasminogen activator for Occluded arteries), indicated that troponin elevation in the context of an acute coronary syndrome was of greater long-term prognostic importance in patients with renal impairment than in the normal population.

Mild troponin elevation is common in patients with asymptomatic end-stage renal disease. This has raised the possibility that these high-risk patients could be risk stratified according to troponin. In such patients, elevation in troponin may reflect microinfarctions or LVH.

One large study found that dialysis patients with elevated troponin were more likely to have severe angiographic coronary disease.

Why do patients on haemodialysis have an elevated risk of cardiovascular events?

Hypertension is the single most important risk factor for the development of cardio- and cerebrovascular complications. Despite the universally recognised detrimental effect of hypertension in dialysis patients, 60–70% of patients remain hypertensive while undergoing HD. Extracellular fluid expansion is the most important contributory factor, which can be limited by strict adherence to fluid restriction or by using prolonged daily haemodialysis (e.g. for 12 hours overnight). Although an expansion of extracellular volume accounts for persistent (or resistant) hypertension in many haemodialysis patients, some remain hypertensive despite reaching their 'dry weight'. It has been suggested that these patients have inappropriate activation of the renin–angiotensin system, which leads to an increase in peripheral vascular resistance, and hence MAP. Increased activity of the sympathetic system has also been demonstrated in HD patients. In addition, administration of exogenous EPO may cause exacerbation of hypertension in dialysis patients.

Other vascular risk factors specific to dialysis patients include an elevation of calcium and phosphate (due to hyperparathyroidism) which can result in soft tissue calcification. In particular, calcification of the media of arteries is observed. Dialysis patients may also have evidence of chronic inflammation (raised CRP and ferritin) and this inflammatory milieu may also drive atherosclerosis.

Traditional risk factors such as smoking and diabetes contribute to vascular disease in dialysis patients. Some patients have ESRF secondary to renovascular disease or diabetic nephropathy and will therefore already have significantly diseased blood vessels before starting dialysis.

The role of an elevated cholesterol/LDL in the progression of vascular disease in dialysis patients is unclear and as yet, studies have not shown an obvious survival benefit from the use of statins in dialysis patients.

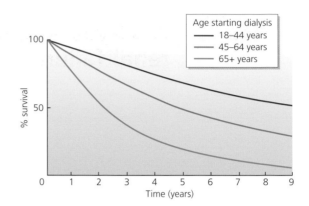

Figure 26.3 Patient survival on dialysis. Based on UK Renal Registry figures 1997–2005.

CASE REVIEW

A 58-year-old man with ESRF on dialysis has persistent problems with fluid overload and as a result has chronic hypertension. He subsequently presents with a severe headache whilst on dialysis and has focal neurological signs. A CT head demonstrates intracerebral haemorrhage. He is managed on a neurointensive care unit and makes a good recovery. Three years later he develops hypotension during dialysis and is found to have had a myocardial infarction.

KEY POINTS

- Although dialysis keeps patients alive, it cannot fully recapitulate the function of the kidneys and patients accrue a number of morbidities which inevitably limit their life expectancy:
  - a 20 year old starting dialysis has a 70% 5-year survival
  - a 40 year old starting dialysis has a 40% 5-year survival
  - a 60 year old starting dialysis has a 25% 5-year survival.

Survival curves are shown in Figure 26.3.

- The main causes of mortality are vascular disease, either cardiovascular or cerebrovascular.
- Hypertension is the single most important risk factor for the development of cardio- and cerebrovascular complications; 60–70% of haemodialysis patients are hypertensive, often due to extracellular fluid expansion.
- Long-term uncontrolled hypertension causes LVH which is an independent risk factor for cardiomyopathy, cardiac failure, ischaemic heart disease and death.
- Poorly controlled tertiary hyperparathyroidism with chronic hypercalcaemia also leads to medial calcification of arteries.

- Once vascular disease is established, intradialysis hypotension can precipitate angina, myocardial infarction or CVA so such acute events frequently occur on the dialysis unit. Cardiac events can be silent so it is important to keep this in mind when reviewing haemodialysis patients with persistently low blood pressure post dialysis sessions.
- Troponin-I elevation in a setting of suspected acute coronary syndromes in patients with ESRF is of substantial prognostic importance.
- Other complications of long-term dialysis include an increased risk of infection and malignancy. In addition, some patients develop β2-microglobulin amyloidosis, although this is becoming increasingly rare. This presents with carpal tunnel syndrome, arthropathy and bone disease.

A 54-year-old man with end-stage renal failure

Mr Gerald Byrne is a 54-year-old man who is approaching ESRF (eGFR 16 mL/min/1.73 m²) and has been seen in the renal 'low-clearance' clinic. Having read some of the literature given to him in clinic and attended a dialysis education session, he has decided to opt for peritoneal dialysis (PD) as his preferred form of renal replacement therapy.

Are there any factors which might make Mr Byrne unsuitable for peritoneal dialysis?

• Previous abdominal surgery, with possibility of adhesions; hence poor drainage and inefficient dialysis.
• Poor manual dexterity, e.g. due to arthritis in the hands or a neurological disorder which may render the patient physically unable to perform exchanges.
• Blindness.
• Inadequate home/social circumstances (need lots of space for large amount of fluid, and a clean room set aside for exchanges).
• Poor mental dexterity/inability to grasp importance or method of aseptic technique. If the patient is unable to appreciate this then the risk of developing peritonitis is high.
• Obesity: makes likelihood of adequate volume exchanges low.
• Abdominal hernias: can be repaired at time of placement of PD catheter, but frequently recur.
• Stomas: increase risk of infection
• Severe inflammatory bowel disease.
• Patients with severe COPD may find that respiration is impaired during large-volume dwells.

Are there any reasons why peritoneal dialysis might be a better option for Mr Byrne than haemodialysis?

• For patients who are well motivated and value their independence, PD is a better option than HD. PD patients do not need to travel to the dialysis unit three times a week and can perform exchanges at home or even in work (some employers will put aside a 'clean room' for storage of fluid and exchanges at work).
• PD can also be the best form of dialysis for patients with poor cardiovascular function, e.g. diabetics, who often have difficulty tolerating HD and can become hypotensive and cardiovascularly unstable during HD sessions.
• In some patients (often those who have been on HD previously), vascular access is limited because of central vein stenoses or occlusion. In these patients, PD may be the only option.
• There is some evidence to suggest that PD may prolong residual renal function compared to HD.

Mr Byrne lives 2 hours drive from his nearest HD unit and is keen to try PD in order to maintain his independence and to continue in full-time employment. He has no contraindications to PD and is therefore listed for insertion of a catheter as he is considered to be within 2 months of requiring renal replacement therapy.

Mr Byrne asks what the procedure will involve and whether he will require a general anaesthetic.

What do you tell him?

Peritoneal dialysis catheters can be inserted under local anaesthetic, and this is done routinely in some renal units with a specific interest in PD, in uncomplicated patients with 'virgin' abdomens. The procedure is often performed by a nephrologist rather than a surgeon. In more difficult cases or in units where there is no nephrologist with the required expertise, PD catheters are placed by surgeons, under a general anaesthetic.

Nephrology: Clinical Cases Uncovered. By M. Clatworthy. Published 2010 by Blackwell Publishing.

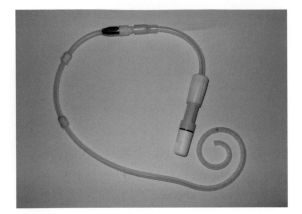

Figure 27.1 A tenckhoff PD catheter.

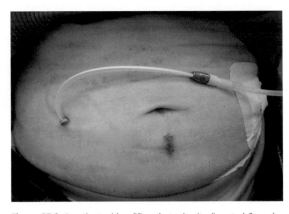

Figure 27.2 A patient with a PD catheter in-situ (inserted 6 weeks previously). Exit site looks slightly erythematous. The paramedian insertion incision is seen below the umbilicus.

There are a number of different designs of catheter available, for example Tenckhoff or Toronto-Western catheters (Figure 27.1).

The insertion procedure involves a paramedian incision through which the catheter is placed into the abdominal cavity between the visceral and parietal peritoneum (Figure 27.2). The intraperitoneal portion may be straight or curved and has small holes distally through which the fluid flows. Curved catheters are said to minimise discomfort which can occur if a strong jet of fluid is produced as the fluid enters the peritoneal cavity. The proximal, extraperitoneal part of the catheter is then tunnelled under the skin laterally so that the proximal cuff of the catheter lies in the tunnel, at least 2 cm from the exit site. The distal cuff should be embedded in the musculature of the anterior abdominal wall. The tunnel and cuffs reduce the risk of bacteria finding their way into the

Table 27.1 Composition of PD exchange fluid

Component	Concentration
Sodium (mmol/L)	132–134
Potassium (mmol/L)	0–2
Calcium (mmol/L)	0–1.75
Magnesium (mmol/L)	0.25–0.75
Chloride (mmol/L)	95–106
Lactate (mmol/L)	35–40
Glucose (g/dL)	1.36–3.86 (dextrose anhydrous) 1.5–4.25 (dextrose monohydrate)
Amino acids	1%
Ph	5.2–5.5
Osmolality (mOsm)	358–511

peritoneal cavity. The insertion procedure is usually covered with prophylactic antibiotics, for example a one-off bolus of vancomycin and gentamicin.

Following PD catheter insertion, the peritoneal cavity is usually rested for at least 1 month to allow adequate healing and to reduce the risk of developing a leak. The catheter can be flushed immediately postoperatively with a low-volume flush but a large-volume dwell is not placed until the peritoneum has healed. During this time the patient should receive appropriate training in readiness to use the catheter.

Mr Byrne's catheter is placed under general anaesthetic by the surgeons without difficulty. Four weeks later his wound appears well healed.

What regimen of peritoneal dialysis exchanges would you prescribe initially and once he is established on peritoneal dialysis?
Composition of fluids

Peritoneal dialysis fluid needs to be similar in composition to interstitial fluid, and hypertonic to plasma in order to achieve fluid removal (Table 27.1 shows typical composition of PD fluid). Several osmotic agents were initially evaluated but glucose was found to be the safest and most effective. Glucose solutions of differing strengths are used, depending on how much ultrafiltration is required. Bags of differing glucose concentrations are colour coded for clarity, which patients find very helpful (Figure 27.3).

- Yellow – 1.36%
- Green – 2.27%
- Orange – 3.86%

Prolonged exposure of the peritoneal membrane to glucose-containing solutions causes damage and a reduction in permeability over time. In addition, glucose is absorbed from the peritoneal cavity during a dwell. This means that UF is not maintained throughout the whole period of the dwell (Figure 27.4). The use of glucose-containing dialysis solutions is associated with a number of adverse metabolic effects, including obesity, glucose intolerance, hyperinsulinaemia, reduced peripheral sensitivity to insulin, and hyperlipidaemia. Therefore, newer solutions have been developed to avoid these unwanted effects, for example icodextrin and amino acid-containing solutions. Icodextrin is a glucose polymer, which is not absorbed to the same extent as glucose during exchange. It exerts a colloid rather than a crystalloid osmotic effect and is particularly effective in producing sustained UF during prolonged dwells. Amino acid-containing dialysis solutions are also available, e.g. Nutrineal, Extraneal. The osmotic and dialysis efficacy is similar to glucose but there are no adverse effects on peritoneal permeability and they may also alleviate the malnutrition sometimes present in patients with ESRF.

Volume of fluid

Initially, relatively small volume exchanges are used, for example, 1 litre. The volume of each exchange is gradu-ally increased provided the patient is not in too much discomfort and there are no obvious leaks. Once a patient is established, a typical exchange involves the instillation of 2 litres of fluid.

Administration of fluid

There are two ways of instilling fluid into the peritoneal cavity.

- *Manual method or continuous ambulatory peritoneal dialysis (CAPD):* this involves the patient or carer manually connecting a bag of PD fluid to the dialysis catheter via a transfer set and instilling the fluid into the peritoneal cavity using gravity, e.g. bag placed on table above the level of the bed/chair. The fluid is then drained out (again using gravity) after a dwell period of several hours, e.g. bag is placed on the floor. This procedure is repeated 3–4 times a day (Figure 27.5).

- *Automated method or automated peritoneal dialysis (APD):* this refers to all forms of PD employing a mechanical device to assist in the delivery and drainage of the dialysate. The various therapeutic regimens encompassed by APD are continuous cyclic PD (CCPD), intermittent PD (IPD), nightly intermittent PD (NIPD) and tidal PD (TPD). The most obvious advantage of APD is that it eliminates the need for intensive manual involvement, reducing the work to two procedures daily – setting up the dialysis machine, and connecting and disconnecting the patient and dismantling the machine. It is a home-based therapy carried out by the patient or carer overnight, which may be more convenient than CAPD because it allows freedom from all procedures during the day.

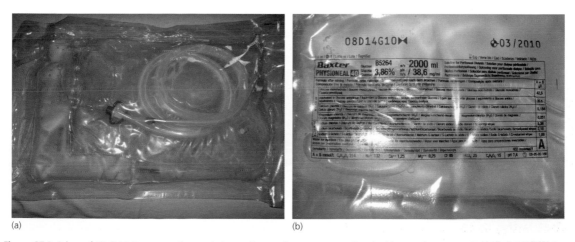

(a)   (b)

Figure 27.3 A bag of PD fluid. Bags are colour coded according to glucose concentration. In this case the orange cap indicates 3.86% glucose (a). The front of the bag confirms the type of fluid and glucose concentration (b).

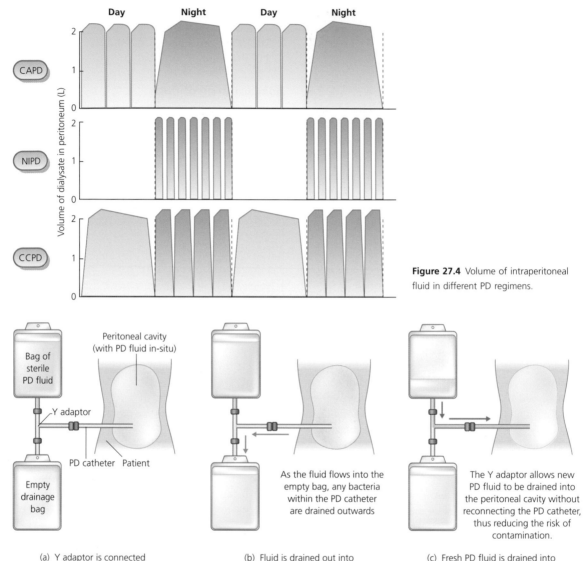

Figure 27.4 Volume of intraperitoneal fluid in different PD regimens.

Figure 27.5 Drainage of fluid into and out of the peritoneal cavity.

Mr Byrne is started on CAPD and is initially asked to perform three 1-litre exchanges/day. Two days later he comes up to the renal unit because the PD fluid is not draining freely from his peritoneal cavity. He has put in 1 litre of dialysate but has only drained 500 mL. He is otherwise asymptomatic. The PD sister has organised a plain abdominal film (Figure 27.6).

What is the likely cause of his fluid drainage problems?

The X-ray shows that the PD catheter is poorly positioned. It is coiled and lies in the upper abdomen. In addition, there is faecal loading. Both of these factors are likely to contribute to the impaired drainage of PD fluid from his abdomen. Other causes of poor drainage include blockage of the catheter tip by omentum or occlusion by fibrin clots.

How would you manage this gentleman?

Provided he is well (no pulmonary oedema or symptomatic uraemia) and his bloods are satisfactory (i.e. not dangerously hyperkalaemic), you should attempt to treat his constipation. This may be achieved with simple

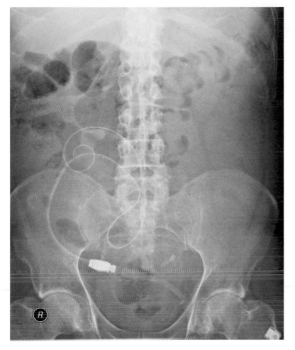

Figure 27.6 Mr Byrne's abdominal X-ray. The tip of the PD catheter lies in the right, upper abdomen. There is also faecal loading evident in the descending colon.

Table 27.2 Complications after PD catheter insertion

Complications	Action
Operative complications	
Exit site haemorrhage	Pressure bandage
Intraperitoneal haemorrhage	Lavage PD fluid
Perforation of hollow viscus	Laparotomy
Postinsertion complications	
Catheter tip migration	Treat constipation; laparoscopic catheter manipulation; surgery
Exit site infections	Antibiotics, cuff exteriorization
Leakage of PD fluid	Stop PD; antibiotic cover. If recurrence, catheter replacement
Pleural leak with effusion	Stop PD; drain effusion if large

laxatives (e.g. lactulose) but often requires more aggressive therapy (e.g. Picolax). A good response to laxatives can actually cause significant movement of the PD catheter into a more satisfactory position and can make a big difference to drainage.

Mr Byrne is asymptomatic and his bloods are stable with a K+ of 4.0mmol/L. He has a good response to Picolax, but continues to have difficulties with fluid drainage. His repeat X-ray shows little improvement in catheter position.

What would you advise next?
This is unlikely to resolve without repositioning of the PD catheter. He should therefore be referred to the surgeons for laproscopic repositioning of PD catheter. If the surgeons feel that the omentum is significantly contributing to the obstruction, then an omentectomy can be performed.

The PD catheter is repositioned laproscopically, and the abdominal X-ray performed post procedure shows an adequately positioned catheter which now drains without difficulty.

What other complications may arise following peritoneal dialysis catheter insertion?
Complications can be divided into immediate operative complications, such as bleeding or perforation, and postinsertion complications, such as catheter tip migration (summarised in Table 27.2).

CASE REVIEW

A 54-year-old man with ESRF is seen in predialysis clinic. Following appropriate education, he opts for peritoneal dialysis as his preferred form of RRT. A PD catheter is inserted under a general anaesthetic. The wound is allowed to heal for 4 weeks but following this his PD catheter does not drain well post dwell. An abdominal film is performed and shows that he is constipated and that the catheter tip does not lie in the pelvis. He is given laxatives but this does not improve catheter position so he undergoes a laparoscopic repositioning of the catheter. Following this, the catheter drains well.

KEY POINTS

- When a patient is approaching ESRF they need to be properly informed of the types of renal replacement available to them. There are four options:
  - haemodialysis
  - peritoneal dialysis
  - transplantation
  - conservative management (may be appropriate if elderly with multiple co-morbidities).
- Although transplantation offers the best option in terms of quality of life and survival for most patients with ESRF, organ supply is the limiting factor. Most patients remain on the transplant waiting list for a number of years before an organ becomes available. As a mode of dialysis, PD has a number of advantages over HD, particularly because the patient can perform exchanges at home and it allows continued independence.
- Peritoneal dialysis catheter insertion is usually performed as a day case and has a low complication rate. The best position for the catheter tip is in the true pelvis. Migration of the catheter out of the pelvis is frequently observed on abdominal radiographs taken for various reasons in patients with a functioning catheter. While about 20% of catheters translocate to the upper abdomen, only one-fifth of these translocated catheters become obstructed.
- Slow drainage due to catheter translocation or occlusion of the tip by bowel or a fibrin clot occurs from time to time in some patients. Constipation is a common cause of this complication, so many PD patients are given regular laxatives in an attempt to avoid constipation. For fibrin clots, the addition of heparin, 500 units/L of dialysis solution, is usually successful in restoring good catheter function.

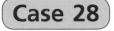

Case 28 A 50-year-old man on peritoneal dialysis with abdominal pain

Mr Robert Quinnel, a 50-year-old patient with ESRF on PD, contacts the PD clinic complaining of abdominal pain and nausea. The PD sister arranges for him to come up to the Medical Admissions Unit for assessment.

What questions would you ask Mr Quinnel?

• Abdominal pain: site, onset, character, severity, radiation, exacerbating and relieving factors of pain.
• Associated features: vomiting, diarrhoea, bowels open? Passing flatus?
• Is the PD fluid clear or cloudy following a dwell?
• Has the PD catheter exit site been mucky/discharging, red or painful?
• Similar episodes previously? Any previous history of PD peritonitis?
• Any other systemic symptoms, e.g. fever, rigors, sweats.
• Any contacts with similar symptoms? Any unusual foods? May be an infective gastroenteritis or food poisoning.
• What is his PD regimen (number of exchanges, size of exchanges, type of fluid, how much UF (i.e. fluid removal with each exchange)?
• Past medical history: how long has he had renal failure for? How long has he been on PD? Has he received any other forms of RRT? Any abdominal problems or abdominal operations previously?
• What medications is he on?

Mr Quinnel developed ESRF due to IgA nephropathy 11 years ago. He was on PD for just 6 months before he received a cadaveric renal transplant. His allograft lasted for 10 years but finally failed 9 months ago. He has been maintained on PD since then without difficulty and has not had peritonitis. His current PD regimen involves four exchanges/24 hours, 2 litre 'yellow' bags (1.36% (low)

Nephrology: Clinical Cases Uncovered. By M. Clatworthy.
Published 2010 by Blackwell Publishing.

glucose). He allows each of the three daytime bags to dwell for 4 hours, and the fourth bag for 12 hours overnight. He has good UF (that is, the volume of fluid which is removed with each exchange; see case 28) and tends to drain out around 400 mL more than he put in. He has also had problems with hypertension and hyperlipidaemia, both of which are being medically managed.

His current symptoms of abdominal pain and nausea have been going on for around 24 hours. He describes a diffuse abdominal ache which is gradually getting worse and is exacerbated by movement. It has been associated with anorexia and nausea and he also feels very hot and sweaty. He opened his bowels this morning and noticed that his motions were slightly loose. The fluid drained from his overnight dwell this morning was very cloudy, and he has brought it in for you to look at (Figure 28.1).

What is the most likely diagnosis?

If a patient on PD presents with abdominal pain, the principal concern is that they have developed PD peritonitis. Although Mr Quinnel may develop abdominal pain secondary to any other cause of an acute abdomen, PD peritonitis is the most likely diagnosis, particularly given the cloudy PD fluid he has drained from his abdomen. Other diagnoses, such as perforation with faecal peritonitis or pancreatitis, should be kept in mind.

On examination, Mr Quinnel's temperature is 38.5°C. Other observations are as follows: pulse 85 bpm and regular, BP 145/60 mmHg, RR 19, O_2 saturations are 98% on air. The PD catheter exit site does not look erythematous or obviously infected. His abdomen is diffusely tender with peritonism to percussion, and rebound but no guarding. Bowel sounds are present and of normal character. Examination was otherwise unremarkable.

Investigations are shown below.

Hb 12.1 g/dL, WBC 13.2 × 10^9/L, Neutrophils 11.6 × 10^9/L, Lymphocytes 0.68 × 10^9/L, Platelets 261 × 10^9/L

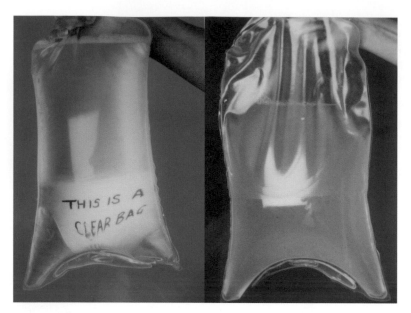

Figure 28.1 PD peritonitis. Left panel shows a normal, clear bag of fluid post-drainage. Right panel shows Mr Quinnel's cloudy fluid bag, consistent with PD peritonitis.

Clotting normal
U+E: Na 134 mmol/L, K 4.9 mmol/L, Urea 30 mmol/L, Creatinine 1129
CRP 158 mg/L
Amylase and LFT: NAD
Albumin 30 g/dL
Glucose 5.2 mmol/L
cCa 2.5 mmol/L, PO$_4$ 1.1 mmol/L

PD fluid (exchange performed in clinic on day of presentation and fluid sent off):

Nucleated cell count 0.3 × 10^9/L
CAPD fluid microscopy: macroscopic appearance – clear
Cell count <100 × 10^6/L
Gram stain: gram-positive cocci (chains) seen

What do these investigations suggest?

Mr Quinnel has a neutrophil leucocytosis and an elevated CRP, both of which are suggestive of a current bacterial infection. He is lymphopaenic, which can occur during a severe bacterial infection. The U+E are consistent with his known ESRF. A normal amylase makes pancreatitis unlikely.

The presence of gram-positive cocci on microscopy of the PD fluid is consistent with a diagnosis of PD peritonitis. The cell count within the PD fluid is usually elevated in cases of peritonitis, although if the patient presents early (as in this case), counts may rise in subsequent fluid samples. Bacteria enter the peritoneal cavity via the line or fluid, due to poor aseptic technique by the patient during exchanges, a split or breach in the catheter or a tunnel/exit site infection. If there is perforation or faecal peritonitis, gram negatives or a mixed population are more likely to be identified.

What are the most common organisms causing peritoneal dialysis peritonitis?

The organisms commonly isolated from PD fluid are shown in Table 28.1. Gram-positive organisms cause up to 75% of all episodes of peritonitis; of these, *Staphylococcus epidermidis* infections are usually mild and easily treated with appropriate antibiotic therapy. *Staph. aureus* is associated with a much more severe presentation and may be life-threatening. Occasionally they may progress to abscess formation. Of the gram-negative organisms, pseudomonas infections are similarly serious. They are difficult to eradicate and lead to irreversible damage to the peritoneal membrane such that it is no longer useful for dialysis. Fungal peritonitis is uncommon, is generally caused by candida species and usually requires catheter removal.

Culture-negative peritonitis accounts for 10–30% of all episodes. This may be due to antibiotic administration prior to culture or poor microbiological technique, or can occur secondary to peritoneal irritants, e.g.

Table 28.1 Causative organisms in PD peritonitis

Organism	Frequency (% total)
Culture negative	10–30
Coagulase-negative staphylococci	20–25
Staph. aureus	10–15
Other gram-positive cocci	10–15
Pseudomonas	5
Enterococcus	1–5
Other gram negatives	10–15
Mixed growth	1–5
Fungal	1–5

chemicals, dialysis fluid components, endotoxins and antiseptics.

What treatment should Mr Quinnel be started on?

Most renal units have specific PD peritonitis protocols that provide the best empirical treatment, based on known previous cultures, until sensitivities are available. This usually involves the administration of intraperitoneal (IP) antibiotics, for example vancomycin or ceftazidime, which provide antimicrobial activity against most gram-positive bacteria. In addition, there should be some provision for gram-negative organisms if vancomycin is used, for example, oral ciprofloxacin.

Mr Quinnel is given 2g of vancomycin IP (the vancomycin is injected into the bag of PD fluid which the patient then drains into the abdominal cavity) and is commenced on ciprofloxacin 500mg po bd. His abdominal pain improves over the next few days. His subsequent PD fluid results are shown below.

Day 2 PD fluid: nucleated cell count 7×10^9/L (97% neutrophils, 1% lymphocytes, 2% monocytes)
Day 3 PD fluid: nucleated cell count 3.5×10^9/L (94% neut, 2% lymph, 4% mono)
CAPD fluid culture:
Streptococcus epidermidis: heavy growth
Sensitivities: penicillin S, vancomycin S
Blood cultures negative.

How often would you measure his vancomycin levels and how long would you keep Mr Quinnel on this treatment?

Vancomycin is renally cleared, so following a bolus IP, levels are likely to be adequate for 2–3 days. Measure levels on day 2 following administration. Treatment should be continued for at least 2 weeks.

If uncomplicated, PD peritonitis can be managed as an outpatient, with frequent review and assessment of clinical status. Provided the patient is not systemically unwell (hypotension, tachycardia, severe peritonism), blood and fluid can be taken for culture, antibiotics given and arrangements made to review within a couple of days.

In most cases of peritonitis the symptoms begin to resolve rapidly after the initiation of treatment and disappear within 2–3 days. During this period the cell counts in the effluent decrease and bacterial cultures become negative. Persistence of symptoms is indicative of a complicated cause or a possible resistant organism. These patients require further investigation and often catheter removal.

Overall, the outcome of PD peritonitis is quite good. Complete cure is achieved in around 85% of cases without recourse to catheter removal. Catheter removal is required in up to 15% of cases. The condition can be serious, though, and mortality rates are reported to be around 1–3%.

Prevention of peritonitis is of critical importance. Careful selection of patients and meticulous training is paramount. The incidence of Staph. aureus infections may be reduced by applying mupirocin at the exit site and eradication of nasal carriage.

Mr Quinnel's peritonitis clears well with a 2-week course of IP vancomycin. Four years after this presentation with PD peritonitis, he is reviewed routinely in PD clinic. He has had two other episodes of peritonitis in the intervening years. He now has little UF with his exchanges and complains of intermittent colicky abdominal pain and weight loss.

His dialysis adequacy is also suboptimal, with a weekly Kt/V of 0.9. (see case 26 for explanation of dialysis adequacy. In patients on PD, UK Renal Association guidelines suggest a target Kt/V of 1.7/week)

A CT abdomen is performed and is shown in Figure 28.2.

What complication has occurred?

Encapsulating peritoneal sclerosis (EPS). This is a well-recognised complication of long-term PD which is estimated to occur in 1–5% of patients on PD. Macroscopic

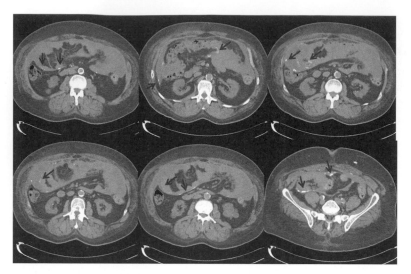

Figure 28.2 CT abdomen showing early peritoneal sclerosis. Peritoneal calcification (*arrows*) present throughout the abdomen.

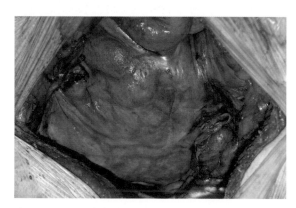

Figure 28.3 Tanned, thickened peritoneum encasing loops of bowel in a patient with EPS.

changes in the peritoneum can be seen after relatively short periods of PD, particularly 'tanning' of the peritoneum. Patients who remain on PD for a number of years can develop more extensive peritoneal thickening (Figure 28.3). Clinical features include abdominal pain and swelling secondary to bowel obstruction, blood-stained effluent and UF failure. Radiological features include peritoneal thickening and calcification (Figure 28.4a), with the development of the so-called 'abdominal cocoon' which may contain fluid collections (Figure 28.4b). Histopathological derangements include loss of mesothelium, gross interstitial thickening within the peritoneal membrane, with a variable inflammatory infiltrate. Risk factors include multiple episodes of peritonitis and time on dialysis. The main treatment is to stop PD and switch to HD, although this does not always halt progression and certainly does not reverse changes. Other treatment strategies include immunosuppression, tamoxifen and surgery. The latter involves a long, painstaking operation in which the surgeon carefully unpicks the thickened peritoneum from around the bowel. Patients are often malnourished due to recurrent subacute obstruction, and frequently require nutritional support.

Even with treatment, the prognosis of EPS is poor, with mortality reaching 90% in some series. Given the grim outlook, it has been suggested that patients who remain on PD for more than 5 years should be routinely screened by CT scanning in order to identify changes consistent with EPS. PD should then be discontinued in these patients before the development of severe symptoms.

Mr Quinnel is switched to HD and the PD catheter removed. His abdominal pain improves, although he is eating much less and losing weight. One month later he re-presents with bowel obstruction. This is conservatively managed with a wide-bore NG tube and parenteral nutrition. Peritoneolysis is performed but unfortunately he dies 1 week postoperatively from overwhelming sepsis.

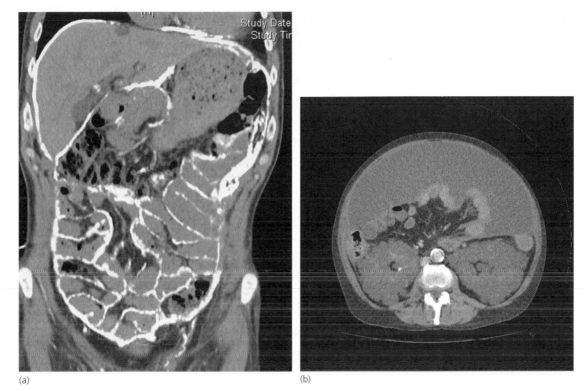

(a)   (b)

Figure 28.4 Radiological appearances in advanced EPS. (a) Non-contrast CT scan of a patient who had been on PD for 19 years. There is extensive calcification (bright white signal) surrounding all loops of bowel. (b) Non-contrast CT scan demonstrating a large fluid collection anteriorly (dark grey) within layers of thickened peritoneum, which compresses the bowel loops. This patient had ESRF secondary to polycystic kidney disease and had been on PD for 6 years prior to presentation.

CASE REVIEW

A 50-year-old man on PD presents with fever, abdominal pain and cloudy PD fluid post drainage. On examination, he is febrile and his abdomen is peritonitic. Investigations show elevated inflammatory markers and white cell count in blood and neutrophils and gram-positive cocci in the PD fluid from which *Strepotococcus epidermidis* is cultured.

He is treated with vancomycin and recovers well. Four years later he develops encapsulating peritoneal sclerosis. This is managed by switching him to haemodialysis. Although some of his abdominal symptoms improve, he re-presents with obstruction and dies following a peritonectomy.

KEY POINTS

- Peritonitis remains one of the most common and serious complications of PD. The earliest clinical sign of infection is turbidity of the drained effluent post dwell. Other features include abdominal pain, change in bowel habit and nausea and vomiting. The generally accepted definition of peritonitis in CAPD entails any two of the

three features: signs or symptoms, cloudy dialysate with more than $100\,\text{cells/mm}^3$, and the presence of micro-organisms in the dialysate.
- Cloudy effluent is not necessarily diagnostic of infective peritonitis. It can be due to blood, fibrin, intra-abdominal pathology, diarrhoea and eosinophilic peritonitis. The

Continued

latter is a syndrome including cloudy effluent in an asymptomatic patient with persistently negative cultures. It occurs in the early stages of CAPD and tends to resolve spontaneously within weeks. It is thought to occur secondary to an 'allergy' to some component of the fluid or administration kit.

- The main route of infection of the peritoneal cavity (30–40%) is through the lumen of the catheter, followed by periluminal factors (i.e. from around the outside of the catheter and the exit site; 20–30%). The risk of infection via these routes is increased in patients who are chronic nasal or skin carriers of *Staphylococcus aureus*. Other less common routes of infection are transcolonic (20–25%) and haematogenous (5%).
- Coagulase-negative staphylococci are the major causative organisms in CAPD peritonitis. They tend to adhere to and grow on polymer surfaces, producing an extracellular, slimy matrix or biofilm which becomes embedded with organisms.
- Fungal peritonitis is much rarer. Patients are usually acutely ill with severe abdominal pain and may deteriorate rapidly or die if catheter removal is delayed.
- Overall, the outcome of PD peritonitis is quite good. Complete cure is achieved in around 85% of cases without recourse to catheter removal.
- Encapsulating peritoneal sclerosis is a well-recognised complication of long-term peritoneal dialysis which is estimated to occur in 1–5% of patients on PD. It is characterised by peritoneal tanning and thickening. Clinical features include abdominal pain and swelling secondary to bowel obstruction, blood-stained effluent, UF failure, and abdominal masses due to distinct fluid collections. It can be treated surgically by peritoneolysis but has a poor prognosis.

Case 29 A 49-year-old man with chronic kidney disease

Mr Paul Bennet, a 49-year-old electrician, presented to the renal services 1 month ago with near ESRF. Investigations showed no obvious cause for his kidney failure, with an US showing two 8 cm kidneys with thin cortices and no evidence of hydronephrosis. His eGFR is now around 18 mL/min/1.73 m² so he is referred to the predialysis/low clearance clinic to discuss the different forms of renal replacement therapy (RRT).

The patient asks what is likely to happen to his kidney function, and if there is any treatment for kidney failure.

What do you tell him?

It is likely that Mr Bennet's renal function will continue to decline and that he will require RRT within the next 6 months. There are three forms of RRT available for patients with ESRF:

- haemodialysis
- peritoneal dialysis
- renal transplantation.

Mr Bennet attends a predialysis education session and decides he will probably opt for peritoneal dialysis. He is keen to continue working and is worried about the impact that dialysis will have on his life. Mr Bennet would like to know more about transplantation.

What are the types of donor from which a transplant kidney might be obtained for Mr Bennet?

- Deceased donor
  - Heart beating: donors meet criteria for brainstem death (Box 29.1). They are often in neuro-ITU, typically post-road traffic accident or intracerebral haemorrhage.
  - Non-heart beating (also known as deceased cardiac death or asystolic donors)

> ### Box 29.1 Criteria for brainstem death
>
> **Irreversibility**
> - No sedating, paralyzing or toxic drug
> - No gross electrolyte or endocrine disturbance
> - No profound hypothermia
>
> **Absent cerebral function**
> - No seizures or posturing
> - No response to pain in cranial nerve distribution
> - Absent brainstem function
> - Apnoea in response to acidosis and hypercarbia
> - No papillary or corneal reflex
> - No oculocephalic or vestibular reflex
> - No tracheobronchial reflex

- Living donor
  - Related: most commonly parent to child or sibling to sibling
  - Unrelated: usually spouse to spouse, most commonly wife to husband. Occasionally close friends will donate kidneys
  - Altruistic: recently introduced in the UK (2007). Members of the general public may decide that they wish to give a kidney to someone on the waiting list. The same work-up applies as with any other living donor, with particular emphasis on lack of psychiatric condition and on ensuring the individual is fully aware of the implications of their action

Currently the main issue in transplantation is a shortage of organ donors. There are over 7000 patients on the renal transplant list awaiting a kidney in the UK. The average waiting time for a patient on the deceased donor list is around 3 years, but it may be much longer. The number of heart-beating donors in the UK has remained relatively constant at 750–800 per annum. In an attempt to increase the supply of organs, many more living and non-heart beating donors are being identified.

Nephrology: Clinical Cases Uncovered. By M. Clatworthy.
Published 2010 by Blackwell Publishing.

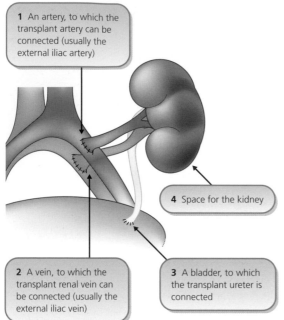

1 An artery, to which the transplant artery can be connected (usually the external iliac artery)

4 Space for the kidney

2 A vein, to which the transplant renal vein can be connected (usually the external iliac vein)

3 A bladder, to which the transplant ureter is connected

Figure 29.1 Technical requirements for transplantation.

Mr Bennet is informed that he may be worked up for consideration for a deceased donor kidney but the current waiting time in the UK is around 3 years. You inform him that the alternative option is receiving a kidney from a live donor, if there is someone suitable amongst his family and friends.

What are the processes involved in transplant work-up?

Basic transplant work-up includes the following.

1. Assess for problems which make the patient *immunologically difficult* to transplant, particularly any sensitising events (blood transfusion and pregnancy, especially if multiple partners).

2. Assess for problems which make the patient *technically difficult* to transplant. There are four basic technical ('plumbing') requirements for transplantation (Figure 29.1).

- An artery (usually the external iliac artery), to which the transplant renal artery will be anastomosed.
- A vein (usually the external iliac vein), to which the transplant renal vein will be anastomosed.
- A bladder, to which the transplant ureter will be anastomosed.
- Some space for the kidney.

These requirements can be compromised if the patient has:

- severe peripheral vascular disease which can make the arterial anastomosis difficult. Therefore the patient's lower limb pulses should be carefully assessed, including auscultation of the femoral artery for a bruit
- a history of venous thromboembolic disease, particularly clots in the lower limb veins. Patients on chronic haemodialysis may also have had numerous lines inserted into their femoral veins which can lead to stenosis and thrombosis
- a history of urological problems, including congenital bladder malformations or reflux. If these issues are not resolved prior to transplantation, then the problem may recur and damage the transplanted kidney. In addition, patients who have had ESRF for a number of years often have negligible urine output. In such cases, the bladder may shrink to the size of a walnut and will be difficult to find intraoperatively and will only hold small volumes post transplant. Intraoperatively, the patient is catheterised and methylene blue dye is added to normal saline and infused into the bladder to assist the surgeon in identifying it.
- Space is rarely a problem, because the kidneys are usually placed extraperitoneally in one or other iliac fossa. The exception is in patients with polycystic kidney disease, in which the native kidneys can becomes so enlarged that they extend into the lower abdomen. In some cases they need to be removed prior to transplantation.

3. Assess for problems which make the patient an *anaesthetic risk*. Patients with CKD are at increased risk of atherosclerosis and of coronary, cerebral and peripheral vascular disease. An ECG and CXR should be performed in all patients. Most will also need some form of stress test (either an exercise tolerance test or an isotope perfusion study) and an echocardiogram to assess LV function. If these are abnormal, then the patient will need to be referred for further cardiological assessment, often coronary angiography.

4. Assess for problems which put the patient at increased risk of *immunosuppression-related side-effects*. If a patient has ESRF secondary to renal inflammation then they may have had a significant net dose of immunosuppression (e.g. cyclophosphamide or even biological agents). Such patients may not require as heavy immunosuppression. In particular, lymphocyte-depleting agents should be avoided. Immunosuppression also increases the risk of developing a malignancy and enhances the progression of existing cancers. Thus, most centres would agree that patients with a history of malignancy must be cancer free for at least 5 years prior to transplantation.

Mr Bennet is assessed and appears to be a good candidate for transplantation. He is non-sensitised, had no past medical history prior to his presentation with ESRF and has an excellent exercise tolerance (can walk an unlimited distance and jogs twice a week for >2 miles). His pulses are easily palpable and there are no bruits. ECG and CXR are normal and he is within 6 months of requiring dialysis and can therefore be activated on the national deceased donor waiting list. Given the lengthy wait for a deceased donor kidney for the average patient with ESRF, the patient's wife (who has come to the clinic with him) says that she would like to give one of her kidneys to her husband.

What are the main factors to consider in working up a living donor?

Fitness of donor

Donating a kidney involves a significant operation, lasting around 3–4 hours, and a general anaesthetic. If the donor has any pre-existing medical condition which would place them at high risk of complications during an anaesthetic, e.g. previous MI, poor LV function, then they would not be considered for donation. In many centres, donor nephrectomy is now undertaken laparoscopically. Although a technically more challenging procedure, the donor tends to recover much more quickly and may be discharged within 3–4 days of the procedure. As well as physical considerations, the transplant physicians and surgeons must also be sure that the donor is mentally and emotionally sound and understands the implications of the procedure. They must also be certain that there is no coercion involved in donation.

Adequacy of donor renal function

The donation will involve the donor losing one kidney. Therefore it is important to ensure that the donor has adequate renal function to allow for this. Pre-existing medical conditions such as diabetes mellitus or hypertension which can lead to chronic kidney disease are a relative contraindication to donation. Initially, a US scan of the renal tract is performed to ensure that the donor has two kidneys. The urine is dipsticked to rule out microscopic haematuria or proteinuria which may indicate underlying renal disease. Renal function is measured by serum creatinine, creatinine clearance and calculated GFR, together with the split function. If the renal function is sufficient to allow halving of the GFR and some decline in renal function with age, then the donor is considered suitable. They will then undergo an MRI scan to accurately delineate the renal anatomy, and to define the number of vessels supplying each kidney. This assists the surgeons undertaking the nephrectomy to decide which kidney is technically most amenable to removal; for example, a kidney with three renal arteries is technically more challenging to remove than a kidney with a single renal artery.

Compatibility

ABO

AB antigens are found on the surface of red cells and endothelial cells. Individuals who are blood group A have A antigens on their blood cells and circulating anti-B antibodies present in their serum. Blood group B individuals have B antigen on red cells and anti-A antibodies. Blood group O individuals have neither A nor B antigens on their RBC and therefore have both anti-A and -B antibodies. Blood group AB individuals have both A and B antigens on the surface of RBC and neither anti-A nor anti-B antibodies. Thus, if a blood group A individual were to donate a kidney to a blood group B individual, the circulating anti-A antibody in the recipient would immediately bind to the endothelium, activating complement and phagocytes, damaging the endothelium and causing occlusion of the vessels and immediate infarction of the kidney (Figure 29.2). For this reason blood group incompatible transplantation is not routinely undertaken. More recently, with a shortage of donors, the issue of ABO-incompatible transplantation has been revisited. The recipient can undergo a desensitisation treatment in which antibodies are removed by plasma exchange and the patient receives much heavier immunosuppression.

HLA

The human leucocyte antigens (HLA) are highly polymorphic glycoproteins found on the surface of cells. They are divided into class I and class II molecules. Class I molecules are found on the surface of all cells, and class II on the surface of antigen-presenting cells. They are encoded by a cluster of genes found on chromosome 6 called the major histocompatibility complex genes (Figure 29.3). In humans there are three MHC class I genes (A, B and C) and three MHC class II genes (DP, DQ and DR). Given that an individual has two copies of each gene, the maximum number of mismatches that can occur between two individuals is 12, i.e. two A mismatches, two B mismatches, etc. However, in renal transplantation only A, B and DR mismatches are considered, so the maximum number of mismatches possible is six. Such a mismatch would be described as a 2-2-2 mismatch (2 A, 2 B and 2 DR mismatches). The best mismatch would be a 0-0-0 mismatch. The more mismatches that

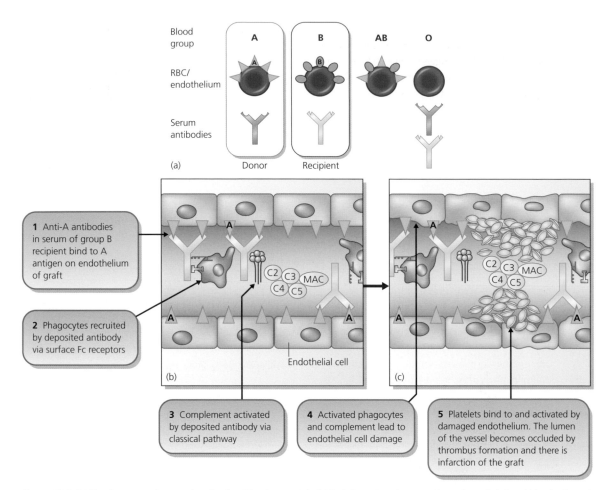

1 Anti-A antibodies in serum of group B recipient bind to A antigen on endothelium of graft

2 Phagocytes recruited by deposited antibody via surface Fc receptors

3 Complement activated by deposited antibody via classical pathway

4 Activated phagocytes and complement lead to endothelial cell damage

5 Platelets bind to and activated by damaged endothelium. The lumen of the vessel becomes occluded by thrombus formation and there is infarction of the graft

Figure 29.2 (a) Blood group antigens and antibodies. Blood group A individuals have A antigens on the surface of their red blood cells and endothelial cells, and circulating anti-B antibodies (and vice versa for blood group B individuals). AB individuals have both A and B antigens and no AB antibodies. Blood group O individuals have neither A nor B antigens, but circulating antibodies to both antigens. (b) Hyperacute rejection. If a blood group A donor gives a kidney to a blood group B recipient, the pre-formed anti-A antibodies will bind to the endothelium in the graft causing hyperacute rejection.

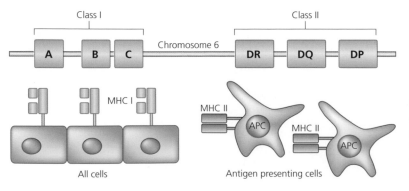

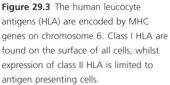

Figure 29.3 The human leucocyte antigens (HLA) are encoded by MHC genes on chromosome 6. Class I HLA are found on the surface of all cells, whilst expression of class II HLA is limited to antigen presenting cells.

are present, the more likely it is that the allograft will be recognised as foreign and rejected. This is reflected in allograft survival data which suggest that ≈80% of those patients receiving a 0-0-0 mismatched kidney will still have a functioning allograft at 5 years compared with ≈55% of those receiving a 2-2-2 mismatched kidney (Figure 29.4). DR mismatches are more significant than A or B mismatches, so every effort is made to avoid DR mismatches.

Mr Bennet's wife is seen in the living transplant assessment clinic and is found to be in good health. She has two normal-sized kidneys and a creatinine clearance of 104 and is therefore fit enough to be a donor. Both she and her husband are blood group O and are therefore compatible. The HLA mismatch is also favourable (1-1-0). The patient's GFR is now 8 mL/min/1.73 m² and he therefore requires RRT. Following appropriate consent and organisation, he and his wife are admitted for living donor transplantation.

How long would you expect Mr and Mrs Bennet to be in hospital for?

Patients undergoing laproscopic nephrectomy recover very quickly post-operatively. They are often back on their feet the day after the operation and can be discharged as early as day 3 post-operatively. A rise in creatinine is to be expected as their GFR will have been roughly halved.

Renal transplantation involves a 3–4 hour operation and on average, patients stay in hospital for 7–10 days.

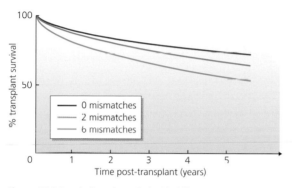

Figure 29.4 Renal allograft survival with different HLA mismatches.

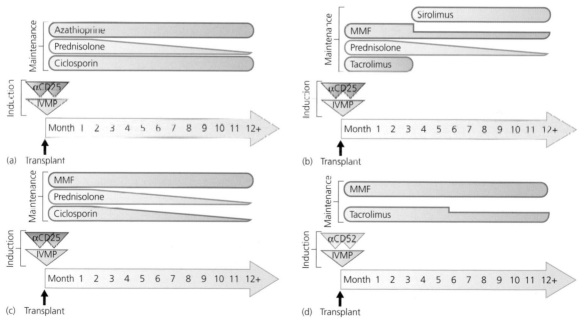

Figure 29.5 Immunosuppressive regimens in renal transplantation. A variety of different regimens can be used, but in general they involve the use of intravenous induction agents (methyl prednisolone and mono- or polyclonal antibodies) followed by oral maintenance therapy. (a) regimen 1 – methyl prednisolone and anti-CD25 followed by triple therapy with azathioprine, prednisolone and ciclosporin. (b) Regimen 2 – induction as for 1, but MMF is used instead of azathioprine and tacrolimus instead of ciclosporin. At 3 months the tacrolimus is stopped and replaced by sirolimus, thus minimizing CNI toxicity. (c) Regimen 3 – Induction as for 1, ciclosporin weaned with high dose MMF cover in order to reduce CNI exposure. (d) Regimen 4 – Lymphocyte depleting agent used at induction (anti-CD52, alemtuzumab) allowing a steroid-free maintenance regimen.

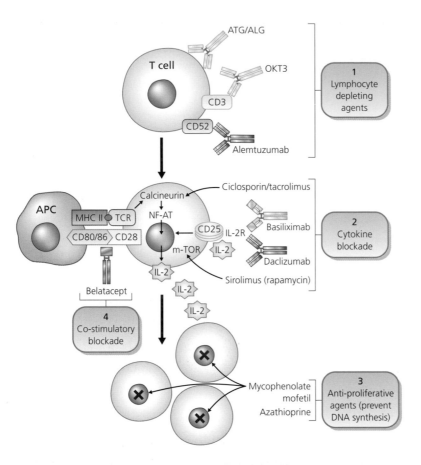

Induction agents:

1 Anti-CD25 antibodies - block IL-2 binding to its receptor (basiliximab/daclizumab)

2 Anti-CD52 antibody - binds to T and B lymphocytes, leading to depletion (alemtuzumab)

3 Anti-thymocyte globulin/anti-lymphocyte globulin - bind to T lymphocytes, leading to depletion

Maintenance agents:

1 Calcineurin inhibitors - act downstream of T cell receptor, reduce activation of nuclear factor of activated T cells (NFAT), a transcription factor which promotes IL-2 production (ciclosporin/tacrolimus)

2 Anti-proliferative agents - inhibit DNA synthesis, thus reduce lymphocyte proliferation (azathioprine/MMF)

3 Signalling blockade - acts downstream of IL-2R by inhibiting MTORC1. This inhibits protein synthesis and proliferation (sirolimus (rapamycin))

Figure 29.6 Mechanism of action of immunosuppressive agents. Agents either (1) Deplete lymphocytes (particularly T cells). (2, 3) Prevent T cell proliferation by blocking the production or action of IL-2 (the main cytokine driving T cell proliferation) or by preventing the synthesis of new DNA. (4) Inhibit T cell activation by antigen presenting cells.

Those who have been on dialysis for prolonged periods and have significant co-morbidities may develop complications which keep them in for longer.

Mr Bennet's wife has an uncomplicated donor nephrectomy and is discharged on day 4 post-operatively. Mr Bennet also does very well postoperatively and is discharged on day 7 with a creatinine of 110 μmol/L. His discharge medications include immunosuppressants, septrin for PCP prophylaxis,

valganciclovir as CMV prophylaxis, ranitidine 150 mg/bd as gastric protection and aspirin 75 mg.

Post-operatively, what immunosuppressants should Mr Bennet receive?

Immediately following transplantation, the patient is at high risk of developing acute rejection; hence this high-risk period is covered with relatively intense

Table 29.1 Side-effects of immunosuppressant agents used in transplantation

	SRL	CyA	Tac	MMF	Aza	Pred
Nephrotoxicity	−	++	++	−	−	−
Hypertension	−	+	+	−	−	+
Dyslipidaemia	+++	++	+	−	−	+
Diabetogenic	−	+	+++	−	−	++
Hyperuricaemia	−	+	+	−	−	−
Neurotoxicity	−	++	+	−	−	+
Anaemia	+	−	−	+	+	−
Leucopaenia	+	−	−	+	+	−
Thrombocytopaenia	+	−	−	+	+	−
Skin and gums	+	++	−	−	−	+
Osteoporosis	−	+	+	−	−	++
GI upset	+	−	−	+++	−	−

SRL, Sirolimus; CyA, ciclosporin A; Tac, tacrolimus; MMF, mycophenolate mofetil; Aza, azathioprine; Pred, prednisolone.

induction immunosuppression. This usually includes intravenous corticosteroids in combination with a biological agent (polyclonal or monoclonal antibodies). Some centres (particularly in North America) use a lymphocyte-depleting antibody such as anti-thymocyte globulin (ATG) or anti-lymphocyte globulin (ALG) or the monoclonal antibody alemtuzumab (CAMPATH-1H). In the UK, many centres use anti-CD25 monoclonal antibodies (daclizumab or basiliximab).

Following induction therapy the patient requires maintenance immunosupression (Figure 29.5). In contrast to induction agents, these are administered orally, and typically consist of triple therapy (a combination of prednisolone, a calcineurin inhibitor such as ciclosporin or tacrolimus, and an anti-proliferative agent such as azathioprine or mycophenolate mofetil). The mechanisms of action of these drugs are summarised in Figure 29.6.

> Mr Bennet is at low immunological risk and is given IV methyl prednisolone at induction together with an anti-CD25 antibody on days 0 and 3 postoperatively. He is also commenced on maintenance therapy in the form of prednisolone 20 mg po od, azathioprine 100 mg od and ciclosporin 250 mg po bd.

The patient asks whether there are any side-effects of the immunosuppressant tablets he is taking

Immunosuppressants must be sufficiently potent to inhibit the recipient's immune response to the allograft. Inevitably, this is associated with inhibition of the immune system's intended function – defence against infection and tumour surveillance. Immunosuppressant side-effects can be divided into generic, i.e. associated with any drug which inhibits the immune system, and specific, those associated with a particular immunosuppressant.

- Generic
  - Infection: particularly CMV, PCP, candida, BK nephropathy
  - Malignancy – post-transplant lymphoproliferative disorder (PTLD), skin malignancies (SCC>BCC), solid organ tumours
- Specific
  - Corticosteroids: glucose intolerance/diabetes mellitus, hypertension, weight gain, thinning of skin, poor wound healing, osteoporosis, gastric ulceration
  - Calcineurin inhibitors (ciclosporin/tacrolimus): nephrotoxic

○ Ciclosporin: gingival hypertrophy, hirsuitism, coarsening of facial features, hypertension, gout
○ Tacrolimus: diabetes mellitus
○ Azathioprine: cytopaenias
○ MMF: GI upset, particularly diarrhoea

○ Sirolimus: poor wound healing, rashes, mouth ulcers

Immunosuppressant side-effects are summarised in Table 29.1.

CASE REVIEW

This man presented to his GP with minimal symptoms but investigations showed near end-stage chronic kidney disease. This scenario is not unusual as unfortunately, patients with CKD can remain relatively asymptomatic and present with poor renal function and two small kidneys, the cause of which remains unclear. The patient was assessed for transplantation and received a living donor kidney transplant from his wife. He is discharged on a combination of immunosuppressants and prophylactic antimicrobials.

KEY POINTS

- In a patient with ESRF, there are a number of treatment options including conservative management, haemodialysis, peritoneal dialysis and renal transplantation.
- For younger patients or those with few co-morbidities, renal transplantation is the treatment of choice and offers significant benefits over dialysis in terms of survival and quality of life.
- Currently, the main barrier to transplantation is lack of organs and this issue has been addressed in a number of ways, including the use of non-heart beating donors or more marginal donors (i.e. older donors with known co-morbidities such as hypertension), and the use of living donors.
- In the case of living donor kidney transplantation, ABO incompatibility or the presence of donor-specific HLA antibodies were previously contraindications to living donation, but a number of centres now offer desensitisation programmes in which antibodies are removed by plasma exchange prior to transplantation.
- All patients must receive immunosuppression post transplantation to prevent rejection; this can be divided into induction and maintenance phases.
- Induction therapy is given at the time of transplantation and includes IV corticosteroids and a therapeutic antibody (either an anti-CD25 or a lymphocyte-depleting antibody).
- Maintenance involves triple or dual therapy with a combination of oral corticosteroids, a calcineurin inhibitor (ciclosporin or tacrolimus) and an anti-proliferative agent (azathioprine or mycophenolate mofetil).

Case 30 A 38-year-old man with a rise in creatinine 2 weeks post renal transplant

Mr Shane Parker, a 38-year-old man on haemodialysis, is admitted for a non-heart beating kidney transplant. He has ESRF secondary to IgA nephropathy and has been on dialysis for 18 months. He has no significant residual urine output and his last dialysis session was performed the day before admission. Blood tests performed on admission were satisfactory (in particular, K+ was within the normal range), and ECG and CXR were unchanged from previously. He therefore undergoes transplantation; the operation is uncomplicated and includes the insertion of a ureteric stent. He returns to the ward 4 hours later after a short period in recovery. The allograft is a 1 1 0 mismatch (see case 29, p. 195) and the donor is CMV seropositive and recipient CMV seronegative. Postoperatively his urine output is poor (30 mL/h).

How would you manage this man?

Oliguria immediately post transplant can be due to:
- Pre-renal causes:
  - renal artery thrombosis
  - renal vein thrombosis (leading to reduced perfusion)
  - hypotension secondary to hypovolaemia or acidosis
- Renal causes:
  - acute tubular necrosis (ATN)
  - hyperacute rejection (antibody-incompatible transplants)
- Post-renal causes:
  - ureteric obstruction (uncommon if ureteric stent used)
  - catheter obstruction

Appropriate measures include the following.
- Careful history and examination – Airway, Breathing, Circulation: tachycardia/hypotension may indicate hypovolaemia, haemorrhage or graft infarction. Excess

Nephrology: Clinical Cases Uncovered. By M. Clatworthy.
Published 2010 by Blackwell Publishing.

pain/swelling of graft? Renal artery and vein thrombosis lead to rapid infarction of the graft. If the graft is infarcted, patients can become very acidotic and unwell as tissue necrosis occurs. Transplants are very occasionally salvageable if thrombosis is immediately identified and patients are returned to theatre for thrombectomy. Both arterial and venous thrombosis are uncommon and usually lead to graft loss.
- Fluid resuscitation: Mr Parker should be given intravenous fluids until he is intravascularly volume replete. Most patients will have a central line inserted by the anaesthetist in theatre, so measurement of CVP should be possible to guide fluid replacement. Aim for a CVP of 8–10 cm H_2O. CVP is measured by connecting the patient's central venous catheter to an infusion set which is connected to a small-diameter water column. The CVP is usually measured from the midaxillary line. Normal measurement is between 5 and 10 cm H_2O.
- Urgent US scan to exclude obstruction/thrombosis. The US should also be able to identify significant haematomas.

It is important to note that transplant oliguria may not be obvious in renal transplant recipients who have a significant residual native urine output. In such cases, the patient may return from theatre passing good volumes of urine, all of which originate from their own kidneys. It is therefore important to ascertain the patient's pretransplant urine output.

Mr Parker is relatively comfortable and his pain is controlled with patient-controlled analgesia (PCA). Pulse is 89 bpm and BP120/70 mmHg. His abdomen is soft, and mildly tender over the graft, which does not seem obviously swollen. His CVP is 7 cm H_2O. A 500 mL bolus of normal saline is given. CVP post fluid increases to 10 cm H_2O. An urgent US scan shows an unobstructed transplant kidney with good arterial and venous waveforms, and reasonable perfusion throughout the parenchyma. He remains oliguric with a urine output of 20-30 mL/h.

Box 30.1 Warm and cold ischaemia time

- Warm ischaemic time: period between circulatory arrest and commencement of cold storage. For obvious reasons, this is longer in non-heart beating donors than in heart beating donors
- Cold ischaemic time: refers to the period of cold storage when the kidney is taken out of the donor, flushed with a preservation fluid (e.g. University of Wisconsin solution or Collins solution) and then placed on ice in a sterile container for transport. Alternatively kidneys may be placed on a machine and perfused with cold preservation solution until anastomosed to the recipient. If the cold ischaemic time (CIT) exceeds 20 hours, then graft outcome is worse than those with a CIT of <20 hours. Most transplant centres would not use a kidney with a CIT of >30 hours.

Box 30.2 Risk factors for delayed graft function

- Donor factors
  - Higher donor age
  - Hypertension
  - Acute renal impairment
  - Treatment with nephrotoxins
  - Prolonged donor hypotension
  - Marked catecholamine storm during brainstem coning
- Allograft factors
  - Prolonged warm ischaemic time
  - Prolonged cold ischaemic time
  - Prolonged anastomosis time
- Recipient factors

What is the most likely cause of his oliguria?

He is euvolaemic and has no obvious technical issues (arterial/venous thrombosis or obstruction) on US scan. Therefore, the most likely diagnosis is delayed graft function (DGF) secondary to ATN. He may need further haemodialysis post transplant whilst his allograft recovers. DGF is relatively common and occurs in around 30–50% of heart-beating donor kidneys and 50–70% of non-heart beating donor kidneys but is rare in living donor kidneys. Risk factors for DGF are prolonged warm or cold ischaemia times (Box 30.1), increasing donor age and co-morbidity. A full list of risk factors for DGF is shown in Box 30.2. Note, not all DGF is due to ATN and all other causes (as listed above) should be excluded first.

Acute tubular necrosis in transplant kidneys, as in native kidneys, is characterised by the presence of tatty-

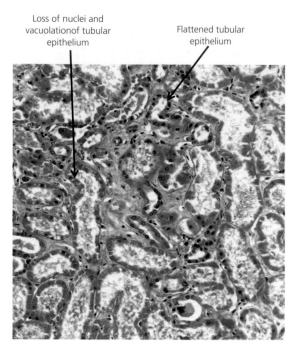

Figure 30.1 Renal transplant biopsy showing ATN.

looking tubular cells, many of which lack nuclei and begin to slough off into the tubular lumen (Figure 30.1). The recovery of ATN in transplant kidneys (as in native kidneys) is variable and may take days to weeks, or very occasionally a number of months. Diagnosis is confirmed by biopsy. The recovery of ATN is slowed by the presence of nephrotoxins, principally calcineurin inhibitors (CNI) in the case of transplant kidneys (e.g. ciclosporin or tacrolimus). Therefore, patients are often run on half-doses of CNI whilst they have ATN.

Mr Parker recovers well from his operation. He receives induction therapy with an intravenous anti-CD25 antibody (see case 30) and intravenous methyl prednisolone. This is followed by oral tacrolimus (half-dose due to presumed ATN), mycophenolate mofetil and prednisolone. He needs one dialysis session on day 2 post-operatively for hyperkalaemia, but by day 3 is sitting out in his chair and is eating and drinking. On day 5 his urine output is a little improved (500 mL/24 h) but the urea and potassium necessitate a further session of dialysis.

What investigation does Mr Parker need next?

If there is no significant improvement in Mr Parker's transplant function over the next 24–48 hours then he should undergo a US-guided renal transplant biopsy.

This is technically easier than a native renal biopsy because the transplant lies much closer to the surface, and is performed with the patient in the supine position (Figure 30.2). A renal transplant biopsy is usually performed if there is DGF for greater than 6 days and is required to confirm ATN as the cause of persistent DGF and to exclude acute rejection. ATN is a risk factor for the development of acute cellular rejection, so biopsies may show both pathologies.

On day 6 post-operatively, Mr Parker's urine output significantly increases to 1500 mL and the creatinine plateaus. On day 7, his creatinine falls by 50 μmol/L so the decision is made to hold off a biopsy. On day 8 his creatinine falls by a further 100 μmol/L to 478 μmol/L. He is therefore discharged with a plan to follow him up in clinic in 2 days. Discharge medications are shown below.

Prednisolone 20 mg od
Mycophenolate mofetil 500 mg bd
Tacrolimus 5 mg bd
Valganciclovir (CMV prophylaxis, dose to be adjusted according to GFR as renally cleared)
Ranitidine 150 mg bd (gastric protection whilst on steroids)
Aspirin 75 mg
Co-trimoxazole 480 mg Mon, Weds, Fri
Amphotericin lozenges 10 mg qds

At the next clinic visit he is well, with a creatinine of 230 μmol/L. He is seen every 2–3 days in clinic and

continues to make progress with a best baseline creatinine of 137 μmol/L.

On day 16 post transplant, clinic blood tests show a creatinine of 242 μmol/L. He feels completely well and is passing good volumes of urine. BP is 136/85 mmHg.

What is the most likely cause of his rise in creatinine?

The differential diagnosis is:
- Calcineurin inhibitor toxicity: high tacrolimus levels are nephrotoxic and can cause a decline in renal function. Typical changes are identifiable on biopsy.
- Immunological issues: in the first 3 weeks post transplant the patient is at high risk of acute rejection, particularly acute cellular rejection.
- Technical issues ('plumbing trouble'):
    - renal artery and renal vein thrombosis tend to present much earlier than this and result in complete loss of transplant function (as described above), so this is unlikely in this case
    - obstruction secondary to ureteric stenosis is unusual at this stage given that ureteric stents are placed in many transplant centres and remain *in situ* until 4–8 weeks post-operatively, thus preventing ureteric obstruction.
- Recurrent disease: reports on the frequency of recurrent IgA nephropathy in transplantation vary, but it is thought to be around 30%.

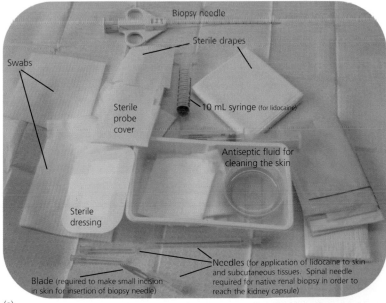

Figure 30.2 (a) Equipment needed for a renal biopsy.

(a)

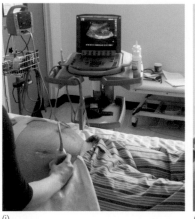

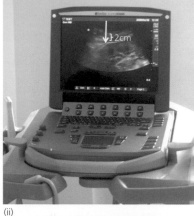

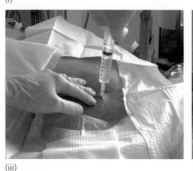

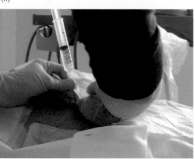

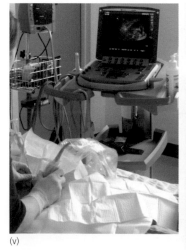

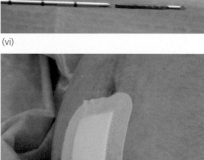

(b)

Figure 30.2 (b) Performing a renal transplant biopsy. (i) The patient is placed supine and the renal transplant localised by ultrasound (in the right iliac fossa in this case). (ii) The operator visualises the kidney in two planes and marks the skin at a point directly above the upper pole of the kidney (*arrow*). They are also able to determine the distance between the skin and the kidney capsule (2 cm in this case.) (iii–iv) Lidocaine is placed into the skin and subcutaneous tissues to anaesthetise the area. (v) Biopsy needle in inserted onto the capsule of the kidney under US guidance. (vi) A good core of renal tissue is obtained. (vii) A dressing is placed over the biopsy site.

• BK nephropathy: BK virus is a member of the Polyomaviridae family (other members of this family include JC virus, which causes progressive multifocal leucoencephalopathy, and simian virus (SV) 40). It is a double-stranded DNA virus and infection is almost universal in adults. Following transplantation, the virus can reactivate in urothelium, causing a florid interstitial nephritis. Urine shows decoy cells and the renal biopsy can be

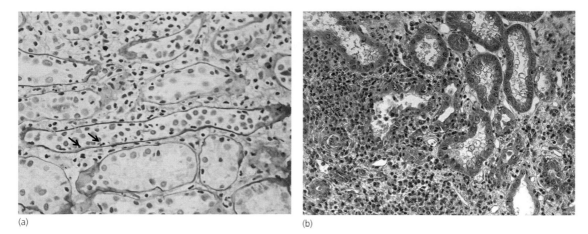

(a)   (b)

Figure 30.3 Renal transplant biopsy showing acute cellular rejection with tubulitis. (a) Tubular walls are infiltrated with mononuclear cells. These have much darker nuclei (*black arrows*) than tubular cells (*green arrow*). More than four mononuclear cells per tubule is considered significant. (b) Marked mononuclear cell infiltrate present within the interstitium.

stained with an antibody to the SV40 antigen, which picks up one of the viral antigens common to this family of viruses. BK can be detected in the blood by PCR in some cases. The treatment is to reduce immunosuppression. Other treatments suggested include ciprofloxacin, cidofovir and leflunamide, although there is no good trial evidence for any of them.

At 2 weeks post transplant, in a patient with a ureteric stent *in situ*, rejection and CNI toxicity are the main concerns. BK nephropathy can occur this early, but it would be less likely.

What investigations would you perform?

- Repeat U+E to verify the rise in creatinine
- Urine dipstick: if nitrites and leucocyte positive, then suggestive of a UTI.
- MSU: if any suggestion of UTI.
- Ultrasound transplant kidney to exclude obstruction and confirm normal perfusion.
- Tacrolimus levels.

If all the above are normal, then this patient needs an urgent transplant renal biopsy to exclude rejection.

Mr Parker's urine dipstick shows a trace protein and blood 1+ but is otherwise negative. Ultrasound shows a morphologically normal kidney with no hydronephrosis and good perfusion throughout. Tacrolimus level is within the target range (10 ng/mL). He proceeds to a renal transplant biopsy (Figure 30.3a).

What does this show?

This shows acute cellular rejection with normal glomeruli, a lymphocytic interstitial infiltrate and tubulitis. Acute cellular rejection is graded according to the Banff criteria, grade Ia being the least severe and grade III the most severe.

Following transplantation, organ rejection is still a significant concern. There are four types of rejection recognised, summarised in Table 30.1.

How would you treat him?

The treatment for acute cellular rejection (as in this case) is intravenous methyl prednisolone. Most centres would give 3×1 g boluses on consecutive days; 80–90% of episodes of acute cellular rejection will respond to corticosteroids. If the patient's creatinine does not fall in response to corticosteroids then further treatment with a lymphocyte-depleting agent such as ATG is undertaken.

The patient is treated with 3 g of methyl prednisolone and his creatinine falls to 160 μmol/L by day 4 post commencement of IV steroids. He is followed up twice a week for the next 2 weeks and weekly thereafter and does not have any further problems. The ureteric stent is removed at 6 weeks without difficulty and he settles to a baseline creatinine of 130 μmol/L.

The patient asks whether this episode of rejection will have an adverse effect on his graft in the longer term.

Table 30.1 Types of transplant rejection

	Hyperacute	Acute cellular	Acute humoral (antibody-mediated)	'Chronic'*
Timing	Immediate	Weeks 1–12	Weeks 1–12	Month 1 onwards
Immune mediators	Preformed antibody, complement	T cells	Antibody	Immune + non-immune mechanisms
Standard treatment	None (graft nephrectomy)	IV methyl prednisolone, ATG (if unresponsive to steroids)	Plasma exchange, increase in maintenance immunosuppression	Control BP, minimise exposure to CNIs
Other treatments	—	Alemtuzumab (if steroid resistant)	IV immunoglobulin, rituximab (anti-CD20), ATG, eculizumab (anti-C5)	Rituximab (for chronic AMR)

*Chronic rejection no longer exists as an entity. The latest Banff classification (2007) distinguishes chronic antibody-mediated rejection and 'tubular atrophy and interstitial fibrosis'.

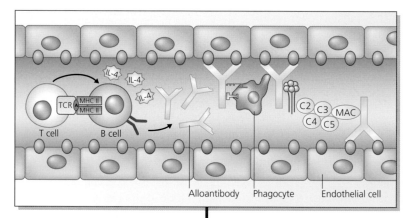

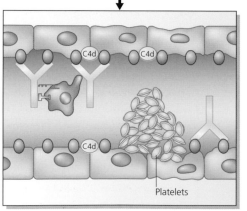

(a)

Figure 30.4 (a) Acute antibody-mediated rejection. Upper panel: alloreactive B and T cells interact. CD4 T cells provide help to B cells (e.g. through production of IL-4, the principle cytokine required to drive B cell activation). These B cells produce alloantibody which binds to antigens on the surface of graft endothelial cells. Deposited antibody activates complement and phagocytes. Lower panel: complement and phagocytes mediate endothelial cell damage, which in turn promotes platelet activation and thrombus formation within the graft. Complement activation is evidenced by the presence of C4d on endothelial cells (particularly those of peritubular capillaries).

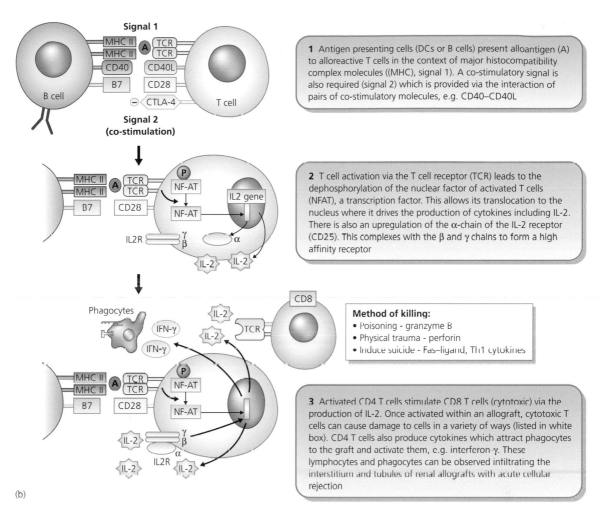

1 Antigen presenting cells (DCs or B cells) present alloantigen (A) to alloreactive T cells in the context of major histocompatibility complex molecules ((MHC), signal 1). A co-stimulatory signal is also required (signal 2) which is provided via the interaction of pairs of co-stimulatory molecules, e.g. CD40–CD40L

2 T cell activation via the T cell receptor (TCR) leads to the dephosphorylation of the nuclear factor of activated T cells (NFAT), a transcription factor. This allows its translocation to the nucleus where it drives the production of cytokines including IL-2. There is also an upregulation of the α-chain of the IL-2 receptor (CD25). This complexes with the β and γ chains to form a high affinity receptor

Method of killing:
- Poisoning - granzyme B
- Physical trauma - perforin
- Induce suicide - Fas–ligand, Th1 cytokines

3 Activated CD4 T cells stimulate CD8 T cells (cytotoxic) via the production of IL-2. Once activated within an allograft, cytotoxic T cells can cause damage to cells in a variety of ways (listed in white box). CD4 T cells also produce cytokines which attract phagocytes to the graft and activate them, e.g. interferon-γ. These lymphocytes and phagocytes can be observed infiltrating the interstitium and tubules of renal allografts with acute cellular rejection

(b)

Figure 30.4 (b) Acute cellular rejection.

What do you tell him?

Evidence suggests that provided an episode of acute cellular rejection is promptly treated and responds fully to such treatment then there are no long-term adverse effects on allograft function. However, recurrent episodes of acute cellular rejection are associated with worse allograft outcomes, as are episodes of acute humoral rejection.

What are the immunological mechanisms underlying transplant rejection?

The immunological mechanisms in the different types of transplant rejection are summarised in Figure 30.4. Hyperacute rejection occurs almost immediately post transplant (within minutes to hours) in recipients who have preformed donor-specific antibodies (typically ABO or HLA). It results in graft thrombosis and infarction.

The most common type of rejection in the current transplant era is acute cellular rejection. This occurs when there is presentation of donor antigen to recipient CD4 T cells by antigen-presenting cells (dendritic cells, B cells and macrophages), which may be donor or recipient derived. In transplantation direct and indirect antigen presentation are distinguished (see Box 30.3). Activated CD4 T cells can then provide help to CD8 (cytotoxic) T cells, phagocytes and B cells, leading to graft infiltration with these cells and the characteristic biopsy changes of acute rejection (Figure 30.4b).

Box 30.3 Antigen presentation in transplantation

- Direct antigen presentation: donor antigen presented in the context of donor MHC molecule (5–10% of recipient's T cell repertoire may recognise foreign MHC, therefore this is very important in transplant rejection).
- Indirect antigen presentation: donor antigen presented in the context of recipient MHC.

Acute antibody-mediated (humoral) rejection occurs when allograft-specific antibodies develop. These will bind to endothelium and activate complement via the classic pathway, thus leading to C4d deposition (a marker of humoral rejection on transplant biopsies). Deposited antibody will also activate phagocytes with Fc receptors, including neutrophils. Other changes seen include neutrophil infiltration into glomeruli (>5/glomerulus) and endothelialitis (Figure 30.4a).

Previously, the term 'chronic rejection' was used to describe gradual attrition of graft function over months to years. However, in the most recent Banff classification of rejection, this term was abandoned in order to distinguish chronic antibody-mediated rejection (as evidenced by vascular changes and persistent C4d staining on biopsy) from interstitial fibrosis and tubular atrophy (which can be caused by a number of factors, including chronic hypertension and CNI toxicity).

Table 30.2 Post-transplant complications

	Early	Intermediate	Late
Technical	Renal vein thrombosis Renal artery thrombosis Lymphocoele Haematoma Urinary leak	Renal artery stenosis Ureteric stenosis	–
Immunological	Acute cellular rejection Acute humoral rejection	Chronic rejection	Chronic rejection

Immunosuppression associated	Specific
	Generic
	  – Infection
		Specific
		Generic
		  – Infection
		  – Malignancy
			Specific
			Generic
			  – Infection
			  – Malignancy

Cardiovascular		Atherosclerosis	Atherosclerosis

CASE REVIEW

A 38-year-old man with ESRF secondary to IgA nephropathy, on maintenance haemodialysis, receives a non-heart beating cadaveric renal transplant. The graft does not function immediately. A US scan shows normal perfusion and no hydronephrosis. At day 6 his urine output significantly increases and his creatinine continues to fall over the next week. He returns to clinic at day 16 post transplant, well, but with a rise in creatinine. A US scan of the transplant is normal and his tacrolimus levels are within the desired range. He therefore undergoes a renal transplant biopsy. This shows acute cellular rejection. He is treated with three pulses of intravenous methylprednisolone, and responds well to this.

KEY POINTS

- Renal transplantation is a moderate-sized operation, which takes around 3–4 hours.
- The patient's post-transplant urine output must be interpreted in the light of their native urine output.
- If the patient is oliguric immediately post transplant, then vascular issues must be urgently excluded with a US scan. If this does not show any evidence of arterial or venous thrombosis or obstruction then the most likely cause is ATN. The patient should be adequately hydrated with intravenous fluids and may require renal support (haemodialysis/filtration).
- Post-transplant ATN is more common in non-heart beating donor kidneys than in heart-beating donor kidneys and is rare in living donor kidneys. It is exacerbated by CNI toxicity.
- A rise in creatinine in the first few weeks post transplant should be considered to be acute rejection until proven

otherwise. Other diagnoses should be sought and excluded, including UTI, CNI toxicity and obstruction.
- Acute rejection is diagnosed by biopsying the transplant kidney. Treatment is with intravenous corticosteroids, which is effective in 80–90% of cases. If this does not result in an improvement in allograft function, then patients should be treated with a lymphocyte-depleting agent, such as ATG.
- Overall, acute cellular rejection has a good prognosis, with many patients returning to their baseline creatinine. More severe cellular rejection or acute humoral rejection has a worse prognosis and recurrent episodes may limit overall allograft survival.
- A summary of post-transplant complications is shown in Table 30.2.

Case 31 A 45-year-old man with a renal transplant and fever

Mr Gavin Edwards is a 45-year-old man who has end-stage kidney disease secondary to ADPKD. He had a renal transplant 8 months ago which has been functioning well (last creatinine in clinic 125 μmol/L). He has attended his GP complaining of fevers and night sweats and has been referred to the transplant clinic for further assessment.

What are the most common causes of fever in a transplant recipient?

The most likely cause of fever in a transplant recipient is infection. Transplant recipients must take maintenance immunosuppression in order to prevent allograft rejection, so they are at increased risk of a number of infections (detailed in Box 31.1). Post-transplant immunosuppression (usually a calcineurin inhibitor, steroids and an antiproliferative) has significant effects on T lymphocytes, so many of the opportunistic infections seen are similar to those observed in patients with HIV, particularly cytomegalovirus (CMV) and *Pneumocystis jiroveci* (previously *P. carinii*).

Malignancy (particularly lymphoma) can also present with fever. Immunosuppression increases the risk of malignancy, particularly malignancies which are driven by oncoviruses. These include skin malignancies (human papilloma virus (HPV)), lymphoma (Epstein–Barr virus (EBV)) and Kaposi's sarcoma (human herpes virus (HHV)-8). Overall, the frequency of malignancy is at least three times higher in transplant recipients compared with the normal population (detailed in Box 31.2). Skin malignancies are 50–100 times more common (depending on sun exposure). Solid organ malignancies are also increased. In renal transplant recipients, susceptibility to cancer is also dependent on age (more common in older individuals). Roughly speaking, a transplant recipient's risk of developing a malignancy is similar to a 'normal' individual 20–30 years older than them.

Occasionally, patients with severe rejection can have a fever, but this is usually associated with graft pain and tenderness.

What additional questions would you ask the patient?

The assessment should be aimed at identifying the cause of the fever, which is most probably infection but could be malignancy. CMV infection and UTI are the most frequently encountered infections, therefore reasonable questions include the following.

• Duration of fevers and any additional symptoms.
• Symptoms consistent with CMV include malaise, lethargy, GI upset (abdominal pain, diarrhoea secondary to colitis), respiratory symptoms (CMV pneumonitis).
• Urinary symptoms (dysuria, frequency, cloudy/offensive urine); check that the vesicoureteric stent has definitely been removed.
• Pulmonary symptoms suggestive of lower respiratory tract infection (cough, sputum, shortness of breath, haemoptysis). Patients with PCP will frequently complain of severe dyspnoea on minimal exertion.
• Symptoms suggestive of a more unusual site of infection, e.g. bone, sinuses.
• Symptoms suggestive of lymphoma (weight loss, night sweats, appearance of enlarged lymph nodes).
• Travel history which may indicate a more unusual cause of infection, e.g. malaria.

It is also useful to determine Mr Edwards' and the donor's CMV serostatus. Patients are usually described as CMV positive if a CMV-specific IgG is detectable in blood. This indicates that they have previously been infected. Following infection, there is initially a rise in IgM followed by a rise in IgG, which remains detectable in the long term. If a CMV-seronegative recipient (R-) receives a transplant from a CMV-seropositive donor (D+) then they may get primary infection whilst immunosuppressed. In patients with evidence of previous exposure to CMV (R+), the virus can reactivate post

Nephrology: Clinical Cases Uncovered. By M. Clatworthy.
Published 2010 by Blackwell Publishing.

Box 31.1 Infections post-transplantation

- Viral
  - CMV
  - BK virus
- Bacterial
  - Including wound (early), chest infection (early), UTI, sinusitis, dental abscess, endocarditis
  - Mycobacterial infection. Individuals at risk of reactivation or primary infection should be placed on prophylaxis
- Fungal
  - *Pneumocystis Jiroveci* Pneumonia
  - *Candida albicans* (including oesophagitis)
- Protozoal
  - *Toxoplasma gondii*

Box 31.2 Malignancy post-transplantation

- Oncovirus associated
  - Post-transplant lymphoproliferative disorder (PTLD) – due to EBV
  - Kaposi's sarcoma – associated with HHV-8
  - Skin malignancies (non-melanotic, SCC > BCC) – associated with HPV
- Non-oncovirus associated
  - Renal – 5× increase in risk
  - Breast – 3× increase in risk in women <35years
  - Colon – 2.5× increase in risk

Table 31.1 Donor and recipient CMV serostatus and infection

Donor serostatus	Recipient serostatus	Incidence of CMV viraemia in the absence of prophylaxis
+	−	75%
+	+	55%
−	+	25%
−	−	<1%

transplant or they may become reinfected with a different strain if the donor is seropositive (Table 31.1). Infection or reactivation can be symptomatic or asymptomatic (in the latter case, the virus is detected by screening the recipients blood for viral DNA or antigens).

Mr Edwards' medications should be noted, in particular the dose and type of immunosuppressive agents (induction, maintenance and any requirement for intensification of immunosuppression due to rejection).

Lymphocyte-depleting induction agents such as ATG are associated with an increased risk of CMV infection. Some patients may also have received heavy immunosuppression for their primary renal disease (e.g. vasculitis or SLE). Overall, the heavier the immunosuppression, the more likely that CMV will develop.

Mr Edwards tells you that he has been unwell for around 3 weeks. He has felt increasingly tired and lethargic. In the past week he has also been getting fever, mainly occurring at night time associated with sweats. He is off his food and has lost around half a stone in weight. He is not coughing up any sputum, nor has he had any urinary or GI symptoms. Reviewing his records, you see that he was CMV seronegative and his donor was CMV seropositive. He received valganciclovir prophylaxis for the first 3 months post transplant, but has not been taking it since. Mr Edwards received an anti-CD25 antibody (non-lymphocyte depleting) at induction followed by prednisolone, mycophenolate mofetil 500mg bd and ciclosporin 200mg bd. He has not had any rejection episodes requiring treatment.

What features are important to seek during clinical examination?

Signs consistent with infection or malignancy should be sought, including the following.

- Lymphadenopathy (full and careful search, including in axillae and groin).
- Anaemia (conjunctival pallor).
- Generic signs of infection (fever, tachycardia, hypotension).
- Organ/system-specific signs of infection.
  - Area of cellulites.
  - Enlarged/erythematous joint.
  - Sinus tenderness.
  - Poor dentition/tooth abscess.
  - CVS: splinter haemorrhages, Osler's nodes, Janeway lesions, Roth spots, new murmur.
  - Chest: raised RR, crepitations, bronchial breathing. Patients with PCP will significantly desaturate following exercise (a useful test is to measure O_2 saturations, then get them to walk up and down the ward briskly, then measure again).
  - Abdomen: hepatosplenomegaly, bladder tenderness, masses.

Mr Edwards looks washed out, but not acutely unwell. Temperature is 38.2°C with reduced skin turgor. His pulse is 92bpm and regular. Blood pressure is 120/75mmHg, JVP is not visible, and cardiovascular examination is otherwise normal. O₂ saturations are 98% on air. Chest is clear with no signs of pneumonia. His abdomen is soft and the allograft is non-tender. There is no hepatomegaly but the spleen is just palpable. He has a 1 × 1 cm lymph node palpable in the left inguinal region but no other lymphadenopathy.

What investigations would you request?

- Blood tests
  - Full blood count
  - U + E
  - LFT
  - Albumin
  - Glucose
  - Inflammatory markers (CRP/ESR)
  - Blood cultures
  - CMV PCR
  - EBV serology
- Urine tests
  - Dipstick
  - Urine for M, C + S
- ECG
- CXR: to assess for any evidence of infection or hilar lymphadenopathy. Patients with PCP have few CXR changes early on in spite of significant hypoxia

The investigations show:

Hb 11.1 g/dL, WBC 6.2 × 10⁹/L, Platelets 147 × 10⁹/L
Clotting: normal
U + E: Na 145 mmol/L, K 4.4 mmol/L, Urea 10.3 mmol/L,
 Creatinine 140 μmol/L
ESR 48 mm/h, CRP 146 mg/L, LFT and calcium: normal
Albumin 28 g/L
Ciclosporin level 230 mg/mL
Urine dipstick: 1+ protein. Negative for nitrites, blood,
 leucocytes and glucose
Urine microscopy: no bacteria on gram stain. <100 cells/mm³
ECG normal
CXR demonstrates a normal cardiac size and clear lung fields
Blood and urine cultures, CMV PCR and viral serology
 awaited

How would you interpret these results?

The investigations show mild anaemia and borderline low platelets. This may be due to marrow suppression secondary to anti-rejection agents (usually azathioprine and MMF) but can occur in CMV infection.

Mr Edwards' transplant function is slightly worse than usual (creatinine normally 125, now 140 μmol/L) but this is not severe enough to indicate a primary transplant problem such as UTI or rejection. It is more likely that there is mild dehydration and that this will improve with fluid replacement.

Inflammatory markers, particularly CRP, are elevated, making an infection likely. Urine studies and CXR do not point towards focal infection in the lungs or urinary tract.

The most likely diagnosis given the presentation and the results of the investigations is CMV infection.

What general treatment measures should you begin?

- He is clinically dehydrated and should therefore be given fluid resuscitation, probably intravenously.
- Fevers can be symptomatically managed with an antipyretic, e.g. paracetamol.

Mr Edwards' microbiology results are returned to you. They show negative blood and urine cultures, but a blood CMV PCR demonstrates 115,000 viral copies/mL.

What treatment would you begin?

Cytomegalovirus should be treated as follows.

- Reduction in immunosupression: the development of a CMV infection suggests that the patient is relatively overimmunosuppressed. Therefore his maintenance immunosuppression should be reduced. Usually the target trough level of CNI is reduced and the antiproliferative agent (azathioprine and MMF) reduced or stopped.
- Specific treatment for CMV: intravenous ganciclovir is the treatment of choice. In some patients with low viral titres or with reactivation rather than primary disease, high-dose oral valganciclovir can be used. Valganciclovir is a pro-drug which is converted in the liver to ganciclovir. Ganciclovir must be phosphorylated in order to generate its active metabolite ganciclovir triphosphate. Phosphorylation is dependent in part on a CMV-synthesised enzyme UL97 phosphotransferase (Figure 31.1). Thus the virus may become resistant to ganciclovir if it mutates to produce a non-functional enzyme.
- Other options for patients with refractory or resistant disease include foscarnet, cidofovir and intravenous CMV immune globulin.

Mr Edwards is started on intravenous ganciclovir. It is likely that this treatment will be required for a number of weeks, so a tunnelled central line is inserted. His mycophenolate mofetil is stopped for the duration of his ganciclovir treatment.

What are the side-effects associated with this intravenous ganciclovir?

Ganciclovir is associated with marrow suppression (therefore watch for pancytopaenia) and renal impairment. Administration over a number of weeks involves the use of a central line or long line. This has associated morbidity, including line infections.

The patient asks whether the CMV infection will have any long-term detrimental effects on his transplant function.

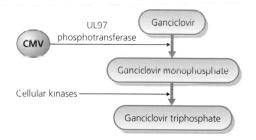

Figure 31.1 Ganciclovir must be phosphorylated in order to convert it into its active form. This is achieved by a CMV-synthesised enzyme UL97 phosphotransferase followed by the patient's own cellular kinases.

What would you tell him?

Cytomegalovirus infection can be associated with an acute decline in allograft function, even in the absence of rejection. In such cases, the virus may be detectable on transplant biopsy, with typical 'owl eye' inclusion bodies within the nuclei of infected cells. CMV-specific antibodies can also be used in immunohistochemical staining of biopsy material (Figure 31.2).

Studies suggest that CMV infection (either symptomatic or asymptomatic) can have an adverse effect on both patient and allograft survival. CMV infection has been associated with an increase in:

• acute rejection
• chronic allograft nephropathy (CMV infection induces fibrosis and vascular thickening in animal models of transplantation). Such chronic changes together with an increase in acute rejection reduce overall long-term allograft survival
• cardiovascular complications, thus reducing patient survival
• post transplant diabetes mellitus.

The patient responds well to ganciclovir treatment. He is feeling much improved, is now afebrile, his appetite has improved and his night sweats have vanished. Three weeks later the virus is no longer detectable in his blood. He is placed back on prophylaxis with valganciclovir for a further 3 months.

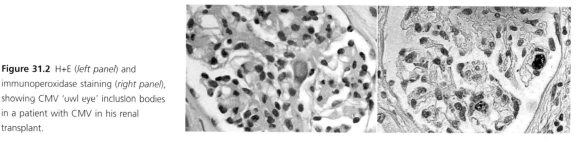

Figure 31.2 H+E (*left panel*) and immunoperoxidase staining (*right panel*), showing CMV 'owl eye' inclusion bodies in a patient with CMV in his renal transplant.

CASE REVIEW

A 45-year-old man presents with fevers and night sweats 8 months post renal transplant. Examination does not reveal any lymphadenopathy or focal signs of infection. Investigations demonstrate a CMV titre of around 115,000 copies/mL of blood. His immunosuppression is reduced and he is treated with intravenous ganciclovir, followed by 3 months of oral valganciclovir prophylaxis.

KEY POINTS

- Fever post-transplant usually occurs secondary to infection. Other possibilities include malignancy (particularly PTLD) and severe acute rejection.
- Cytomegalovirus is a γ herpes virus and is one of the most common infections encountered post transplant. The likelihood of infection post transplant is dependent on whether the recipient has had previous CMV infection and therefore has immunological memory for the virus. Immune memory is detected by looking for the presence of CMV-specific antibody (IgG).
- Around 50% of adults in the UK are CMV immune. In those transplant recipients who are CMV antibody negative (seronegative) who receive an allograft from a CMV-seropositive donor, 60% will develop a symptomatic CMV infection post transplant in the absence of prophylaxis. Thus, most transplant centres would give CMV prophylaxis to this high-risk group of recipients in the form of oral valganciclovir.
- Cytomegalovirus infection can be relatively asymptomatic and be picked up only by routine screening by blood PCR. Symptoms associated with CMV include fever, sweats, lethargy and weight loss. CMV can affect the gut (CMV colitis), the eyes (CMV retinitis, 'brush fire'), the lungs (CMV pneumonitis) and the allograft. It is diagnosed by the detection of viraemia (by quantitative PCR on blood samples or by detecting CMV pp65 antigen in the blood) or by the identification of classic inclusion bodies on biopsy or bronchoalveolar lavage.
- Cytomegalovirus infection can be associated with an acute decline in allograft function, even in the absence of rejection. In such cases, the virus may be detectable on transplant biopsy, with typical 'owl eye' inclusion bodies within the nuclei of infected cells. CMV-specific antibodies can also be used in immunohistochemical staining of biopsy material (see Figure 31.2).
- Other infections classically encountered post transplantation include urinary tract infections and *Pneumocystis jiroveci*.
- An important differential in a transplant patient with fever is PTLD. PTLD is rare in the first year post transplant (0.1% of transplants) but can occur. It is driven by Epstein–Barr virus (oncogenic) and is more likely if patients have received lymphocyte-depleting agents, such as ATG, at induction.

MCQs

For each situation, choose the options you feel are most correct.

1 *In a patient with acute renal failure (acute kidney injury), which of the following is an indication for urgent dialysis?*

a. Pericardial rub
b. Anuria
c. Peripheral oedema
d. Urea >50 mmol/L
e. K⁺ 6.4 mmol/L
f. Creatinine >900 µmol/L

2 *A patient with acute renal failure has a K⁺ of 7.0 mmol/L and ECG changes. Which of the following is the most appropriate immediate management step?*

a. 10 u insulin in 50 mL 50% dextrose intravenously
b. 10 mL 10% calcium gluconate intravenously
c. 40 mg intravenous furosemide
d. 1 mg intravenous adrenaline (epinephrine)
e. Oral calcium resonium

3 *Which of the following features suggest that renal failure is acute rather than chronic?*

a. A normal renal function 1 month previously
b. Anaemia
c. Hypocalcaemia
d. Normal-sized kidneys on US examination
e. Acute-onset anuria
f. Vomiting

4 *Which of the following investigations should be performed routinely in patients with ARF?*

a. Urine dipstick
b. Urine microscopy
c. Urine electrolytes
d. US renal tract
e. CT abdomen
f. PTH

5 *Which of the following are useful in managing fluid balance in a patient with ARF?*

a. Daily weights
b. Input-output charts
c. Daily urea levels
d. Urinary Na losses
e. Repeated clinical examination

6 *Which fluid regimen is most appropriate in a patient with ARF secondary to ATN, who is currently euvolaemic?*

a. Free fluids orally
b. Match intake to output
c. Provide a total (oral + IV) of 3 litres in 24 hours
d. Match intake to output +500 mL
e. 500 mL fluid challenges until his urine output improves

7 *In a patient with ARF and red cells casts in the urine, which of the following diagnoses should be considered?*

a. Acute tubular necrosis
b. Acute glomerulonephritis
c. Obstruction
d. Rhabdomyolysis
e. Acute interstitial nephritis

Nephrology: Clinical Cases Uncovered. By M. Clatworthy.
Published 2010 by Blackwell Publishing.

PART 3: SELF-ASSESSMENT

8 *With regard to SLE, which of the following statements are correct?*

a. It is usually a monogenic disorder characterised by ANA and immune complex deposition.
b. Lupus pernio is one of the typical dermatological manifestations.
c. Ninety-five percent of patients are ANA positive and 40% are anti-Sm antibody positive.
d. C3 levels are usually lower than C4 levels.
e. Renal biopsy typically shows 'full-house' immunostaining.

9 *Which of the following can present with a pulmonary-renal syndrome?*

a. Membranous GN
b. FSGS
c. Goodpasture's disease
d. ANCA-associated vasculitis
e. Minimal change GN
f. Rhabdomyolysis
g. SLE

10 *With regard to anti-GBM disease, which of the following are true?*

a. Patients may present with nephrotic syndrome.
b. Pulmonary haemorrhage is rare in non-smokers.
c. Fluid overload may precipitate pulmonary haemorrhage.
d. Antibodies specifically recognise the a3 chain of type I collagen.
e. Renal failure is usually reversible.
f. Treatment includes plasma exchange.

11 *With regard to AAV, which of the following are true?*

a. Clinical features may be non-specific and variable, leading to delayed diagnosis.
b. Patients who are pANCA positive will usually have proteinase-3 specific autoantibodies.
c. Patients with pulmonary haemorrhage should not receive plasma exchange.
d. Untreated, it has a 1-year mortality rate of 80–90%.
e. Once remission is achieved, relapse is uncommon, occurring in less than 10% of patients.

12 *With regard to IgA nephropathy, which of the following are true?*

a. It is the most common primary GN in adults.
b. It is rarely associated with elevated systemic IgA levels.
c. It never presents as nephrotic syndrome.
d. Approximately 20% of patients present with ARF.
e. Flares can be precipitated by heavy exercise.
f. It can be associated with Crohn's disease.

13 *With regard to a renal biopsy, which of the following is true?*

a. It should not be performed if platelet count is 100×10^9/L.
b. There is a 1 in 100 risk of microscopic haematuria post biopsy.
c. There is no risk of losing the kidney post biopsy.
d. There is a 1 in 200 risk of requiring a blood transfusion post biopsy.
e. Blood pressure has no effect on the risk of bleeding post biopsy.

14 *Which of the following are true in relation to an adult with nephrotic syndrome?*

a. A renal biopsy is mandatory.
b. Their protein intake should be restricted.
c. A low-potassium diet would be useful.
d. Diuretics will not be effective in managing oedema.
e. The most likely underlying diagnosis is minimal change GN.
f. The patient should be referred to a nephrologist.

15 *Which of the following glomerulonephritides commonly present with nephrotic syndrome?*

a. Minimal change GN
b. IgA nephropathy
c. Lupus nephritis
d. Membranous GN
e. Post-streptococcal GN
f. FSGS

16 *With regard to membranous GN, which of the following are true?*

a. Two-thirds of cases have secondary causes.
b. It is the most common cause of nephrotic syndrome in adults.
c. Fifty percent go into complete remission spontaneously.
d. Ten percent develop progressive renal impairment.
e. It can be associated with NSAID use,
f. It is the most common biopsy finding in patients with lupus nephritis.

17 *A patient with nephrotic syndrome secondary to FSGS is readmitted 6 days post biopsy complaining of loin pain and haematuria. What is the most likely diagnosis?*

a. Pyelonephritis
b. Renal vein thrombosis
c. Perinephric haematoma
d. Renal stone
e. Cyst rupture

18 *With regard to FSGS, which of the following are true?*

a. It commonly presents as nephritic syndrome.
b. It can be associated with obesity and HIV infection.
c. Primary FSGS has a benign prognosis with <5% of patients progressing to ESRF.
d. It does not recur in renal transplants.
e. There are familial forms, caused by mutations in nephrin and podocin.

19 *With regard to minimal change GN, which of the following is true?*

a. It is the least common cause of nephrotic syndrome in children.
b. Around 90% of children with minimal change GN are responsive to corticosteroids.
c. Children never require a renal biopsy to confirm the diagnosis.
d. It is not associated with an increased risk of thromboembolism.
e. Around 20% of children will relapse after an initial response to steroids.

20 *Which of the following are cause of a metabolic acidosis with a high anion gap?*

a. Renal tubular acidosis
b. Diabetic ketoacidosis
c. Respiratory failure
d. Myocardial infarction
e. Salicylate overdose
f. Diarrhoea

21 *An 18-year-old girl is admitted with a suspected salicylate overdose. Her bloods are as follows:*
Na+ 136 mmol/L, K+ 5.0 mmol/L, Urea 10.3 mmol/L, Creatinine 118 µmol/L, Cl⁻ 102 mmol/L
ABG: pH 7.10 (7.35–7.45), pO2 19.6 kPa (8–12), pCO2 3.6 kPa (4–6), HCO₃⁻ 12 mmol/L (22–28)
What is the anion gap?

a. 10
b. 12
c. 18
d. 27
e. 30

22 *Which of the following suggest a distal rather than proximal RTA?*

a. Variable urine acidification
b. Normal K+
c. Plasma bicarbonate of <10 mmol/L
d. Plasma bicarbonate of 20 mmol/L
e. Glycosuria
f. Aminoaciduria
g. Nephrocalcinosis

23 *With regard to rhabdomyolysis, which of the following statements is true?*

a. Patients present with an elevated creatine kinase, a low potassium and a low calcium.
b. Urine is dark brown in colour but is dipstick negative for blood.
c. In patients with renal involvement, alkalinisation of the urine may inhibit myoglobin cast formation.
d. Peak CK level has no effect on the likelihood of developing renal impairment.
e. Most patients end up with long-term renal impairment.

24 *With regard to patients with hyponatraemia, which of the following statements is true?*

a. A serum sodium of 125–130 mmol/L is associated with the development of seizures.
b. In a patient with a serum sodium of 110 mmol/L, correction should be undertaken as quickly as possible with the use of hypertonic saline.
c. A patient with Addison's disease may have hyponatraemia and intravascular volume depletion.
d. In a patient with hyponatraemia secondary to SIADH, the urine osmolality is usually <500 mosmol/kg.
e. Hyponatraemia secondary to SIADH can be caused by demeclocycline.

25 *Which of the following bacteria is the most common cause of UTI encountered in general practice?*

a. Klebsiella
b. Enterobacter
c. Enterococcus
d. *E. coli*
e. Proteus

26 *Which of the following is the most common renal stone?*

a. Calcium phosphate stone
b. Calcium oxalate stone
c. Triple (calcium, ammonium, phosphate) stone
d. Uric acid/urate stone
e. Cystine stone

27 *Which of the following symptoms are typical of a patient with hypercalcaemia?*

a. Polydipsia
b. Abdominal pain
c. Paraesthesia
d. Dyspepsia
e. Seizures

28 *Which of the following are a common cause of fever in renal transplant recipients?*

a. PTLD
b. BK nephropathy
c. CMV infection
d. UTI
e. Influenza infection
f. HIV

29 *With regard to adult polycystic kidney disease, which of the following is true?*

a. It is usually autosomal recessive.
b. Five percent have cysts in the liver as well as the kidneys.
c. The classic valvular lesion seen is tricuspid regurgitation.
d. Some patients have berry aneurysms and intestinal diverticulae.
e. ACEI inhibit the progression of renal cyst formation.

30 *Which of the following are secondary causes of hypertension?*

a. Cushing's disease
b. Renal artery stenosis
c. Phaeochromocytoma
d. Addison's disease
e. All of the above

31 *With regard to a patient with ESRF requiring RRT, which of the following statements are true?*

a. A 40 year old starting haemodialysis has around a 50% 5-year survival.
b. Those patients receiving a renal transplant have the same 5-year survival as those who remain on dialysis but a better quality of life.
c. Haemodialysis is the preferred form of renal replacement therapy for diabetics.
d. A colostomy is a contraindication to peritoneal dialysis.
e. In a patient starting haemodialysis the AVF can usually be used 2 weeks after formation.

32 *With regard to transplant immunosuppression, which of the following statements are true?*

a. Tacrolimus acts by inhibiting calcineurin and is associated with gingival hypertrophy.
b. The main side-effects of mycophenolate mofetil are diarrhoea and cytopaenias.
c. Anti-CD25 antibodies are frequently used as maintenance agents.
d. Sirolimus is non-nephrotoxic but associated with mouth ulcers, rashes and occasionally pneumonitis.
e. Alemtuzumab is an anti-CD52 antibody, which suppresses T cell proliferation.

33 *The complications of chronic kidney disease include:*

a. Primary hyperparathyroidism
b. Secondary hyperparathyroidism
c. Macrocytic anaemia
d. Accelerated vascular disease
e. Fluid overload and hypertension

1 Clinical presentation

a. Minimal change GN
b. Focal segmental glomerular sclerosis
c. ANCA-associated vasculitis
d. Goodpasture's disease
e. Haemolytic-uraemic syndrome
f. Adult polycystic kidney disease
g. Pre-eclampsia
h. IgA nephropathy
i. Systemic lupus erythematosus
j. Simple urinary tract infection
k. Nephrolithiasis

For each of the clinical presentations described below, select one or more diagnoses from the list given above.

1. A 25-year-old man with acute renal failure and pulmonary haemorrhage.
2. An 18-year-old girl with nephrotic syndrome (5.5 g protein/24-h urine collection; albumin 20 g/L; pitting oedema to knees).
3. A 57-year-old man who presents with a creatinine of 980 μmol/L, haematuria 1+ on urine dipstick, two 7.5 cm kidneys (with cortical thinning) on US.
4. A 42-year-old man with hypertension (BP 150/95 mmHg) and macroscopic haematuria.
5. A 34-year-old woman with hypertension (BP 165/90 mmHg), anaemia (Hb 7.4 g/dL), thrombocytopaenia (platelets 68) and creatinine 169 μmol/L.

2 Examination

a. Membranous nephropathy
b. Systemic amyloidosis
c. SLE
d. Acute tubulointerstitial nephritis
e. ANCA-associated vasculitis
f. Renal cell carcinoma
g. APKD
h. Minimal change GN
i. IgA nephropathy
j. Post-streptococcal GN
k. Hepatitis C with cryoglobulinaemia and mesangiocapillary GN type I
l. Pyelonephritis

Each of the patients described below has renal impairment. Choose the most likely underlying diagnosis from the list given above.

1. A 68-year-old woman with a purpuric skin rash, nasal crusting and bibasal inspiratory crepitations in the lungs. Her observation chart shows that she is febrile.
2. A 22-year-old woman with mouth ulcers and a photosensitivity rash on her neck and forearms. Abdominal examination demonstrates splenomegaly (the spleen can just be tipped).
3. A 45-year-old man with old needle-track scars in the antecubital fossa, livedo reticularis on his thighs and ankle oedema.
4. A 55-year-old man with macroglossia, hepatosplenomegaly and pitting oedema to the mid-thighs.
5. A 59-year-old man with a pansystolic murmur, a fullness in both flanks (right>left), and a palpable liver edge (4 cm below the costal margin).

Nephrology: Clinical Cases Uncovered. By M. Clatworthy.
Published 2010 by Blackwell Publishing.

PART 3: SELF-ASSESSMENT

3 Immunological investigations

a. Goodpasture's disease
b. Hepatitis C with mesangiocapillary GN type I
c. Post-streptococcal GN
d. Microscopic polyangiitis
e. Wegener's granulomatosis
f. Systemic lupus erythematosus
g. IgA nephropathy
h. Membranous GN
i. Atypical HUS
j. FSGS

Match the investigation results below with one or more of the nephroimmunological diagnoses given above.

1. Anti-dsDNA antibodies present in serum
2. Mixed cryoglobulins detectable in serum
3. pANCA detectable, with an MPO ELISA titre of 139
4. Antiglomerular basement membrane antibody detectable with an ELISA titre of 196
5. Borderline low serum C3, significantly low C4

4 Urine appearance and tests

a. Membranous nephropathy
b. Rhabdomyolysis
c. Acute porphyria
d. FSGS
e. Cystitis
f. Transitional cell carcinoma of the bladder
g. ADPKD
h. Minimal change
i. IgA nephropathy
j. Post-streptococcal GN

For each of the following descriptions of urine, select one or more diagnoses from the list above.

1. Frothy or foamy
2. Cloudy
3. Macroscopic haematuria
4. Dark brown with dysmorphic red cells and red cell casts on microscopy
5. Dark brown with blood on dipstick but no red cells on microscopy

5 Radiological investigations

a. Obstructive uropathy secondary to benign prostatic hypertrophy
b. Adult polycystic kidney disease
c. Long-standing primary hyperparathyroidism
d. Chronic renal tubular acidosis
e. Neurogenic/neuropathic bladder secondary to multiple sclerosis
f. Ureteric stricture secondary to renal calculi
g. Chronic IgA nephropathy with eGFR 12 mL/min/1.73 m²
h. Normal kidney
i. Acute tubular necrosis
j. Chronic tubulointerstitial nephritis

For each of the following radiological images, select one or more correct diagnoses from the list above.

1. Similar appearance observed in left kidney.

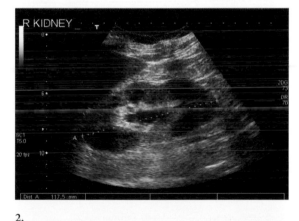

2.

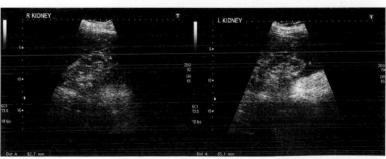

Kidney length = 8.27 cm   Kidney length = 8.51 cm

3.

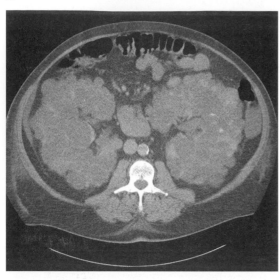

4.

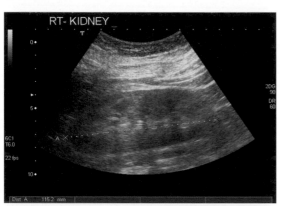

5.

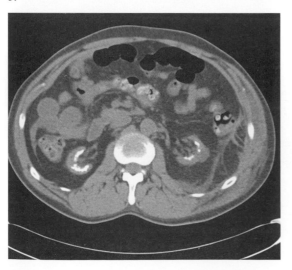

6 Renal biopsy
a. FSGS
b. Amyloid
c. Acute tubular necrosis
d. Lupus nephritis
e. Membranous GN
f. Goodpasture's disease
g. IgA nephropathy
h. Haemolytic-uraemic syndrome
i. ANCA-associated vasculitis
j. Chronic pyelonephritis

For the renal biopsy images shown below, select one or more diagnoses from the list given above.

1.

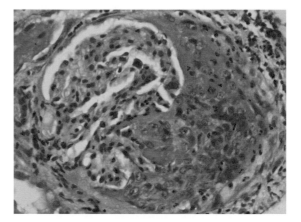

2.

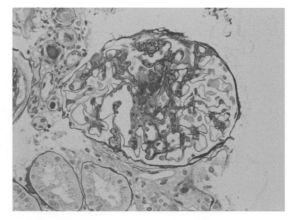

3.

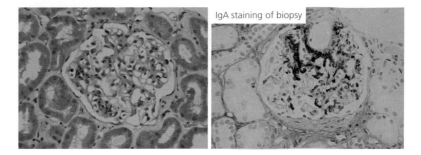

IgA staining of biopsy

4.

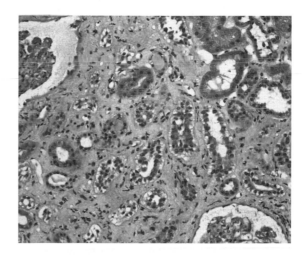

5.

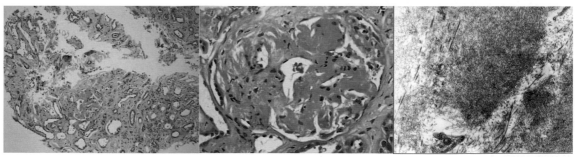

Low power view   High power view   Electron microscopy

7 Biochemical investigations

a. Renal tubular acidosis
b. Addison's disease
c. Hyperparathyroidism
d. Cushing's disease
e. Conn's syndrome
f. Sarcoidosis
g. SIADH
h. Liquorice consumption
i. Myeloma

Match the following biochemical test results with one or more the diagnoses listed above.

Normal ranges

Na 135–145 mmol/L, K 3.5–5.3 mmol/L, Urea 2.5–
   6.7 mmol/L, Creatinine 50–120 μmol/L
Glucose 3.5–5.5 mmol/L
Ca 2.12–2.65 mmol/L, PO_4 0.8–1.45 mmol/L
Alkaline phosphatase (ALP) 30–300 iu/L

Biochemical test results

1. Na 129 mmol/L, K 6.3 mmol/L, U 5.0 mmol/L,
   creatinine 78 μmol/L, glucose 3.0 mmol/L
2. Na 145 mmol/L, K 2.9 mmol/L, U 4.8 mmol/L,
   creatinine 100 μmol/L
3. Na 121 mmol/L, K 3.9 mmol/L, U 2.7 mmol/L,
   creatinine 65 μmol/L
4. Ca 2.95 mmol/L, PO_4 2.42 mmol/L, ALP 200 iu/L
5. Ca 3.04 mmol/L, PO_4 0.51 mmol/L, ALP 459 iu/L

8 Patient management

a. A 25-year-old man with K+ 6.7 and tall tented T waves/widening of QRS on ECG.
b. A 56-year-old man with acute renal failure (Na 141, K 5.2, U 23, creatinine 257) secondary to an ANCA-associated vasculitis.
c. An 18-year-old primagravida, 32 weeks pregnant with BP 160/95 mmHg and proteinuria on dipstick.
d. A 68-year-old lady with acute renal failure (Na 143, K 4.6, U 43, creatinine 556) secondary to an ANCA-associated vasculitis.
e. A 62-year-old man with nephrotic syndrome (Alb 12, 10.2 g protein on 24-h urine collection, oedema to abdominal wall, ascites, small left pleural effusion) secondary to membranous GN.

f. A 45-year-old woman with symptomatic hypocalcaemia and U waves on ECG.
g. A 32-year-old man with acute renal failure (Na 136, K 5.6, U 36, creatinine 396) secondary to Goodpasture's disease.
h. A 56-year-old woman with probable essential hypertension (BP 155/90 on three occasions).
i. A 17-year-old girl with nephrotic syndrome (Alb 22, 8.6 g protein on 24-h urine collection, oedema to mid-thighs) secondary to minimal change GN.
j. A 36-year-old man with BP 150/95 mmHg, creatinine 135 μmol/L (stable for the last 6 months) and microscopic haematuria with IgA nephropathy on biopsy.

Match each of the following management plans with the clinical scenarios listed above.

1. Treat hypertension with labetalol followed by nifedipine if there is persistent high blood pressure.
2. Give IV 10 mL 10% calcium gluconate followed by 50 mL 50% dextrose and 10 units of Actrapid.
3. Restrict fluids, give loop diuretic, an ACEI and prednisolone 60 mg po, od (with a PPI and Calcichew D3).
4. Give three 1 g pulses of methyl prednisolone IV, followed by plasma exchange and intravenous cyclophosphamide (with a prophylactic PPI, Calcichew D3, co-trimoxazole and amphotericin).
5. Restrict fluids, give loop diuretic, an ACEI and anticoagulate with warfarin.
6. Give three 1 g pulses of methyl prednisolone IV, followed by IV cyclophosphamide (with a prophylactic PPI, Calcichew D3, co-trimoxazole and amphotericin).

9 Clinical presentation – transplantation

a. Recurrent primary disease
b. Post-transplant lymphoproliferative disorder
c. CMV infection
d. Acute cellular rejection
e. Lymphocoele
f. Renal vein thrombosis
g. Renal artery stenosis
h. CNI toxicity
i. BK nephropathy
j. Urinary tract infection
k. Delayed graft function secondary to ATN

For each of the post-transplant clinical presentations below, select the most appropriate diagnosis/es from the list above.

1. A 29-year-old man with ESRF secondary to APKD who receives a non-heart beating donor kidney. Following return from theatre, immediately post transplant he is noted to be oliguric (urine output <20 mL/h).

2. A 56-year-old man with ESRF of unknown cause who receives a living donor kidney from his wife. He does well postoperatively and his creatinine falls to 100 μmol/L. Two weeks later he is seen in clinic with a rise in creatinine to 256 μmol/L.

3. A 37-year-old woman with ESRF secondary to IgA nephropathy who received a heart-beating donor kidney 3 months ago. She now presents with fevers (temperature 38.5°C on three occasions).

4. A 45-year-old woman with ESRF secondary to FSGS who received a living donor kidney from her husband 6 months ago. Her baseline creatinine has remained steady since transplant (creatinine 89 μmol/L) but she is hypertensive (BP 150/90 mmHg) with proteinuria 2+ on dipstick.

5. A 55-year-old male with ESRF secondary to diabetic nephropathy presents 9 months post transplant with a BP 160/90 mmHg) and a gradually rising creatinine (130 to 190 μmol/L over a 3-month period). Decoy cells are identified in his urine on microscopy.

---

10 Renal transplant biopsy

a. Three pulses of intravenous methyl prednisolone
b. Reduce maintenance immunosuppression
c. Plasma exchange
d. Intravenous ganciclovir
e. Antithymocyte globulin
f. Increase maintenance immunosuppression
g. Aim for minimal CNI until graft function improves
h. Ciprofloxacin
i. Transplant nephrectomy
j. Switch from tacrolimus to sirolimus

For each of the cases and their renal transplant biopsy images shown below, select the correct management plan from the list above.

1. A 56-year-old man with ESRF of unknown cause biopsied 6 days following a non-heart beating donor kidney transplant (2-0-0 mismatch). His maintenance immunosuppression is prednisolone, ciclosporin and azathioprine.

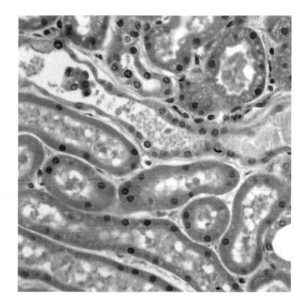

2. A 22-year-old woman with ESRF secondary to IgA nephropathy biopsied 6 weeks following a living donor kidney transplant (2-1-1 mismatch) due to a rise in creatinine with normal US scan. Her maintenance immunosuppression is prednisolone, tacrolimus and mycophenolate mofetil. C4d staining on this biopsy was negative.

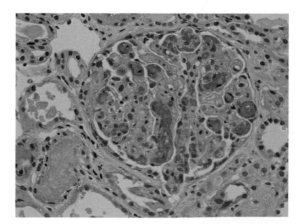

3. A 48-year-old male with ESRF secondary to APKD biopsied 2 weeks following a heart-beating donor kidney transplant (1-1-0 mismatch) due to a rise in creatinine with normal US scan. His maintenance immunosuppression is prednisolone, ciclosporin and azathioprine.

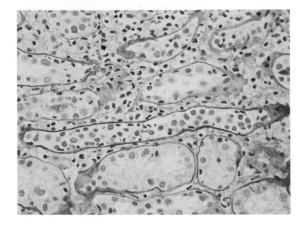

4. A 65-year-old man with ESRF secondary to AAV, biopsied 2 months following a non-heart beating donor transplant (1-0-0 mismatch) because of a rise in creatinine with normal US scan. His maintenance immunosuppression is prednisolone, tacrolimus and mycophenolate mofetil. The biopsy shown is stained with an anti-SV40 HRP antibody.

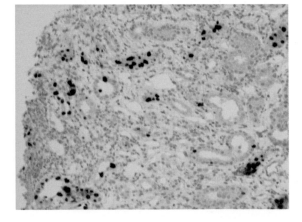

5. A 35-year-old, highly sensitised woman with ESRF secondary to FSGS, biopsied 10 days following a heart-beating donor kidney transplant (1-0-0 mismatch) due to a rise in creatinine with normal US scan. She is mildly febrile (temp 37.8 °C). Her maintenance immunosuppression is prednisolone, tacrolimus and mycophenolate mofetil. The biopsy shown is stained with a C4d HRP antibody.

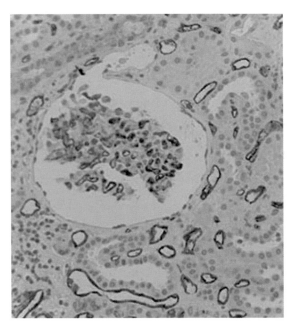

SAQs

1 *A 45-year-old man presents with lethargy and vomiting. Blood tests show a creatinine of 560 μmol/L. One month ago his creatinine was 98 μmol/L. A US scan shows two 12 cm kidneys.*

a. Is this likely to be acute or chronic renal failure? Justify your answer.
b. How would you classify the causes of renal failure?
c. What is the most common cause of acute renal failure?
d. Describe the general management principles of patients with acute renal failure.

2 *A 24-year-old woman presents with oedema, proteinuria (6.7 g in 24 hours) and a serum albumin of 20 g/dL.*

a. What term would you use to describe her clinical presentation?
b. What further investigations would you perform?
c. What are the possible underlying causes of her presentation?
d. What general management measures would you consider?

3 *A 36-year-old man presents with BP 185/100 mmHg, peripheral oedema, oliguria, urine dipstick blood 4+, protein 3+, creatinine 311 μmol/L. US scan shows two 11.5 cm kidneys with normal cortical thickness.*

a. What term would you use to describe his clinical presentation?
b. What are the possible underlying causes of this presentation?
c. What further investigations would you perform?
d. What general management measures would you consider?

4 *A 45-year-old man presents with an episode of loin pain and macroscopic haematuria. BP is 150/85 mmHg and creatinine is 190 μmol/L. He has previously been fit and well. A renal US scan shows multiple cysts in both kidneys.*

a. What is the most likely diagnosis?
b. What other facts would you ascertain when taking a history?
c. What features would you seek on examination?
d. How would you manage this patient?

5 *A 30-year-old man is referred to the nephrology clinic after a pre-employment health screen showed that he was persistently hypertensive (BP 145/90 mmHg) and has blood 2+ on urine dipstick on two occasions (protein/leucocytes/nitrites negative). His creatinine is 100 μmol/L (eGFR 81 mL/min/1.73 m^2) and US of his renal tract demonstrates no obvious abnormalities. A renal immunology screen is negative (ANA, ANCA, anti-GBM, immunoglobulin, complement C3/C4).*

a. What is the most likely diagnosis and who first described this disease?
b. How would you manage this man?
c. Describe the typical renal biopsy findings?
d. What factors might suggest a poorer prognosis in this disease?

Nephrology: Clinical Cases Uncovered. By M. Clatworthy.
Published 2010 by Blackwell Publishing.

6 A 66-year-old woman attends her GP complaining of increasing shortness of breath and wheeze. On examination, there is a bilateral polyphonic expiratory wheeze throughout the precordium. She has previously been fit and well, with no history of asthma. She is prescribed a salbutamol inhaler and a 7-day course of amoxicillin. She returns 3 weeks later with persistent wheeze and has now developed numbness on the ulnar border of the left hand. Investigations are as follows:

Hb 10.2, WBC 11.9 (neutrophils 7.1, lymphocytes 1.9, eosinophils 3.1), platelets 460

Urea 14, creatinine 230

Urine dipstick: blood 3+ protein 2+

FEV_1 2.8L, FVC 4.9L

a. What is the most likely diagnosis?
b. What other clinical features would you seek?
c. How would you confirm the diagnosis?
d. Name two other conditions characterised by acute renal impairment and eosinophilia?

7 A 50-year-old alcoholic is admitted to the emergency department with agitation and confusion. He is mildly dehydrated but not obviously jaundiced. BP is 125/75mmHg and O_2 sats are 95% on air. His investigations are as follows:

pH 7.20, pCO_2 2.9, pO_2 10.8, HCO_3^- 8

Na 141, K^+ 4.0, urea 12, creatinine 130, Cl 106, Glu 11.0

Urine dipstick: no ketones

a. How would you describe this acid–base disturbance?
b. What is your differential diagnosis and which is most likely?
c. Which other investigations may be of use?
d. How would you manage this man?

8 A 56-year-old man attends his GP with lethargy and malaise. Routine bloods show a creatinine of 461 μmol/L (eGFR 12mL/min/1.73 m²). A US renal tract shows that his right kidney is 7.5cm and his left kidney 8cm, both with cortical thinning. There is no obvious dilation of the collecting system.

a. Do you think this man has acute or chronic renal failure? Justify your answer.
b. What is your differential diagnosis as to the most likely underlying cause?
c. How would you classify the severity of his renal failure?
d. What are the main complications observed in this condition?

9 A 58-year-old woman with APKD is referred to the 'low clearance clinic'. She has been followed up in the general nephrology clinic for 20 years, and her blood pressure managed aggressively with a combination of ACEI and a calcium channel blocker. Unfortunately, her renal function has gradually declined and her eGFR is now 15mL/min/1.73 m². It is likely that she will need RRT within the next 6 months.

a. What forms of RRT are available to this patient? Which would be preferable?
b. What factors might make you advise one RRT modality over another?
c. What are the main complications of the different forms of dialysis?
d. Outline your management plan for the next 6 months.

10 A 37-year-old man with ESRF of unknown cause is referred to the transplant assessment clinic. His wife is keen to donate a kidney to him. Transplant work-up shows that the donor is CMV positive and the recipient CMV negative. The HLA mismatch is 2-1-0. The donor is blood group B and the recipient is blood group A.

a. What are meant by the terms 'CMV positive' and 'CMV negative' and what are their implications in this case?
b. What are HLA, and what does a 2-1-0 mismatch refer to?
c. What is the major issue when considering transplantation in this case?
d. How could the problem be overcome?

1. a. Indications for urgent dialysis are factors which may be life-threatening or lead to serious complications. In particular, symptomatic uraemia (pericarditis, encephalopathy), severe pulmonary oedema, severe acidosis or hyperkalaemia (with ECG changes) refractory to medical therapy. Anuria is not an indication for urgent dialysis. It is one of the features of renal failure, but may be reversible if the underlying cause of ARF is treated, e.g. if a urinary catheter is inserted in a patient who is obstructed. Severe, symptomatic pulmonary oedema in a patient with ARF is an indication for urgent dialysis. In contrast, peripheral oedema is not. An absolute urea value is less important than whether the patient is symptomatic as a result of uraemia. An absolute potassium value is not a specific indication for dialysis; rather, whether there are associated ECG changes (tented T waves, prolonged P-R interval, widening of QRS, sine waves) or if the hyperkalaemia is resistant to medical treatment. Creatinine is not toxic in itself, therefore an absolute value is not important in deciding on whether a patient needs dialysis urgently. Higher levels of creatinine at presentation reflect the patient's muscle bulk and dietary red meat intake.

2. b. The first step in management should be to give 10 mL 10% calcium gluconate intravenously, followed by intravenous insulin and dextrose to induce cellular uptake of K^+. Furosemide inhibits the NaK2Cl co-transporter and leads to an increase in urinary sodium and potassium (see Part 1, Figure D) with a corresponding reduction in serum potassium levels. However, in a patient with ARF, the kidney is unlikely to have sufficient tubular function to effectively reduce potassium. Adrenaline (epinephrine) activates $\alpha 2$-adrenoreceptors (causing vasoconstriction) and $\beta 1$-adrenoreceptors (increasing heart rate and force of contraction). Calcium resonium is given orally or rectally and binds potassium within the GI tract, thus preventing its absorption. It is useful in preventing worsening hyperkalaemia but has no place in the immediate acute management of life-threatening hyperkalaemia.

3. a,c. A recent measurement of normal renal function is the best way of confirming that renal failure is acute rather than chronic. Anaemia can occur in both acute (acute inflammation/infection/erythropoietin deficiency) and chronic renal failure (due to erythropoietin deficiency/iron deficiency/chronic disease) and therefore is not helpful in distinguishing the two. Hypocalcaemia due to inadequate hydroxylation of vitamin D by the enzyme 1α-hydroxylase can occur in both acute and chronic renal failure. Normal-sized kidneys on US examination may occur in conditions in which the normal renal tissue is replaced by deposited substrate or cysts rather than undergoing the usual scarring and shrinkage. Examples include diabetic nephropathy, systemic amyloidosis, glycogen storage disorders or polycystic kidney disease. Acute-onset anuria is suggestive of ARF. CKD tends to lead to a gradual decline in urine output over months/years. Vomiting is associated with uraemia in both acute and chronic renal failure. It can also be a precipitating factor for ARF if it is sufficient to cause volume depletion and pre-renal failure.

4. a,b,d. Urine dipstick is helpful in delineating the cause of ARF. Blood and protein (+/− leucocytes) on dipstick are indicative of an active urinary sediment and raise the possibility of a 'renal' cause of ARF, e.g. an acute glomerulonephritis or

Nephrology: Clinical Cases Uncovered. By M. Clatworthy. Published 2010 by Blackwell Publishing.

tubulointerstitial nephritis. The presence of leucocytes and nitrites on dipstick is indicative of infection. Urine microscopy may demonstrate casts (e.g. red cell casts, indicative of glomerulonephritis) or crystals (e.g. in patients with stone disease). Although urine electrolytes (e.g. measurement of urine sodium) can help to distinguish between pre-renal ARF (low urine sodium) and established ATN (high urine sodium due to death/dysfunction of tubular cells and therefore lack of pump activity moving sodium out of the urinary space), in practice by the time the result has returned, the diagnosis is clinically obvious (see case 1, Table 1.1). US renal tract is useful in determining the size of the kidneys (small kidneys with cortical thinning indicate likely CKD over ARF), the presence of cysts (indicating APKD) or a dilated pelvicalyceal system (hydronephrosis, indicating obstruction). A CT abdomen is not usually required in patients with ARF and can exacerbate the problem if contrast is used. PTH levels are measured in patients with CKD rather than ARF.

5. a,b,e. It is important to ensure patients with ARF are well filled in order to optimise the chance of renal recovery; however, an excess of fluid must be avoided in order to minimise the risk of pulmonary oedema. Accurately assessing fluid balance can be achieved by regular clinical examination together with review of the input-output chart and daily weights. Although blood urea levels do increase in patients who are dehydrated, they are not helpful in patients with ARF as they will be elevated as a result of kidney dysfunction. Urine sodium levels are discussed in question 4, and are not useful in this context.

6. d. As discussed in question 5, in patients with ARF the aim is to ensure that the patient is well filled in order to optimise the chance of renal recovery, but to avoid an excess of fluid in an attempt to minimise the risk of pulmonary oedema. In patients who are oliguric, the input must be tailored to match the output (the main elements of which are urine output and insensible losses). In a non-febrile patient, without vomiting and diarrhoea, insensible losses amount to about 500 mL. Thus a reasonable fluid replacement regimen is urine output plus 500 mL.

7. b. Red cell casts on urine microscopy specifically indicate glomerular inflammation

(glomerulonephritis) and are not seen in the other conditions.

8. c,e. SLE only rarely occurs as a monogenic disorder (in patients with deficiencies in complement pathway components such as C1q, C2 and C4). In most cases, SLE is a polygenic disorder, in which polymorphisms in a number of immunologically important genes (such as HLA molecule and Fcγ receptor genes) contribute to disease susceptibility. These polymorphisms occur commonly in the general population and, if present in isolation, do not cause disease. Rather, inheritance of a combination of susceptibility alleles is required for disease development. Typical dermatological manifestations include a malar (butterfly) rash, photosensitivity rashes, discoid lesions and mouth ulcers. Lupus pernio is a characteristic cutaneous manifestation of sarcoid not SLE. SLE is characterised by ANA in 95% of cases, as well as other autoantibodies, such as anti-dsDNA (occurs in 70% of cases) or anti-Sm (occurs in 40% of cases). These autoantibodies form immune complexes, which circulate and become deposited in tissues such as the kidney or skin. Immune complex deposition leads to complement activation (via the classic pathway), hence C4 is usually very low in SLE with a more modest reduction in C3. (See Part 1, Figure L for a summary of the complement system.) Immune complex deposition and complement activation in the kidneys lead to 'full-house' immunostaining, with detectable IgG, IgM, IgA, C1q, C3 and C4.

9. c,d,g. Pulmonary-renal syndrome is characterised by acute renal failure secondary to a rapidly progressive GN, together with pulmonary haemorrhage. A full list of causes is given in case 8, Box 8.2 and includes ANCA-associated vasculitis, Goodpasture's disease (also known as anti-GBM disease) and SLE. Membranous, FSGS and minimal change GN usually present with nephrotic syndrome rather than a pulmonary-renal syndrome. Rhabdomyolysis presents with ARF, but not with pulmonary haemorrhage.

10. b,c,f. Patients with anti-GBM disease (Goodpasture's disease) present with acute renal failure secondary to a rapidly progressive GN (usually a crescentic GN is demonstrated on renal biopsy). A proportion will also have pulmonary haemorrhage. Pulmonary haemorrhage occurs

when there is damage to the alveolar endothelium (which is non-fenestrated and therefore does not usually allow circulating anti-GBM antibodies to gain access to the alveolar basement membrane). Factors leading to alveolar endothelial damage and hence pulmonary haemorrhage include cigarette smoking, exposure to inhaled hydrocarbons, pneumonia/pulmonary infection and pulmonary oedema. The pathogenic antibodies in anti-GBM disease specifically recognise the non-collagenous domain of the a3 chain of type IV collagen. Renal failure is often irreversible, particularly if the patients are oligoanuric at the time of presentation. Those with pulmonary haemorrhage may present earlier and have remediable renal disease. Treatment includes removal of the pathogenic antibody with plasma exchange and immunosuppression to both dampen antibody-associated inflammation (corticosteroids) and reduce further antibody production by depleting T and B cells (cyclophosphamide).

11. a,d Patients with AAV frequently present with non-specific symptoms such as malaise, lethargy, arthralgia, myalgia, fevers and night sweats. This non-specific presentation can often lead to a delayed diagnosis and to some patients being labelled as having functional rather than organic disease. pANCA bind myeloperoxidase and cANCA bind proteinase-3 (see case 5, Figure 5.4). Pulmonary haemorrhage and a creatinine of >500 µmol/L are indications for plasma exchange in patients with AAV. Prior to treatment, 1-year mortality was as high as 90%. With treatment (steroids and cyclophosphamide with maintenance azathioprine) it is now 10–30%. AAV is a relapsing disease. Although around 80–90% will achieve remission, 50–60% will have a relapse within the first year.

12. a,e. IgA nephropathy is the most common primary GN, making up around 30% of all biopsy-proven primary GN in European populations and an even higher proportion in the Far East. Thirty percent of patients with IgA nephropathy have elevated serum IgA levels. IgA nephropathy tends to present in two ways: either with asymptomatic hypertension and microscopic haematuria or with episodes of macroscopic haematuria and loin pain which are frequently precipitated by mucosal infections, but can be precipitated by heavy exercise and

vaccination. Five percent present with ARF and very rarely with nephrotic syndrome. IgA nephropathy can be associated with coeliac disease in some patients.

13. d. See Part 1, Box I for details.

14. a,f. Adults with nephrotic syndrome should undergo a renal biopsy in order to determine the cause (unless there is a significant contraindication, e.g. patient has a single kidney). Dietary protein restriction is not useful, as the patients are already protein deficient due to urinary loss, and in fact this may have a deleterious effect. Potassium levels are not usually abnormally high in patients with nephrotic syndrome, so there is no indication for potassium restriction. Loop diuretics (e.g. furosemide) are useful in treating oedema, but may need to be given intravenously if there is significant gut oedema (which can prevent full absorption of the drug from the GI tract). In adults with nephrotic syndrome, the most common primary GN identified on biopsy is membranous GN. In children it is minimal change GN.

15. a,d,f. Glomerulonephritides presenting with nephrotic syndrome include minimal change, membranous, FSGS and mesangiocapillary GN. Secondary causes include diabetic nephropathy and amyloidosis. IgA nephropathy tends to present with asymptomatic hypertension and microscopic haematuria or episodic macroscopic haematuria. Lupus nephritis and post-streptococcal GN usually present as a nephritic syndrome.

16. b,e. Membranous GN is idiopathic in two-thirds of cases. Associations are shown in case 11, Box 11.1. Prognosis is variable:
   • 25%: spontaneous complete remission (within ~5 y)
   • 25%: partial remission/stable
   • 50%: persistent proteinuria and progressive renal impairment.
   Most patients with lupus nephritis have a diffuse proliferative GN. Membranous GN is seen in around 5% of biopsies and is graded as class V lupus nephritis.

17. b. Nephrotic syndrome is a hypercoagulable state due to a combination of loss of anticoagulant factors in the urine and the presence of severe peripheral oedema which can be associated with significant immobility. In addition, many patients will also be intravascularly volume depleted due to

the use of diuretics. Patients are at risk of thromboembolic disease, with DVT occurring in 25%, PE in 5–10% and renal vein thrombosis in 15–20%. The latter presents with loin pain, haematuria and deteriorating renal function. Because of the high risk of thromboembolism, most nephrologists would advocate full anticoagulation (with warfarin) for patients with an albumin of <20 g/L.

18. b,e. FSGS most commonly presents as nephrotic syndrome. Secondary causes include obesity and HIV infection. Primary FSGS has a relatively poor prognosis with at least 40% progressing to ESRF. In patients with primary FSGS, the recurrence rate post transplant is around 30%. There are a number of familial forms of FSGS (both autosomal dominant and recessive). Mutations have been identified in podocin, nephrin, α-actinin-4 or TRPC6 (see case 13, Table 13.1).

19. b. Minimal change is the most common cause of nephrotic syndrome in children. As in adults, the main complications are infection, thrombosis, hypovolaemia and those related to treatment. Children with nephrotic syndrome do not routinely need to undergo renal biopsy, because the diagnosis is most likely to be minimal change GN. Exceptions include those with haematuria, significant hypertension and renal impairment, all of which are unusual in minimal change GN. More than 90% of children will respond to corticosteroids, although around 70% will have some sort of relapse. Around 5–10% of children will be truly steroid resistant and may go on to develop lesions consistent with FSGS. Some of these will develop ESRF.

20. b,d,e. Metabolic acidosis with a high anion gap occurs due to increased production/reduced clearance of acids. The main causes are:
- lactic acidosis (shock, hypoxia, sepsis, MI)
- ketoacidosis (diabetes, alcohol)
- renal failure
- liver failure
- drugs/toxins (salicylates, ethylene glycol, methanol).

Renal tubular acidosis results in a metabolic acidosis with a normal anion gap. Respiratory failure leads to accumulation of carbon dioxide and a respiratory acidosis.

21. d. The anion gap is calculated by the following formula:

$$(Na^+ + K^+) - (HCO_3^- + Cl^-)$$

In this case:

$$(136 + 5) - (12 + 102) = 27$$

Normal anion gap is 10–18 mmol/L. This represents the unestimated anions which consist of albumin, phosphate and other organic acids. It can help in distinguishing the cause for a metabolic acidosis.

22. c,g. The typical features of distal (type I) and proximal (type II) RTA are summarised in case 22, Table 22.1.

23. c. Rhabdomyolysis can be caused by physical damage to muscle, for example, compression, excessive exercise, prolonged seizure activity or electrocution. The classic clinical picture is of elevated creatine kinase (CK), high K^+ (released from damaged muscle cells), low calcium (bound to damaged muscle) and acute renal impairment. Myoglobin is a muscle protein which is released following damage to muscle fibres. Dark urine which is dipstick positive for blood but contains no red cells or casts on microscopy is likely to be due to myoglobinuria. Treatment is rehydration which may be facilitated by alkalinising the urine. In rhabdomyolysis CK levels are usually raised at least five times the normal range and can be 100 times normal. Levels rise 12 hours after the initial damage and the higher the peak level, the more likely that renal impairment will occur. Patients often require a period of renal support but usually fully recover renal function.

24. c. Mild hyponatraemia is common and usually asymptomatic. If the sodium falls to around 120 mmol/L then there is often restlessness, irritability and confusion. Sodium levels of <110 mmol/L lead to progressive coma and seizures. Serum sodium should be corrected gradually (usually with fluid restriction) as rapid correction can result in central pontine myelinolysis (CPM). When assessing the cause of hyponatraemia, it is important to establish the volume status of the patient. If the patient is hypovolaemic then hyponatraemia may be caused by diuretics or hypoadrenalism (Addison's disease)

(see case 23, Table 23.1). In SIADH there is dilute plasma with osmolalities of <260 mosmol/kg and inappropriately concentrated urine with urine osmolalities of >500 mosmol/kg. SIADH may be caused by intracranial pathology such as head injury or infection, pulmonary pathologies including pneumonia, malignancies and drugs (particularly chlopromamide and chlorpromazine). It is treated with fluid restriction and, in severe cases, demeclocycline.

25. d. The most common bacteria causing UTI are shown in case 17, Table 17.1.

26. b. There are four main types of renal stones:
    • calcium oxalate stones (most common, 60–70% of total)
    • phosphate stones, calcium or triple (calcium, magnesium, ammonium)
    • uric acid/urate stones
    • cystine stones.

27. a,b. The classic presenting symptoms of hypercalcaemia are described in case 3, Box 3.1 ('bones, groans, stones and moans').

28. c,d. The most likely cause of fever in a transplant recipient is infection. Transplant recipients must take maintenance immunosuppression in order to prevent allograft rejection, so they are at increased risk of a number of infections, including UTI, chest infections, CMV and pneumocystis (detailed in case 31, Box 31.1). PTLD is an important differential in a transplant patient with fever but is relatively uncommon (occurs in 2–4% of transplant recipients). It is usually driven by Epstein–Barr virus and is more likely if patients have received lymphocyte-depleting agents, such as ATG, at induction. BK virus is an infection seen in transplant recipients which causes a decline in allograft function (causing interstitial inflammation and fibrosis) but patients do not usually have any systemic symptoms such as fever or sweats. Transplant patients are screened for HIV infection (as well as hepatitis B and C) prior to transplantation.

29. d. Adult polycystic kidney disease (APKD) is also known as autosomal dominant polycystic kidney disease (ADPKD) and is relatively common, occurring in 1 in 800 of caucasian populations. Infantile polycystic kidney disease is autosomal recessive. APKD is characterised by the development of cysts in all parts of the nephron as well as in other organs including the liver (in around 80% of patients), pancreas and ovaries. Other manifestations include mitral valve prolapse, berry aneurysms and intestinal diverticulae. There are currently (2009) no treatments available which have been proven to reduce cyst formation. Patients should be monitored for hypertension, and this should be treated with ACEI where possible.

30. a,b,c. Secondary causes of hypertension are shown in case 15, Box 15.1. Addison's disease is usually associated with hypotension due to excess renal sodium loss, which results in hyponatraemia and intravascular volume depletion.

31. a,d. Overall, patients starting dialysis have around a 10% annual mortality rate. This is even higher in elderly or diabetic patients. Renal transplantation offers benefits in terms of both quality of life and survival. The average 5-year survival following a cadaveric transplant is now 85–90%. Diabetics tend to do particularly badly on haemodialysis, in part because many of them already have significant vascular disease, which dialysis seems to accelerate. There is also some evidence that peritoneal dialysis may be a better option than haemodialysis, at least for younger, fitter diabetics (see case 21). Contraindications to peritoneal dialysis are, broadly speaking, factors which result in inadequate space for fluid exchange or an increased risk of infection and are described in case 27. An arteriovenous fistula usually takes at least 6–8 weeks to mature into a vessel which can easily be needled and from which adequate flows can be achieved.

32. b,d. Tacrolimus is a calcineurin inhibitor and is associated with nephrotoxicity, glucose intolerance/post-transplant diabetes and tremor. Ciclosporin is associated with gingival hypertrophy. Mycophenolate mofetil (MMF) inhibits DNA synthesis and thus lymphocyte proliferation. MMF specifically inhibits the enzyme inosine monophosphate dehydrogenase which is the rate-limiting enzyme in guanosine nucleotide synthesis. The side-effects of MMF include cytopaenias and diarrhoea. Anti-CD25 monoclonal antibodies are given IV and are used as induction agents rather than maintenance agents. Sirolimus inhibits the mammalian target of rapamycin

(mTOR) complex 1. It is non-nephrotoxic and lowers the risk of developing malignancy post transplant. Its side-effects include mouth ulcers, rashes and rarely pneumonitis. Alemtuzumab (CAMPATH-1H) is a humanised, rat monoclonal antibody which binds to CD52 and profoundly depletes lymphocytes including T cells, B cells, macrophages and NK cells. The side-effects of immunosuppressants are summarised in case 29, Table 29.1, and their mechanisms of action in Figure 29.6.

33. b,d,e. Patients with CKD have reduced activity of the renal enzyme 1α-hydroxylase, which leads to a reduction in $1,25(OH)_2$-vitamin D formation, hypocalcaemia, secondary hyperparathyroidism and eventually to tertiary hyperparathyroidism (see Part 1, Figure Fb). Patients with CKD develop anaemia secondary to erythropoietin deficiency as well as iron deficiency. This leads to a normocytic or sometimes microcytic anaemia if there is significant iron deficiency. Accelerated atherosclerosis/vascular disease, hypertension and chronic hypercalcaemia lead to accelerated atherosclerosis and vascular calcification (particularly medial calcification), and an increased risk of coronary artery disease, peripheral vascular disease (PVD) and cerebrovascular accidents. Patients with CKD often experience a gradual reduction in urine output. This leads to intravascular volume overload which increases SV. An increase in SV will lead to a rise in cardiac output ($CO = SV \times HR$). A rise in CO will lead to an increase in mean arterial pressure ($MAP = CO \times TPR$).

EMQs answers

1

1. c,d,i. AAV, SLE and Goodpasture's disease can all present with pulmonary-renal syndrome.

2. a,b. (h,i – a rare presentation for IgA nephropathy, less than 5% of patients with IgA nephropathy present with nephrotic syndrome: i – a small minority of patients with lupus nephritis present with nephrotic syndrome.)

3. h. IgA nephropathy can present, as in this case, with end-stage renal failure.

4. f,h,k

5. e,g,i All three diagnoses may be associated with haemolytic anaemia. Patients with HUS or pre-eclampsia will have a Coombe's test-negative haemolytic anaemia. Patients with SLE will have specific anti-red cell and antiplatelet autoantibodies and will be Coombe's test positive.

2

1. e. Typical features of Wegener's granulomatosis (upper respiratory tract, lower respiratory tract and renal involvement). Purpuric rash is also typical of small vessel vasculitis, although it could occur in cryoglobulinaemia, but the nasal crusting would not be in keeping with this diagnosis.

2. c.

3. k. Livedo reticularis occurs if there is sluggish blood flow in the cutaneous circulation. This typically occurs in cryoglobulinaemia, where the cryoglobulins precipitate in the colder peripheral circulation. Cryoglobulinaemia is associated with hepatitis C infection, but can also occur in SLE. The presence of needle-track scars makes the former diagnosis much more likely. In addition, SLE is less common in men (9:1 female to male ratio). Livedo reticularis can also occur in antiphospholipid syndrome or in SLE patients with anticardiolipin antibodies.

4. b. Although a patient with hepatitis C with cryoglobulinaemia and mesangiocapillary GN type I may have hepatosplenomegaly (if they have Hep C-associated chronic liver disease) and nephrosis/oedema (associated with mesangiocapillary GN), they would not have macroglossia. Systemic amyloidosis causes organomegaly (including macroglossia) and may be associated with nephrotic syndrome and renal impairment.

5. g. APKD is associated with a variety of cardiac valvular lesions, typically mitral valve prolapse. Although both kidneys have cysts on US, progression may be asymmetrical, leading to one kidney being more easily palpable than the other on abdominal examination. A less likely diagnosis is systemic amyloidosis (particularly AL amyloid), which can affect the myocardium, leading to cardiomyopathy and conduction disturbances. It is also associated with organomegaly, including renomegaly. Renal cell carcinoma may lead to a fullness palpable in the flanks, but is unlikely to be bilateral. The liver edge would suggest metastatic disease, and the murmur would be a coincidental finding, therefore this diagnosis is possible but much less likely.

3

1. f.

2. b,f.

3. a,d,e. Generally cANCA is seen in association with the clinical features typical of Wegener's granulomatosis (upper respiratory tract, lower respiratory tract and renal involvement) and pANCA with microscopic polyangiitis (rash and ARF). However, there is some cross-over. Occasionally, some patients with vasculitis (pANCA positive) also have anti-GBM antibodies

Nephrology: Clinical Cases Uncovered. By M. Clatworthy.
Published 2010 by Blackwell Publishing.

(usually of a low titre). These patients tend to have a better renal prognosis than those with 'pure' Goodpasture's disease.

4. a,d (see answer to 3).

5. b,c,f,i. A very low C4 suggests activation of the classic complement pathway, i.e. via antibody as seen in these conditions.

4

1. a,d,h. All three present with nephrotic syndrome and heavy proteinuria which leads to frothy appearance of urine.

2. e. Urine is cloudy or mucky when there is a UTI, and will also probably be dipstick + for nitrite and leucocytes.

3. f,g (i, less commonly). Macroscopic haematuria occurs in these conditions.

4. i,j. Description consistent with glomerular haematuria as seen in these glomerulonephritides.

5. b. Myoglobin makes urine dark brown and gives a false positive for blood on urine dipstick but with no red cells on microscopy.

5

1. a,e. This is a US renal tract showing hydronephrosis of the kidney with a dilated pelvicalyceal system. Hydronephrosis suggests obstruction of the renal tract and can occur secondary to lesions within the lumen (calculi, haematoma, ureteric/bladder tumours), lesions within the wall (ureteric stricture, TB/stones), neurogenic bladder, pelviureteric muscular dysfunction, urethral stricture (gonococcal/instrumentation, pinhole meatus) or lesions outside the urinary tract causing compression and hence obstruction (retroperitoneal tumours or fibrosis, abdominal aortic aneurysm, pelvic tumours, prostatic obstruction). Lesions in the bladder or distal to it (e.g. neuropathic bladder, prostatic hypertrophy) cause bilateral hydronephrosis. Ureteric stenosis is unlikely to be bilateral, and therefore usually causes only unilateral hydronephrosis.

2. g,j (rarely e) This is a US renal tract showing a small kidney with cortical thinning, suggestive of chronic kidney disease. Some patients with chronic obstruction (such as in E) may develop small shrunken kidneys at end stage without obvious dilation of the pelvicalyceal system.

3. b. A CT abdomen showing polycystic kidneys.

4. h,i. A US showing a normal-sized kidney with no hydronephrosis and reasonable corticomedullary differentiation.

5. c,d. A CT abdomen showing medullary nephrocalcinosis. This can be caused by any condition in which there is chronic hypercalcaemia and hypercalciuria (e.g. primary hyperparathyroidism, sarcoidosis), in renal tubular acidosis, primary hyperoxaluria, renal tuberculosis and medullary sponge kidney.

6

1. d,f,g,i. This biopsy shows a glomerulus with a cellular crescent occupying part of the tuft, i.e. a crescentic GN. This can be caused by all the four causes listed or may occur as a primary condition.

2. a. Focal and segmental sclerosis of glomeruli, typical of FSGS.

3. g. This renal biopsy shows mesangial proliferation, with marked mesangial IgA staining.

4. j (g, if chronic). This biopsy shows tubular atrophy and interstitial fibrosis. This can occur secondary to any chronic pathology and does not give any particular information about the underlying cause. Patients who present with advanced CKD of a variety of causes e.g. IgA nephropathy, chronic pyelonephritis, etc., and small kidneys on US have this sort of unhelpful appearance of an end-stage kidney on biopsy. There may also be areas of thyroidisation.

5. b. Appearances typical of renal amyloid with deposition of eosinophilic (pink) proteinaceous material in the kidney, particularly in the glomerulus (shown in high power, middle panel). The diagnosis is confirmed by the presence of apple-green birefringence under polarised light following Congo red staining or by identification of typical fibrils on EM (right panel).

7

1. b. Typical features of Addison's with hyponatraemia, hyperkalaemia and hypoglycaemia.

2. a,d,e,h. Hypokalaemia can occur due to renal potassium loss (loop and thiazide diuretics, renal tubular acidosis or excess aldosterone), GI potassium loss (diarrhoea, laxative abuse, villous adenoma) or if there is alkalosis when hydrogen ions are transported out of cells at the expense of K^+

flowing in. Liquorice is made from the root of *Glycyrrhiza glabra* and contains glycyrrhetinic acid which has mineralocorticoid activity.

3. g. Significant hyponatraemia may occur in SIADH or Addison's disease but the low/normal K$^+$ makes the latter diagnosis unlikely.

4. i. Hypercalcaemia with normal phosphate and ALP is most probably due to myeloma.

5. c. Hypercalcaemia with low phosphate and elevated ALP is most probably due to primary hyperparathyroidism. Sarcoidosis can cause this picture, but is more usually associated with high phosphate as well as calcium.

8

1. c. These are the agents of choice in pregnancy. In non-pregnant patients, ACEI or ARB would be first choice in a patient with proteinuria.

2. a. Calcium gluconate inhibits the development of cardiac arrhythmias, insulin causes a redistribution of K$^+$ to the intracellular compartment.

3. i. Manage oedema with fluid restriction and diuretic, proteinuria with an ACEI and in most cases (>90%), minimal change GN is responsive to corticosteroids.

4. d,g. Patients with AAV who present with a creatinine of >500 μmol/L or with pulmonary haemorrhage should receive plasma exchange.

5. e. Nephrotic patients with an albumin <20 should be anticoagulated to prevent venous thromboembolism. Patients with membranous GN are at particular risk of this complication.

6. b. AAV without pulmonary haemorrhage and with a presenting creatinine <500 mmol/L does not require additional plasma exchange.

9

1. f,k. Oliguria post transplant can be due to a variety of causes, some catastrophic and graft threatening (renal artery/vein thrombosis, hyperacute rejection), but is more commonly due to ATN.

2. a,d,e,h,j. A rise in creatinine 2 weeks post transplant can be caused by a variety of pathologies. The main concern is acute rejection but CNI toxicity, transplant pyelonephritis and compression by a large lymphocoele can also lead to a decline in allograft function. A US scan, urine dipstick and CNI level

should allow the rapid exclusion of these other pathologies.

3. b,c,j.

4. a,g,h.

5. i. Decoy cells (urothelial cells with abnormal nuclei) are typical of BK nephropathy. BK virus causes a severe interstitial inflammation and thus decline in allograft function. It can also be associated with the development of ureteric stenosis. Patients do not typically have any systemic features of infection such as fever.

10

1. g. The biopsy shows ATN. This is a common cause of delayed graft function and should be managed with supportive therapy (including dialysis) and any exposure to CNI minimised, as this can delay recovery.

2. c,j. This biopsy shows a thrombotic microangiopathy. This can represent recurrent primary disease, but more often occurs in association with tacrolimus, ciclosporin or sirolimus. Patients should be treated with plasma exchange and the likely offending drug stopped.

3. a,f. This biopsy shows acute cellular rejection which is usually treated with intravenous methylprednisolone. If a patient develops ACR then their compliance with maintenance immunosuppression should be checked, and if there appear to be no issues with compliance then maintenance immunosuppression may be increased to prevent further rejection episodes.

4. b,h. This biopsy shows BK nephropathy with interstitial inflammation and tubular epithelial cells with abnormal nuclei. BK nephropathy is considered to be a sign of overimmunosuppression, so the dose of maintenance agents should be trimmed and consideration given to running on dual therapy. There are some case reports and series suggesting that ciprofloxacin may be useful in BK nephropathy, although there are currently no randomised controlled trial data.

5. a,c,e. This biopsy shows acute humoral rejection which is usually treated with plasma exchange (in order to remove donor-specific antibody) and ATG (causes profound lymphocyte depletion). Many centres will also give methylprednisolone.

PART 3: SELF-ASSESSMENT

SAQs answers

1

a. Given the normal creatinine on a recent blood test and the presence of normal-sized kidneys on ultrasound, this is most likely to be acute renal failure. Most causes of chronic kidney disease lead to small, shrunken kidneys with thin cortices.

b. The causes of ARF are usually classified as pre-renal (e.g. volume depletion), renal (e.g. glomerulonephritis) and post-renal (obstruction).

c. The most common cause of ARF is pre-renal failure, which if left untreated will progress to ATN. ATN occurs if there is persistent hypotension/hypovolaemia +/− exposure to nephrotoxins or sepsis. Histologically, ATN is manifest as ragged, dying tubular cells which lose their nuclei and begin to slough off into the tubular lumen. Pre-renal failure/ATN accounts for 70–80% of cases of ARF.

d. The general management of a patient with ARF includes:
   • correct any volume depletion with intravenous fluids
   • careful monitoring of fluid balance (urine output/fluid intake chart + daily weights + regular clinical examination) in order to maintain euvolaemia
   • stop nephrotoxins (e.g. gentamicin, ACEI, NSAID)
   • consider gastric protection with PPI (due to increased risk of GI bleeds)
   • treat the underlying cause of ARF (e.g. cause of volume depletion or relieve obstruction).

2

a. This patient has the classic features of nephrotic syndrome (>3.5 g proteinuria/24 h, oedema and hypoalbuminaemia). Other features, which occur more variably, include hypertension and hypercholesterolaemia.

b. The patient should have a US of the renal tract and provided there are no contraindications, she should proceed to a renal biopsy in order to determine the histological diagnosis. A screen for conditions which can cause secondary GN associated with nephrotic syndrome should also be performed (see c.)

c. Nephrotic syndrome can occur in primary glomerulonephritides (typically minimal change GN, membranous GN, FSGS and mesangiocapillary GN) or secondary to diabetes mellitus, amyloid, SLE, hepatitis B/C, HIV. These diagnoses should be excluded. For SLE measure ANA, dsDNA, IgG, C3/C4, screen for infections hepatitis B/C and HIV by serological investigations and PCR. Plasma cell dyscrasias such as AL amyloidosis may be associated with an elevated serum paraprotein or elevated serum/urine free light chains.

d. General management measures for patients with nephrotic syndrome include the following.
   • Diuretics, in an attempt to reduce the oedema. Typically loop diuretics are used, e.g. furosemide, and often high doses will be needed, e.g. 80–150 mg. If the patient has established oedema this may include gut mucosal oedema, making oral diuretics ineffective and necessitating the use of intravenous diuretics. Whilst using diuretics, the patient should be fluid restricted, e.g. 1 L/day.
   • Antiproteinuric agents: regardless of the cause of nephrosis, ACEI or ARB should be started in an attempt to reduce proteinuria.
   • Blood pressure control: if the ACEI/ARB does not render the patient normotensive then add in additional agents.
   • Consider anticoagulation: nephrotic syndrome is associated with an increased risk of thromboembolic disease. If the serum albumin is <20 g/L then most nephrologists would consider

Nephrology: Clinical Cases Uncovered. By M. Clatworthy.
Published 2010 by Blackwell Publishing.

formal anticoagulation with warfarin. If >20 g/L then start on aspirin.

3

a. This case shows the typical features of nephritic syndrome. This is characterised by acute renal dysfunction, micro/macroscopic haematuria, hypertension, proteinuria and oedema.

b. There are many causes of nephritic syndrome, all of which result in glomerular inflammation (GN). These include:
   - primary glomerulonephritides
     ○ IgA nephropathy
     ○ membranoproliferative GN
     ○ idiopathic rapidly progressive/crescentic GN
   - secondary glomerulonephritides
     ○ postinfectious GN
     ○ Goodpasture's disease (antiglomerular basement membrane antibody disease)
     ○ SLE
     ○ vasculitides, e.g. ANCA-associated (Wegener's granulomatosis, microscopic polyangiitis), polyarteritis nodosum
     ○ cryoglobulinaemia.

c. Useful blood tests include a renal immunology screen, to assess for the presence of systemic autoimmune disease, in particular:
   - SLE: associated with ANA, anti-dsDNA, low complement (C3/C4), high IgG, anticardiolipin antibody, anti-Sm antibody
   - vasculitis: associated with ANCA
   - Goodpasture's disease: associated with anti-GBM antibodies
   - cryoglobulinaemia: associated with rheumatoid factor, cryoglobulins and low C3/C4
   - C3 nephritic factor: associated with mesangiocapillary GN and low C3.
   Throat swabs should be performed, as well as quantification of ASO titres and anti-DNAseB antibody titres, which will allow confirmation of a recent streptococcal infection. The patient should also proceed to a US-guided renal biopsy as quickly as possible, in order to determine the precise type and cause of glomerular inflammation.

d. As with any cause of acute renal failure:
   - correct any volume depletion with intravenous fluids
   - careful monitoring of fluid balance (urine output/fluid intake chart + daily weights + regular clinical examination) in order to maintain euvolaemia
   - stop nephrotoxins (e.g. gentamicin, ACEI, NSAID)
   - consider gastric protection with PPI (due to increased risk of GI bleeds)
   - treat the underlying cause. This depends on the pathology identified on renal biopsy, but frequently involves the administration of immunosuppressants.

4

a. Adult polycystic kidney disease. This is relatively common, affecting around 1 in 800 individuals in caucasian populations. The presence of >2 cysts in both kidneys at this age is highly suggestive of APKD. Other renal cystic diseases include von Hippel–Lindau syndrome and tuberose sclerosis, but these are less likely in a man of this age with no past medical history.

b. APKD can also be associated with valvular heart disease, diverticular disease and berry aneurysms. Any history consistent with these associated features of APKD, including history of stroke/cerebral haemorrhage, should be sought. Some patients also develop coronary artery aneurysms. It is important to take a family history as APKD is an autosomal dominant condition. New mutations occur in only 5% of cases, although many patients will not be aware of a positive family history of disease. Mutations in the PKD1 gene (chromosome 16p) occur in 85% and PKD2 (chromosome 4q) in 10% of cases.

c. On examination there may be signs associated with chronic hypertension, e.g. retinopathy, left ventricular hypertrophy (hyperdynamic, heaving apex beat +/− systolic flow murmur), signs consistent with valvular pathology (mitral valve prolapse, MR, AR) or signs consistent with cysts in other organs (e.g. hepatomegaly).

d. It is important to control blood pressure, ideally with ACEI or ARB. There are currently no treatments which have been shown to reduce cyst formation or progression in a randomised controlled trial. However, there are ongoing studies aimed at determining whether a combination of ACEI and ARB can reduce the rate of increase of kidney volume as well as decline in renal function. Other agents being evaluated include sirolimus, tolvaptan (ADH analogue) and octreotide.

If the patient progresses to end-stage kidney disease then RRT should be provided. The development of cysts can cause the kidneys to become so big that a nephrectomy may be required before transplantation to make room for the allograft.

As with all genetic diseases, it is important to provide counselling for the patient and other family members who may potentially be affected. Screening (using abdominal US) is useful in young adults. If there are no cysts present at the age of 30 years, then the APKD is unlikely, but cannot be completely excluded before this age.

5

a. The most likely diagnosis is IgA nephropathy. This was first described by Berger in the late 1960s and is sometimes called Berger's disease. It is the most common GN in adults and has a male preponderance (2 : 1 M : F ratio). The classic presentation is as described in this case, a male in his 20s–30s with asymptomatic microscopic haematuria +/− hypertension. Patients diagnosed under the age of 25 years tend to present with episodic macroscopic haematuria (often precipitated by mucosal infections; see case 6). The main differential diagnosis for a patient with persistent microscopic haematuria is thin membrane disease but this is much less common than IgA nephropathy.

b. The management of IgA nephropathy depends on the clinical presentation. Urine dipstick abnormalities will spontaneously resolve in 10–25% of patients who present with microscopic haematuria (as in this case). Thus, in such a patient, many nephrologists would take a watching brief and would not even perform a confirmatory biopsy at this stage. This is because a renal biopsy carries significant risks and provided the renal function is stable, management would not be altered by a confirmatory biopsy. General management measures include control of blood pressure (often present) and proteinuria (less frequently present), for example using an ACEI or ARB, and regular review in nephrology clinic with monitoring of BP, urine dipstick and renal function. Provided these factors are stable then no further management is required. If renal function begins to decline or there is an increase in proteinuria then a confirmatory renal

biopsy should be undertaken. A number of immunosuppressive regimens have been trialled, including corticosteroids +/− chlorambucil, cyclophosphamide, azathioprine or mycophenolate mofetil, but there is little consensus opinion. Generally, more aggressive treatment is reserved for patients with heavy proteinuria +/− progressive renal dysfunction and severe lesions on biopsy.

c. IgA nephropathy can only be diagnosed with certainty by performing a renal biopsy. Typical biopsy appearances include:
   - mesangial cell proliferation
   - mesangial matrix proliferation
   - mesangial deposition of IgA on immunostaining
   - glomerulosclerosis (in patients with advanced disease).

d. Overall, 20–40% of patients with IgA nephropathy progress to ESRF over 10–20 years. Poor prognostic features include older age, heavy proteinuria, renal impairment at the time of presentation, persistent hypertension, male sex and a crescentic GN on biopsy. The higher the proportion of glomeruli containing crescents, the worse the prognosis.

6

a. The most likely diagnosis is Churg–Strauss syndrome (sometimes termed 'allergic granulomatosis and angiitis'). The syndrome was first described by Jacob Churg and Lotte Strauss at Mount Sinai Hospital in New York, 1951. The patient's presentation is typical: late-onset asthma, a peripheral eosinophilia and peripheral nerve involvement. It is the rarest of the small vessel vasculitides, Wegener's granulomatosis and microscopic polyangiitis being more common. The disease usually has three phases: an early phase characterised by rhinitis and adult-onset asthma, an eosinophilic phase (characterised by peripheral eosinophilia and organ infiltration with eosinophils), and a severe late phase characterised by organ-threatening eosinophilic vasculitis.

b. Other clinical features include:
   - a history of systemic symptoms such as fever, night sweats, lethargy and weight loss
   - a history of allergic rhinitis
   - a history of dyspepsia, indicative of eosinophilic gastritis
   - a purpuric rash on examination

- symptoms or signs indicative of neurological involvement, including a peripheral neuropathy or mononeuritis multiplex
- signs consistent with myocardial involvement (eosinophilic cardiomyopathy), e.g. poor LV function, valvular regurgitation and arrhythmias
- anterior uveitis or retinal vasculitis.

The American College of Rheumatology outlines six diagnostic criteria for Churg–Strauss.

1. Late-onset asthma
2. >10% eosinophils in the blood
3. Mono- or polyneuropathy
4. Non-fixed pulmonary infiltrates
5. Abnormalities of paranasal sinuses
6. Extravascular eosinophils on biopsy

However, these features occur variably and should be an aid to diagnosis and not applied rigidly. As with all the small vessel vasculitides, the diagnosis is frequently delayed and difficult.

c. The diagnosis should be confirmed histologically by biopsying an affected organ. In this case, a renal biopsy should suffice and would show an eosinophilic small to medium vessel vasculitis, often with fibrinoid necrosis, as well as eosinophilic infiltration of the interstitium. Other organs sometimes biopsied include the lungs, gastric mucosa and nerves. Additional useful investigations include ESR and CRP (elevated), and ANCA; 50–70% of patients are ANCA positive and this is usually a pANCA (i.e. reacts with myeloperoxidase). Studies suggest that patients who are ANCA negative are more likely to have severe cardiac involvement.

Most patients respond rapidly to corticosteroids.

d. Other conditions which give rise to eosinophilia and renal impairment include:
- interstitial nephritis (usually secondary to drugs)
- cholesterol emboli (occur in vasculopaths, usually following instrumentation or thrombolysis). Can be associated with fever, renal impairment and a purpuric rash in the extremities.

Both conditions can give rise to eosinophiluria.

7

a. This is a metabolic acidosis with a high anion gap. When interpreting arterial blood gases, start with pH, then look at pCO$_2$, then look at bicarbonate.
1. Look at the pH. Is the patient acidotic (pH <7.35) or alkalotic (>7.45)?

2. Look at the pCO$_2$. Is CO$_2$ consistent with the pH? Remember CO$_2$ is an acidic gas ($CO_2 + H_2O \leftrightarrow H_2O_2 \leftrightarrow H^+ + HCO_3^-$). In the case of acidosis, if the primary problem is respiratory then the CO$_2$ will be elevated.
3. Look at the bicarbonate. This gives information about the metabolic component of the acid–base disturbance.

In this case pH <7.35 therefore this is acidosis. pCO$_2$ is low, therefore the primary problem is metabolic. The HCO$_3^-$ is low, confirming that this is a metabolic acidosis.

$$\text{Anion gap} = (Na^+ + K^+) - (HCO_3^- + Cl^-)$$
$$= 141 + 4.0 - (8 + 106)$$
$$= 145 - 114$$
$$= 31$$

Normal anion gap is 10–18 mmol/L which represents the unestimated anions in the blood which consist of albumin, phosphate and other organic acids.

b. Metabolic acidosis with a high anion gap occurs due to increased production/reduced clearance of acids.
- Lactic acidosis (shock, hypoxia, sepsis)
- Ketoacidosis (diabetes, alcohol)
- Renal failure
- Liver failure
- Drugs/toxins (salicylates, ethylene glycol, methanol)

In this particular case, pO$_2$ is normal, urea + creatinine values do not suggest renal failure, he is not jaundiced (therefore liver failure unlikely), blood sugars are not grossly elevated and there are no ketones detectable on urine dipstick (therefore this is not diabetic ketoacidosis). Thus, the most likely diagnosis is ingestion of drugs or toxins, particularly ethylene glycol (anti-freeze).

c. Ethylene glycol is metabolised by the hepatic enzyme alcohol dehydrogenase to glycoaldehyde, then glycolate, then oxalate. Oxalate precipitates in the urine as calcium oxalate crystals. Diamond-shaped calcium oxalate crystals may be identified by urine microscopy (although this tends to occur late in the process). In addition, most anti-freeze solutions contain a fluorescein dye in order to help mechanics identify the source of radiator leaks. If the urine is placed under a UV lamp in the dark, then there may be sufficient fluorescein dye to cause fluorescence, clinching the diagnosis (a frequent manoeuvre in televised hospital dramas such as ER!).

d. The enzyme alcohol dehydrogenase preferentially metabolises ethanol. Therefore, historically, an ethanol infusion was given to block the formation of oxalate crystals. A specific pharmacological inhibitor of alcohol dehydrogenase is now available, and is usually used instead of ethanol. In patients who are severely acidotic, haemodialysis or filtration may be required.

8

a. This man has CKD, as evidenced by the presence of small kidneys with thin cortices, suggesting a long-standing, irreversible process.
b. The most common causes of CKD in the UK are:
   • diabetic nephropathy
   • hypertensive nephropathy
   • APKD
   • chronic glomerulonephritides
   • chronic pyelonephritis/reflux nephropathy
   • obstructive uropathy
   • renovascular disease.
c. The man has CKD stage 5 (see table below) and is therefore likely to need RRT in the near future.

CKD stage	eGFR (mL/min/1.73 m²)	Other features
1	90+	Normal renal function but urine dipstick abnormalities or known structural abnormality of renal tract or diagnosis of genetic kidney disease
2	60–89	Mildly reduced renal function plus urine/structural abnormalities or diagnosis of genetic kidney disease
3	30–59	Moderately reduced renal function
4	15–29	Severely reduced renal function
5	<15	End-stage renal failure

d. The complications of CKD are:
   1. Anaemia, due to erythropoietin deficiency.
   2. CKD-BMD: CKD leads to bone and mineral abnormalities at three levels, together termed CKD-BMD.

• Renal bone disease: native vitamin D (cholecalciferol) is hydroxylated first by the liver to 25-hydroxy vitamin D, and second (principally) by the kidneys to the active hormone 1,25 dihydroxyvitamin D3 (calcitriol). Low circulating calcitriol levels are characteristic of patients with kidney failure, because the loss of functioning nephrons leads to loss of the activating enzyme 1α-hydroxylase. Calcitriol deficiency leads to decreased intestinal calcium absorption, hypocalcaemia and impaired mineralisation of bone, manifesting as 'renal rickets' in children and osteomalacia in adults.
• Hyperphosphataemia, abnormalities of calcium metabolism and secondary hyperparathyroidism: healthy kidneys excrete phosphate, so in CKD phosphate accumulates. To compensate for this, two hormones are released which increase phosphate excretion by the kidneys: PTH, by the parathyroid glands, and FGF23, released by bone cells. However, FGF23 stops 1α-hydroxylase in the kidneys from activating vitamin D, and worsens vitamin D deficiency. Low vitamin D levels lead to further increase in PTH release because parathyroid cells sense both calcium and vitamin D. When these are low, more PTH is released to increase calcium and to try and stimulate vitamin D production. The end result is a spiralling increase in PTH, which releases calcium from bone; this process also weakens bone and increases phosphate. If left untreated, the parathyroid glands become enlarged and stop responding to the normal inhibitory signals. This leads to hypercalcaemia and is termed tertiary hyperparathyroidism.
• Extraskeletal calcification: the abnormalities above lead to the deposition of calcium in soft tissues and arteries.
3. Hypertension secondary to chronic intravascular volume overload.
4. Accelerated atherosclerosis/vascular disease: hypertension and chronic hypercalcaemia lead to accelerated atherosclerosis and vascular calcification, and an increased risk of coronary artery disease, PVD and cerebrovascular accidents.
5. Metabolic acidosis: the kidneys excrete the daily acid load generated by amino acid metabolism. As the kidneys fail, patients develop a progressive metabolic acidosis. Chronic acidosis can promote

renal bone disease and leads to muscle wasting and malnutrition.

9

a. There are four options for a patient approaching ESRF.

- Conservative management: appropriate for the very elderly and infirm who would not tolerate chronic dialysis
- Haemodialysis
- Peritoneal dialysis
- Renal transplantation

Pre-emptive (i.e. before the patient starts dialysis) renal transplantation is the modality of choice and offers advantages in terms of survival and quality of life for the majority of patients. Patients can be placed on the deceased donor kidney waiting list 6 months before dialysis is anticipated to start but they are likely to wait for around 2–3 years before getting a kidney. A better option would be a living donor kidney, if there is a friend or relative willing to donate.

b. Factors which make patients unsuitable for PD include:

- Previous abdominal surgery, with possibility of adhesions, hence poor drainage and inefficient dialysis.
- Poor manual dexterity, e.g. due to arthritis in the hands or a neurological disorder which may render the patient physically unable to perform exchanges.
- Blindness.
- Inadequate home/social circumstances (need lots of space for large amount of fluid, and a clean room set aside for exchanges).
- Poor mental dexterity/inability to grasp importance or method of aseptic technique. If the patient is unable to appreciate this then the risk of developing peritonitis is high.
- Obesity: reduces likelihood of adequate volume exchanges.
- Abdominal hernias: can be repaired at time of placement of PD catheter, but may frequently recur.
- Stomas: increase risk of infection.
- Severe inflammatory bowel disease.
- Patients with severe COPD may find that respiration is impaired during large-volume dwells.

Factors which make HD a less useful RRT option include the following.

- Haemodialysis severely limits independence and quality of life. HD patients need to travel to the (sometimes distant) dialysis unit three times a week. Most HD patients find it difficult to continue in full-time employment with these restrictions.
- Patients with poor cardiovascular function, e.g. diabetics, often have difficulty tolerating HD and can become hypotensive and cardiovascularly unstable during HD sessions.
- In some patients (often those who have been on HD previously), vascular access is limited because of central vein stenoses or occlusion. In these patients, PD may be the only option.

Therefore, a careful history and assessment of the patient should be undertaken in order to allow the best dialysis modality to be chosen.

c. The overall survival of patients on both HD and PD is reduced compared with healthy individuals of the same age and sex. Generic complications of ESRF include an increased risk of cardiovascular disease, infection and malignancy. In addition, there are specific complications associated with both PD and HD.

The complications of peritoneal dialysis include:

- complications associated with PD catheter insertion (e.g. perforation of abdominal viscus, haemorrhage)
- bacterial or fungal peritonitis
- exit site infections
- catheter tip migration
- leakage of PD fluid (including into the pleural cavity)
- hyperglycaemia
- encapsulating peritoneal sclerosis – a complication of long-term PD occurring in 1–5% of patients.

The complications of haemodialysis include:

- complications associated with central line insertion (pneumothorax, haemorrhage/haematoma formation, arterial puncture, mediastinal damage)
- line infection
- infective endocarditis
- AVF complications (thrombosis, development of aneurysmal segment, steal syndrome)
- venous stenoses/thrombosis
- dialysis-associated hypotension
- chronic volume overload with persistent interdialytic hypertension.

d. In the next 6 months the patient should receive appropriate education on the various forms of RRT, to allow them to make an informed decision. If there is a relative or friend available who is willing to donate a kidney, then the transplant work-up for both donor and recipient should be commenced ASAP. In the absence of a living donor, the recipient should begin work-up for placement on the deceased donor waiting list. In such cases, the patient should also be prepared for dialysis. This largely involves establishing appropriate access. If HD is the modality of choice then an AVF should be formed at least 2 months prior to the anticipated date of use to allow it to heal and mature. Similarly, the PD catheter should be placed at least 6 weeks prior to the anticipated start date. In addition to access issues, other complications of CKD should be managed including anaemia, hyperphosphataemia, vitamin D deficiency and hypertension.

10

a. Patients are described as 'CMV positive' if a CMV-specific IgG is detectable in their blood. This indicates that they have previously been infected with CMV (as is the case in around 50% of UK adults, the proportion increasing with increasing age). Following infection, there is initially a rise in IgM but then a rise in IgG, which remains detectable in the long term. If a CMV-seronegative recipient (R-) receives a transplant from a CMV-seropositive donor (D+) then they may get primary infection whilst immunosuppressed. This can be a severe and even life-threatening illness. Thus, such patients are usually given CMV prophylaxis for at least 3 months post transplant with valganciclovir.

b. The HLA are highly polymorphic glycoproteins found on the surface of cells. They are divided into class I and class II molecules. Class I molecules are found on the surface of all cells, and class II on the surface of antigen-presenting cells. They are encoded by a cluster of genes found on chromosome 6 called the major histocompatibility complex genes. In humans there are three MHC class I genes, A, B and C, and three MHC class II genes, DP, DQ and DR. Given that an individual has two copies of each gene, the maximum number of mismatches that can occur between two individuals is 12, i.e. two A mismatches, two B mismatches, etc. However, in renal transplantation, only A, B and DR mismatches are considered, so the maximum number of mismatches possible is six. Such a mismatch would

be described as a 2-2-2 mismatch (two A, two B and two DR mismatches). The best mismatch would be a 0-0-0 mismatch. In this case there are two A, one B and no DR mistmatches. DR mismatches have a more significant deleterious effect on long-term allograft function and survival than A or B mismatches, so every effort is made to avoid DR mismatches.

c. The major issue in this case is that the donor and recipient are ABO blood group incompatible. AB antigens are found on the surface of red cells and endothelial cells. The donor (blood group B) has B antigens on red cells and the recipient (blood group A) has anti-B antibodies. Thus, if a blood group B individual were to donate a kidney to a blood group A individual, the circulating anti-B antibody in the recipient would immediately bind to the vascular endothelium within the transplanted kidney, activating complement and phagocytes, and causing occlusion of the vessels and immediate infarction of the kidney (hyperacute rejection). For this reason blood group-incompatible transplantation is not routinely undertaken.

d. In cases of ABO-incompatible transplantation, the recipient can undergo a desensitisation procedure prior to transplantation. This usually begins at least a month prior to transplantation and involves repeated sessions of plasma exchange (to remove anti-B antibodies) and the administration of immunosuppressive treatment in order to suppress further production of antibody (e.g. rituximab, a B cell-depleting anti-CD20 monoclonal antibody, ATG or intravenous immunoglobulin). Previously, splenectomy was also used. The transplant only goes ahead if antibody titres are at a low level on the planned day of transplant. Patients will then receive additional sessions of plasma exchange post transplant and relatively heavy maintenance immunosupression. Japan has been one of the world leaders in ABO-incompatible transplantation (having started their programme in the late 1980s). Living donation is a major part of their transplant programme because deceased donation (particularly from heart-beating donors) is not considered to be culturally acceptable. Thus, up to 80% of all renal transplants performed in Japan are from living donors. In contrast, in the UK, around 30% of transplants are from living donors. In Japanese centres, allograft outcome post ABO-incompatible transplant is now excellent, with a 94% 2-year survival. Many UK centres are also beginning to undertake ABO-incompatible transplants due to the ever-increasing number of patients awaiting renal transplantation.

An alternative strategy to desensitisation is 'paired donation'. In such schemes, couple A (e.g. the pair described above, with blood group B donor and blood group A recipient) could give the kidney to couple B (with blood group A donor and blood group B recipient) and vice versa. Thus both recipients would receive a blood group-compatible transplant. The UK now operates a paired donation scheme, where each transplant centre submits the details of ABO-incompatible couples to a central databank at UK Transplant. A computerised matching programme then identifies potential paired donations. If the donation goes ahead, then a good deal of organisation is required so that the donor operations start simultaneously (usually in different parts of the country), the organs are then transported as quickly as possible to the recipient's centre where the transplant operation is performed. A number of successful paired donations have now been performed in the UK and there are plans to extend the paired donation scheme to accommodate three-way exchanges in order to maximise the number of possible transplants.

Index of cases by diagnosis

Index

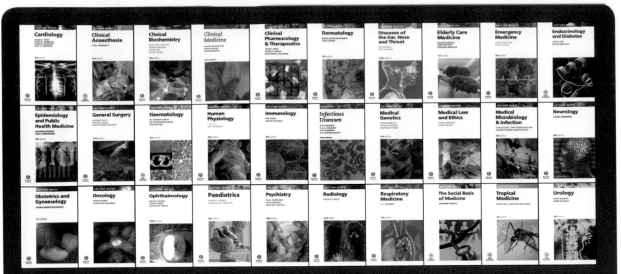
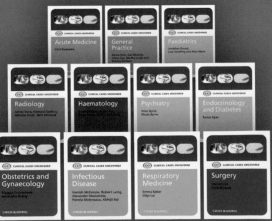
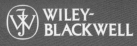